Bovine Ultrasound

Guest Editor

SÉBASTIEN BUCZINSKI, Dr Vét, DÉS, MSc

VETERINARY CLINICS
OF NORTH AMERICA:
FOOD ANIMAL PRACTICE

www.vetfood.theclinics.com

Consulting Editor
ROBERT A. SMITH, DVM, MS

November 2009 • Volume 25 • Number 3

SAUNDERS an imprint of ELSEVIER, Inc.

W.B. SAUNDERS COMPANY
A Division of Elsevier Inc.

1600 John F. Kennedy Boulevard ● Suite 1800 ● Philadelphia, PA 19103-2899

http://www.vetfood.theclinics.com

VETERINARY CLINICS OF NORTH AMERICA: FOOD ANIMAL PRACTICE Volume 25, Number 3
November 2009 ISSN 0749-0720, ISBN-13: 978-1-4377-1284-1, ISBN-10: 1-4377-1284-3

Editor: John Vassallo; j.vassallo@elsevier.com
Developmental Editor: Theresa Collier

Veterinary Clinics of North America: Food Animal Practice (ISSN 0749-0720) is published in March, July, and November by Elsevier Inc., 360 Park Avenue South, New York, NY 10010-1710. Subscription prices are $163.00 per year (domestic individuals), $260.00 per year (domestic institutions), $81.00 per year (domestic students/residents), $189.00 per year (Canadian individuals), $339.00 per year (Canadian institutions), $239.00 per year (international individuals), $339.00 per year (international institutions), and $123.00 per year (international and Canadian students/residents). To receive student/resident rate, orders must be accompanied by name of affiliated institution, date of term, and the *signature* of program/residency coordinator on institution letterhead. Orders will be billed at individual rate until proof of status is received. Foreign air speed delivery is included in all *Clinics* subscription prices. All prices are subject to change without notice. **POSTMASTER:** Send address changes to *Veterinary Clinics of North America: Food Animal Practice*, Elsevier Health Sciences Division, Subscription Customer Service, 3251 Riverport Lane, Maryland Heights, MO 63043. Customer Service (orders, claims, online, change of address): Elsevier Health Sciences Division, Subscription Customer Service, 3251 Riverport Lane, Maryland Heights, MO 63043. Tel: 1-800-654-2452 (U.S. and Canada); 314-447-8871 (outside U.S. and Canada). Fax: 314-447-8029. E-mail: journalscustomerservice-usa@elsevier.com (for print support); journalsonlinesupport-usa@elsevier.com (for online support).

Reprints. For copies of 100 or more, of articles in this publication, please contact the Commercial Reprints Department, Elsevier Inc., 360 Park Avenue South, New York, NY 10010-1710. Tel.: 212-633-3812; Fax: 212-462-1935; E-mail: reprints@elsevier.com.

Veterinary Clinics of North America: Food Animal Practice is covered in *Current Contents/Agriculture, Biology and Environmental Sciences, MEDLINE/PubMed (Index Medicus),* and *Excerpta Medica.*

Printed and bound by CPI Group (UK) Ltd, Croydon, CR0 4YY
Transferred to Digital Print 2011

Contributors

CONSULTING EDITOR

ROBERT A. SMITH, DVM, MS
Diplomate, American Board of Veterinary Practitioners; Veterinary Research and
Consulting Services, LLC, Stillwater, Oklahoma

GUEST EDITOR

SÉBASTIEN BUCZINSKI, Dr Vét, DÉS, MSc
Diplomate, American College of Veterinary Internal Medicine; Clinique Ambulatoire
Bovine/Bovine Ambulatory Clinic, Département des Sciences Cliniques, Faculté de
Médecine Vétérinaire, Université de Montréal, Saint-Hyacinthe, Quebec, Canada

AUTHORS

MARIE BABKINE, DMV, MSc
Diplomate, European College of Bovine Health Management; Clinical Instructor, Centre
Hospitalier Universitaire Vétérinaire, Faculté de Médecine Vétérinaire, Université de
Montréal, Saint-Hyacinthe, Québec, Canada

LAURENT BLOND, Dr Vét, MSc
Diplomate, American College of Veterinary Radiology; Département des Sciences
Cliniques, Faculté de Médecine Vétérinaire, Université de Montréal, Saint-Hyacinthe,
Quebec, Canada

UELI BRAUN, Prof Dr med vet, Dr med vet h c
Diplomate, European College of Bovine Health Management; Department of Farm
Animals, University of Zürich, Zürich, Switzerland

SÉBASTIEN BUCZINSKI, Dr Vét, DÉS, MSc
Diplomate, American College of Veterinary Internal Medicine; Département des Sciences
Cliniques, Clinique Ambulatoire Bovine, Faculté de Médecine Vétérinaire, Université de
Montréal, Saint-Hyacinthe, Quebec, Canada

JILL COLLOTON, DVM
Bovine Practitioner and Ultrasound Instructor, Bovine Services, Edgar, Wisconsin

LUC DESCÔTEAUX, DMV, MSc
Diplomate, American Board of Veterinary Practitioners (Dairy); Professor, Department
of Clinical Studies; and Medical Coordinator, Food Animal Ambulatory Clinic, Faculté
de Médecine Vétérinaire, Université de Montréal, St-Hyacinthe, Québec, Canada

MARTINA FLOECK, DVM
Department for Farm Animals and Veterinary Public Health, Clinic for Ruminants,
University of Veterinary Medicine Vienna, Vienna, Austria

SONJA FRANZ, DVM
Professor, Department for Farm Animals and Veterinary Public Health, Clinic for Ruminants, University of Veterinary Medicine Vienna, Vienna, Austria

GIOVANNI GNEMMI, DVM, PhD
Diplomate, European College of Bovine Health Management; Bovine Practitioner and Ultrasound Instructor, Bovinevet Studio Veterinario Associato, Chiovenda (VB), Italy

MARGARETE HOFMANN-PARISOT, DVM
Assistant Professor, Department for Biomedical Sciences, Institute for Physics and Biostatistics, University of Veterinary Medicine Vienna, Vienna, Austria

JOHANN KOFLER, DVM
Diplomate, European College of Bovine Health Management; Associate Professor of Orthopedics in Large Animals, Clinical Department of Horses and Small Animals, Clinic of Horses, Large Animal Surgery and Orthopedics, University of Veterinary Medicine Vienna, Vienna, Austria

RÉJEAN C. LEFEBVRE, DMV, PhD
Diplomate, American College of Theriogenologists; Département des Sciences Cliniques, Faculté de Médecine Vétérinaire, Université de Montréal, St-Hyacinthe, Quebec, Canada

BEATRICE LEJEUNE, Dr med vet
Clinical Instructor, Clinic for Ruminants, Vetsuisse-Faculty of Bern, Bern, Switzerland

ADRIAN STEINER, Dr med vet, MS, Dr Habil
Diplomate, European College of Veterinary Surgeons; Diplomate, European College of Bovine Health Management; Professor and Head, Clinic for Ruminants, Vetsuisse-Faculty of Bern, Bern, Switzerland

ROBERT J. VAN SAUN, DVM, PhD
Diplomate, American College of Theriogenologists; Diplomate, American College of Veterinary Nutrition; Professor of Veterinary Science and Extension Veterinarian, Department of Veterinary and Biomedical Sciences, Pennsylvania State University, University Park, Pennsylvania

Contents

Ultrasound imaging is a noninvasive and readily available diagnostic modality that meets increasing applications in bovine medicine. This article presents the basis of physical principles of this imaging modality based on the interaction of ultrasound with the tissues, different modes of examination, and ways to obtain good quality images. The main artifacts that may be encountered during ultrasound imaging are also described. Finally, Doppler ultrasound is briefly explained. This article aims to help practitioners perform an optimal ultrasonographic examination.

Ultrasonography is an ideal diagnostic tool for investigating gastrointestinal disorders in cattle. In animals with traumatic reticuloperitonitis, inflammatory fibrinous changes and abscesses can be imaged. Ultrasonography can be used to assess the size, position, and contents of the abomasum. This article describes the ultrasonographic techniques used for examination of the reticulum, rumen, omasum, abomasum, small intestine, and large intestine. The normal findings are presented followed by a description of the most important diseases of these organs.

Ultrasonography is a valuable tool for the diagnosis of liver disease. Discrete or diffuse lesions can be imaged, aspirated, and biopsied under visual guidance. The ultrasonographic examination of the liver is performed on the right side of the standing animal using a real-time 3.5 to 5.0 MHz linear or convex transducer. This imaging modality also can be used to aspirate bile from the gallbladder for the diagnosis of liver flukes. Ultrasonography cannot be used to evaluate liver regions obscured by the lungs, however.

Assessment of the bovine cardiovascular system is challenging because the position of the heart, deep in the thorax, may interfere with clinical findings. With advances in bovine ultrasonography, normal and abnormal findings of the bovine cardiovascular system have been described. Cardiovascular ultrasound can be of valuable help as a noninvasive diagnostic tool, especially when clinical findings are inconclusive. This article presents an up-to-date review of echocardiography and vascular ultrasound in the diagnosis and prognosis of the most common cardiovascular diseases in cattle.

Ultrasonography of the respiratory system is a noninvasive and readily available tool that allows an accurate evaluation of the pleura and some superficial lung lesions. It can aid clinicians in the diagnosis and treatment of various thoracic conditions that affect cattle.

Ultrasonography is a helpful diagnostic tool in cattle with urinary tract disorders. It can be used to diagnose pyelonephritis, urolithiasis, hydronephrosis, renal cysts, renal tumors, amyloidosis, cystitis, bladder paralysis, bladder rupture, bladder neoplasms, and, occasionally, nephrosis, glomerulonephritis, and embolic nephritis. This article describes the anatomy, scanning technique, indications, limitations, normal and pathologic sonographic appearance of the bovine urinary tract. References from horses and humans are included, especially when the sonographic findings in these species may complement the understanding of similar diseases reported in cattle.

Ultrasonography is a noninvasive technique for examining the bovine udder and teats. It is performed in the standing animal using a high frequency scanner (7.5–10.0 MHz) for examination of the teat structures (teat canal, rosette of Fuerstenberg, teat cistern, gland cistern) and a 5.0 MHz probe for examining the glandular parenchyma. Ultrasonography is a helpful tool to diagnose pathologic alterations of the udder such as inflammation, mucosal lesions, tissue proliferation, foreign bodies, milk stones, congenital changes, hematoma, and abscess. However, ultrasonography of the teat allows for the localization and demarcation of the extent of pathologic changes and therefore is an important additional diagnostic examination technique.

In the last 15 years, ultrasonography of the bovine musculoskeletal system has become an established diagnostic method used routinely in many veterinary teaching hospitals worldwide. Ultrasonography is ideal for the evaluation of musculoskeletal disorders because they are often associated with extensive soft tissue swelling and inflammatory exudation. The goal of this article is to encourage veterinarians to use ultrasonography for the evaluation of bovine orthopedic disorders. Not only does ultrasonography improve the likelihood of a definitive diagnosis, added use of the machine helps recoup expenses.

theriogenology. To recognize abnormal tissues, however, the operator must have an excellent knowledge of the ultrasonographic anatomy of the reproductive system. This article discusses the basis of ultrasound technique for male reproductive tract examination. Ultrasound evaluation of physiologic and pathologic conditions of external and internal reproduction organs is proposed.

Umbilical disorders are of great clinical relevance in calves during the early postnatal period. They may be classified as (1) noninfectious disorders such as hernias and urachal cysts, (2) infectious disorders involving extra- and intra-abdominal umbilical structures, or (3) combinations thereof. Supplementing clinical examination, umbilical ultrasonography allows the identification of the structures involved and differentiation of the various disorders with a high diagnostic sensitivity. A specific diagnosis of the umbilical disorder is important, because the treatment regimen, prognosis, and treatment costs completely depend upon the extent of the disease and the structures involved.

Limited published reports of nutritional diseases affecting llamas and alpacas were found in a detailed review of relevant literature sources. Anecdotal clinical experiences and nutritional diseases that have been reported range from those diagnosed in common with other species to diseases having a presentation unique to camelids. Vitamin D–associated rickets and greater susceptibility to hepatic lipidosis and zinc deficiency are distinctive nutritional problems for llamas and alpacas. This article will review commonly encountered nutritional diseases, based on literature reports and clinical experience, in llamas and alpacas.

RELATED INTEREST

Veterinary Clinics of North America: Small Animal Practice (Vol. 39, no. 4)
New Concepts in Diagnostic Imaging
Martha Moon Larson, DVM, MS and Gregory B. Daniel, DVM, MS, *Guest Editors*

THE CLINICS ARE NOW AVAILABLE ONLINE!

Access your subscription at:
www.theclinics.com

Bovine Ultrasound

FORTHCOMING ISSUES

March 2010
Emerging, Re-emerging, and Persistent
Infectious Diseases of Cattle
Sanjay Kapil, DVM, MS, PhD and
David A. Vogel, DVM, PhD
Guest Editors

July 2010
Ophthalmology
David L. Williams, MA, VetMB, PhD
BSc, PhD?
Guest Editor

November 2010
Bovine Respiratory Disease
Victor S. Cortese, DVM, MS, PhD
and Bruce W. Brodersen, DVM, MS, PhD
Guest Editors

RECENT ISSUES

July 2009
Alpaca and Llama Health Management
David E. Anderson, DVM, MS and
Claire E. Whitehead, BVM&S, MS, MRCVS
Guest Editors

March 2009
Bovine Neonatology
Geof W. Smith, DVM, MC, PhD
Guest Editor

July 2008
Field Surgery of Cattle, Part I
David E. Anderson, DVM, MS and
Matt D. Miesner, DVM, MS
Guest Editors

RELATED INTEREST

Veterinary Clinics of North America: Small Animal Practice (Vol. 39, No. 4)
New Concepts in Diagnostic Imaging
Martha Moon Larson, DVM, MS and Gregory B. Daniel, DVM, MS, Guest Editors

THE CLINICS ARE NOW AVAILABLE ONLINE!

Access your subscription at:
www.theclinics.com

Preface

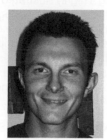

Sébastien Buczinski, Dr Vét, DÉS, MSc
Guest Editor

What do veterinary practitioners, surgeons, internists, and theriogenologists, who are all routinely involved in cattle health management, have in common? Perhaps some items such as a stethoscope, transrectal gloves, and an ultrasound device.

In the early 1980s, ultrasonography began to be used as an important ancillary test at the farm for reproduction monitoring. With continued technologic advances in ultrasound equipment and clinical research performed by pioneers on nonreproductive applications of bovine ultrasonography, this medical imaging technique emerged as a noninvasive, very informative ancillary test with no withdrawal time that can be used for multiple purposes in teaching institutes and by the internist, the surgeon, the theriogenologist, and bovine practitioners in an on-farm setting.

With the numerous interesting published studies on bovine ultrasonography and the absence of an English textbook on extragenital use of bovine ultrasound (the only ones available are written in German[1] and French[2]), it was important to dedicate an issue of the *Veterinary Clinics of North America: Food Animal Practice* to the multiple uses of ultrasound in cattle.

In working with dairy or beef cattle, we are usually trying to practice cost-effective medicine; therefore, any noninvasive tool that can allow a more accurate diagnosis and avoid unnecessary treatment is of primary importance.

Besides the major classical applications of ultrasonography for reproductive tract assessment, it allows one to establish a diagnosis (sometimes a prognosis) and to monitor progression of therapy of the major diseases encountered in bovine practice. For these reasons, it is an interesting ancillary tool that allows a cow-side diagnosis and can spare time and money for the producer or pain for the suffering animal. The information available on the use of ultrasound as an ancillary test continues to grow in peer-reviewed publications concerning experimental and clinical studies. Although it is currently not widely available for the bovine practitioner, some pilot studies concerning the use of Doppler in cattle are now available and show the potential of this function. Therefore, although the ultrasonographic applications presented here are not exhaustive, they aim to present the most useful and practical indications of ultrasonography for veterinarians working with cattle in on-farm or hospital settings.

Vet Clin Food Anim 25 (2009) xi–xii
doi:10.1016/j.cvfa.2009.08.001

This issue could not have been possible without Dr. Robert Smith and his enthusiasm for this topic. I also want to acknowledge John Vassallo for the impressive work that was performed by the editorial team in constructing a highly illustrated issue.

In preparing this issue, I was helped by leaders of bovine ultrasonography throughout the world. I want to acknowledge all of them for their irreplaceable contributions that give a high value to this issue. I am very proud of this issue, and I hope that every veterinarian interested in bovine medicine will enjoy it!

I sincerely hope that this issue of the *Veterinary Clinics of North America: Food Animal Practice* will be of practical help and in every truck of bovine practitioners.

So, on your probes... ready... go!

Sébastien Buczinski, Dr Vét, DÉS, MSc
Clinique Ambulatoire Bovine/Bovine Ambulatory Clinic
Département des Sciences Cliniques
Faculté de Médecine Vétérinaire
Université de Montréal
CP 5000, Saint-Hyacinthe
Quebec J2S 7C6, Canada

E-mail address:
s.buczinski@umontreal.ca

REFERENCES

1. Braun U. Atlas und Lehrbuch der Ultraschalldiagnostik beim Rind. Atlas and textbook of ultrasonographic diagnosis in the cow. Berlin: Parey Buchverlag; 1997 [in German].
2. Buczinski S. Échographie des bovins. [Bovine ultrasonography]. Éditions du Point Vétérinaire. Rueil-Malmaison: Wolters-Kluwer France; 2009 [in French].

Basis of Ultrasound Imaging and the Main Artifacts in Bovine Medicine

Laurent Blond, DrVét, MSc[a],*, Sébastien Buczinski, DrVét, DÉS, MSc[b]

KEYWORDS

• Ultrasound • Physic • Artifact • Bovine • Doppler

Ultrasound has been widely used lately in veterinary medicine. In bovine medicine, ultrasonography was initially used for the examination of the reproductive tract,[1] but many other applications have been described in the last 20 years.[2] Ultrasound imaging has the advantage over radiology of offering better contrast resolution and acquiring slice images of organs in different planes in real time—all with portable and noninvasive and nonionizing equipment. This article is a brief overview of the physical principals, instrumentation, and mode of ultrasound imaging and the main artifacts that can be encountered during a routine examination. Readers are referred to more detailed articles and textbook chapters for in-depth information.[3–6]

PHYSICAL PRINCIPALS

Images are created according to the propagation of ultrasound (sound waves with frequencies beyond what can be perceived by the human ear) within the tissues. Frequency of a sound wave is defined as the number of repetitions of this wave (cycle) per second. One cycle per second = 1 Hz. Ultrasound used for imaging generally has frequencies from 2 to 10 MHz. The wave length is the distance covered by one sound wave during one cycle and determines the penetration power of this sound wave in the tissue (**Fig. 1**).

The propagation speed of sound waves in tissues (velocity) is defined as

$$\text{Velocity (m/sec)} = \text{frequency (Hz)} \times \text{wave length(m)}$$

The velocity of sound in a given tissue is constant and determines the frequency and wave length of the ultrasound to be used for the chosen examination (**Table 1**). For

[a] Département des Sciences Cliniques, Faculté de Médecine Vétérinaire, Université de Montréal, CP 5000, Saint-Hyacinthe, Quebec J2S 6K9, Canada
[b] Clinique Ambulatoire Bovine/Bovine Ambulatory Clinic, Département des Sciences Cliniques, Faculté de Médecine Vétérinaire, Université de Montréal, Saint-Hyacinthe, Quebec, J2S 7C6, Canada
* Corresponding author.
E-mail address: laurent.blond@umontreal.ca (L. Blond).

Vet Clin Food Anim 25 (2009) 553–565
doi:10.1016/j.cvfa.2009.07.002
0749-0720/09/$ – see front matter © 2009 Elsevier Inc. All rights reserved.

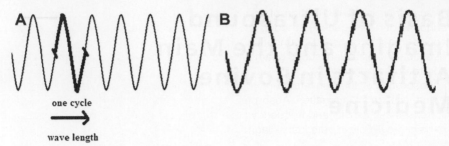

one cycle

wave length

Fig. 1. Schematic representation of sound waves. (A) High-frequency sound wave. The wave length is the distance covered by one sound wave during one cycle (*bold line*). (B) Low frequency sound wave. The wave length is longer.

example, in a given soft tissue organ with constant velocity, ultrasound with a low frequency has a large wave length and allows imaging of deeper structures. On the other hand, a higher frequency improves the resolution of the obtained image but the generated sound waves are rapidly attenuated and the depth of examination is limited. It is important to select the higher possible frequency for the desired depth of examination. Generally the maximum scan depth is 20 to 25 cm. As it travels through the patient, the sound beam is attenuated because of its interactions with tissues. The main interactions of an incident sound wave with matter are reflection, refraction, scattering, and absorption.

Reflection refers to the ultrasound that hits a reflective surface at a perpendicular angle and returns to the transducer. This portion of the sound beam forms the basis of ultrasound images. The proportion of reflected sound waves on tissues is a function of their acoustic impedance defined by the product of the tissue's velocity and density. The amplitude of the reflecting echoes is proportional to the difference of acoustic impedance between two adjacent tissues crossed by the ultrasound. The larger the difference (eg, interface soft tissue–gas), the more of the sound wave that is reflected. There is usually a small difference of acoustic impedance between the abdominal soft tissues. This is ideal because only a small percentage of the waves is reflected, whereas most are transmitted and allow imaging of deeper structures. Reflected sound waves help to image the boundaries between organs. If in a given soft tissue organ there is a focal variation of density, the difference of acoustic impedance with the surrounding parenchyma allows imaging of this focal lesion.

Refraction only occurs when the sound wave passes from one medium to another that has different propagation speeds with an oblique incidence angle. This occurrence results in a change of direction of the transmitted sound wave and may create some artifacts.

Table 1	
Sound velocity in different media	
Medium	**Velocity (m/sec)**
Air	331
Fat	1450
Soft tissue (mean)	1540
Bone	4080

Scattering is the redirection of sound waves in unpredictable directions by rough surfaces or heterogeneous media, such as cellular tissues. Scattering permits ultrasound imaging of tissue boundaries that are not necessarily perpendicular to the direction of the incident sound beam and allows imaging of tissue parenchyma in addition to organ boundaries.

Absorption is the conversion of a portion of the sound beam into heat. It is the primary cause of attenuation. Absorption is higher in bone than in soft tissues. Heating increases as intensity and frequency increase, but the amount of heat generated still remains negligible in veterinary diagnostic ultrasound studies.

THE PROBES

Ultrasound is generated by piezoelectric crystals contained within the probe. After mechanical or electrical impulsion, these crystals change shape and vibrate, emitting a beam of ultrasounds. After stabilization of the crystals, sound waves that are reflected by the tissues and return toward the probe (like echoes) reinduce vibration of the crystals, which then emit electrical impulses that are amplified and transformed in an image by a computer. Different types of probes are available. Most of the probes are real-time sector scanners, which means that the beam shape and resulting screen image are sector shaped or triangular with a sector angle that is commonly 90°. The other probes are linear and give a rectangular image (**Fig. 2**).

Older scanners are mechanical, which means that they generate an ultrasound beam by movement of one or multiple crystals (generally three to four). Rotation or oscillation in a to-and-fro fashion is more common. Modern probes are composed of several elements that contain crystals that do not move. These are called arrays. The elements are fired electronically. Arrays may be formed in several configurations—linear, curvilinear, or annular. Curvilinear probes are curved linear arrays that produce a sector image with a wider field of view than linear probes. Phased array produces an ultrasound beam by firing multiple elements in a precise sequence electronically. This beam can be enlarged or narrowed in different directions, depending on the area of interest. This type of transducer offers a wide field of view despite a small

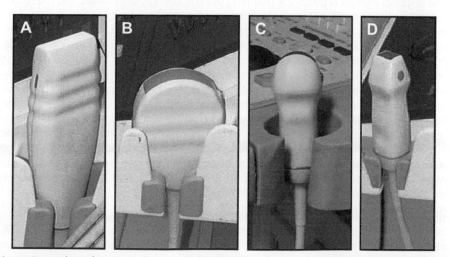

Fig. 2. Examples of available types of probes for ultrasound imaging: (*A*) linear probe, (*B*) curvilinear probe, (*C*) sector scanner, and (*D*) phased array.

size and is convenient for intrathoracic study to image between ribs (eg, cardiac studies).

Sector scanners have limited near field of view compared to linear or curvilinear arrays, but they allow evaluation of deeper structures and structures for which the window of examination is limited. In bovine medicine, commonly used probes are linear or curvilinear with an 3.5 to 8-MHz frequency. Some available probes cover several frequencies at the same time (multifrequency transducers) and go up to 8.5 MHz.

IMAGE CONTROL
B Mode

Images are routinely evaluated in B mode (brightness), which displays the elements of the image according to a gray scale. The level of grays and the intensity of the brightness of the image's dots depend on the amplitude of the reflected echoes. Tissue that transmits most of the echoes is hypoechoic (darker); tissue that reflects most of the echoes is hyperechoic (gray to white). The following tissues are classified from less to the more echoic:

Fluid < muscle < renal cortex < liver < fat < spleen < vessel wall < bone

The position of the image's dot on the screen depends on the delay between the emission of the sound wave and the reception of its echo by the probe. The longer the delays, the lower on the screen the dot is displayed.

To scan an organ in optimal condition, the area of interest must be placed in the center of the screen by placing the probe correctly and adjusting the depth of examination properly. It is important to know that the number of images generated per second (frame per second) decreases with depth, which may be compensated for by increased pulse repetition frequency, which is the number of pulses of sound waves that occur in 1 second. The manipulation of the scanner's control available on most machines is used to obtain uniform image brightness throughout the screen and good image resolution.

Image brightness

If the organ of interest is deep, the returning echo is strongly attenuated and the resulting image of poor quality. This can be compensated for by increasing the amplitude of emitted ultrasonic waves (power) or amplifying the signal of returning echoes (gain). The power control modifies the voltage applied to pulse the piezoelectric crystals, which influence the intensity of the sound beam generated by the transducer. Working with excessive power level is not recommended, however, and it should be set as low as possible. It is better to amplify the returning echoes. To that purpose there are two types of gain: global and differential. Global gain control causes uniform amplification of all returning echoes regardless of their origin. Differential gain is called time-gain compensation and consists of a series of sliders or knobs on the panel control that allow amplification of echoes at a certain depth. This is graphically represented on the screen by a curved line whose slope depends on the gain setting at each depth level. Generally the gain is set at a higher level for the far field and a lower level in the near field to obtain uniform brightness distribution.

Image resolution

There are three types of resolution in ultrasound: lateral, axial, and elevation (**Fig. 3**). Lateral resolution is the capacity to separate two points that are close to each other in the axis perpendicular to the probe. This resolution is influenced by the beam diameter, which is narrowed at the level of the focal zones (usually represented on the right

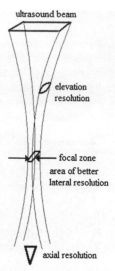

Fig. 3. Representation of the three types of resolution in an ultrasound beam. Elevation resolution is determined by the beam thickness. Lateral resolution is increased where the beam is the narrowest. Axial resolution is along the beam axis and determined by the pulse length.

side of the screen by small triangles). Adjustment of the focal zones decreases the ultrasound beam's width in a given area and allows for increasing lateral resolution. Depending on the type of machine, one or several focal zones may be available. Because higher frequency transducers generate a narrower ultrasound beam, they have better lateral resolution.

Axial resolution is the capacity to separate two elements in the ultrasound beam's axis. In most scanners it is superior to lateral resolution or elevation resolution, and measurements should be taken along the beam axis. Axial resolution is determined by the pulse length, which is usually equal to two or three wavelengths so axial resolution can be increased with increased frequency.

Elevation resolution is the ability to separate two points perpendicular to the ultrasound beam axis and scan plan. It is determined by the beam thickness and is improved with narrower beams and higher frequency.

M Mode

For bovine cardiac assessment M mode may be used.[7,8] This is a diagnostic ultrasound presentation of the temporal changes in echoes in which the depth of echo-producing interfaces on one line is displayed along the vertical axis and time is displayed along the horizontal axis (**Fig. 4**). Recording of motion of the interfaces toward and away from the transducer is then possible. This mode is particularly useful for cardiac chamber and wall measurements.

ARTIFACTS

Artifacts in ultrasound may be divided into two main categories: (1) artifacts related to the operator, such as wrong settings (power, gain, frequency) or poor patient preparation, which impair image quality; (2) artifacts that result from ultrasound interactions

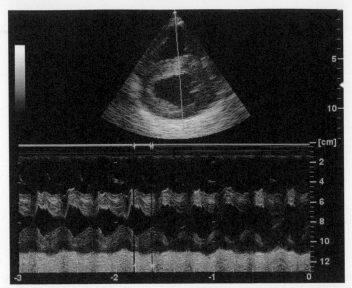

Fig. 4. Example of an M mode image of a calf's heart. The images of the echo-producing interface along the line placed on the upper B mode image are displayed in function of the time, giving a diagram of the motion of the region of interest (*lower image*).

with tissues (absorption, reflection or refraction). If adequately identified, they may be useful in the characterization of a lesion.

Reverberation Artifact

Reverberation artifact is the production of multiple echoes from one ultrasound pulse bouncing back and forth between two or more highly reflective structures in the axis of the sound beam. The air between the probe and the skin is the main cause of reverberation (external reverberation). Reflectors such as intestinal gas and bones are causes for internal reverberation. This artifact is characterized by formation of several hyperechoic lines that are equally spaced and gradually attenuated (**Fig. 5**A).

The comet-tail artifact is a type of reverberation artifact met with small reflective surfaces as gas bubbles or small metallic objects and is characterized by the formation of a narrow beam of closely spaced, discrete, hyperechoic lines (**Fig. 5**B).

Side-lobe Artifact

The emitted ultrasound beam is actually composed of a large primary beam and several secondary beams of variable intensity. When those beams strike highly reflective surfaces, they return to the probe and are interpreted as echoes from the primary beam. Generated images are added to the one coming from the primary beam. It is often seen as hyperechoic lines or dots within a hypo- to anechoic structure (**Fig. 6**) and may mimic material within the urinary bladder or gallbladder, for example. It can be corrected by decreasing the power or the gain.

Slice-thickness Artifact

The ultrasound image is based on the echoes from the structures within the thickness of the ultrasound beam. The ultrasound beam may include in its thickness two

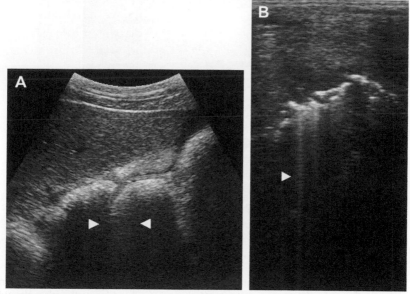

Fig. 5. Reverberation artifacts. (*A*) Gas within the spiral colon is creating reverberation arti- facts (*white arrowheads*) characterized by several hyperechoic lines, equally spaced and gradually attenuated. (*B*) Comet-tail artifact represented by a narrow beam of closely spaced, discrete, hyperechoic lines (*white arrowhead*).

structures of different echogenicity; the more echoic structure appears on a portion of the image (**Fig. 7**). This may be the case when hepatic parenchyma is included in the primary beam thickness when scanning the gallbladder. The echoic parenchyma appears within the hypoechoic bile and may be mistaken with sediments (also known as pseudosludge). Rotation of the probe helps to get rid of this artifact.

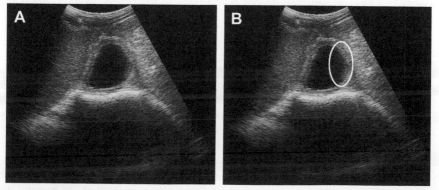

Fig. 6. Grating lobes artifact. (*A*) Transverse image of the gallbladder ventrally to the liver. (*B*) The hyperechoic foci seen within the white ellipse are echoes from secondary beams in- terpreted as coming from the primary beam and imaged within the anechoic structure, mimicking biliary suspension.

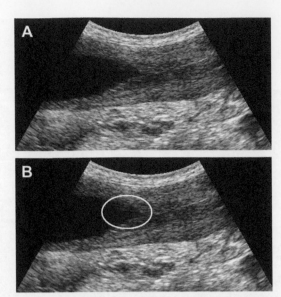

Fig. 7. Slice thickness artifact. (*A*) Longitudinal image of the urinary bladder close to an infected urachal remnant. (*B*) The irregularity of the urinary bladder wall within the white ellipse is not real and actually caused by the fact that part of the urachal canal wall is included in the beam thickness and imaged within the anechoic lumen.

Acoustic Shadowing

Acoustic shadowing appears as an anechoic area distal to a structure that strongly attenuates the ultrasound, such as bone or any mineralized or dense material (eg, metal, wood, fibrosis) (**Fig. 8**). It helps to characterize dystrophic mineralization or calculi.

Edge Shadowing

Edge shadowing is seen distal to the lateral edges of a round or oval structure. It is caused by the refraction of ultrasound on curved interface. These ultrasound waves disperse in a random way and do not come back to the probe, which gives a lack of signal and a black image (**Fig. 9**).

Distal Acoustic Enhancement

Distal acoustic enhancement is caused by augmentation of the amplitude of the echoes (brighter so whiter) distally to a structure with a low attenuation (more often fluid). It is convenient for identifying fluid-filled structures, such as cysts (**Fig. 10**). It may be reduced by decreasing the differential gain at this level.

THE DOPPLER PRINCIPLE

The basis of Doppler effect is the fact that reflected/scattered sound waves from a moving reflector undergo a change of frequency (frequency shift). In general, the magnitude and the direction of this shift provide information regarding the motion of the reflector—usually the red blood cells in veterinary medicine. Doppler ultrasound is used to detect and, if necessary, measure blood flow. The Doppler shift frequency,

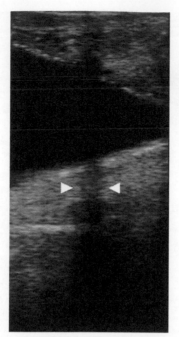

Fig. 8. Acoustic shadowing artifact. The hypoechoic band (*white arrowheads*) superimposed on this image is the result of attenuation of part of the ultrasound beam by a focus of dense material (mineralized or fibrous tissue) in the near field.

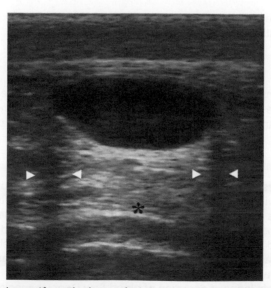

Fig. 9. Edge shadowing artifact. The hypoechoic bands (*white arrowheads*) are the result of the refraction of ultrasound on the curved interface of the jugular vein wall. Distal to the jugular vein there is also increased echogenicity of the tissue secondary to distal acoustic enhancement (*asterisk*).

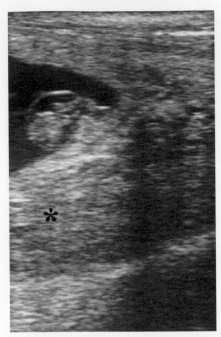

Fig. 10. Distal acoustic enhancement artifact. The increased echogenicity distal to this gravid uterus (*asterisk*) is caused by the augmentation of the amplitude of the echoes distally to allantoic and amniotic fluid with a low attenuation.

which is the difference between transmitted and received frequencies, is expressed by the Doppler equation:

$$Df = \frac{2fv\cos\theta}{c}$$

where f is the transmitted frequency, v is the blood velocity, c is the speed of sound, and θ is the angle between the sound beam and the direction of moving blood. The equation is rearranged by the machine to calculate blood velocity as

$$V = \frac{Dfc}{2f\cos\theta}$$

The angle θ is estimated by the operator by aligning an indicator on a duplex image (B mode image with superimposed Doppler cursor) along the longitudinal axis of the vessel, a process known as angle correction (**Fig. 11**). Because the cosine of 90° is 0, if the ultrasound beam is perpendicular to the direction of blood flow, there is no Doppler shift and an incorrect impression of no flow in the vessel. This angle also should be less than 60° at all times, because the cosine function has a steeper curve above this angle and errors in angle correction are magnified.

There are several forms of depiction of blood flow Doppler imaging: color Doppler, pulsed Doppler, and power Doppler. Color Doppler provides an estimate of the mean velocity of flow within a vessel by color coding the information and displaying it superimposed on the gray-scale image. The flow direction is more often arbitrarily assigned

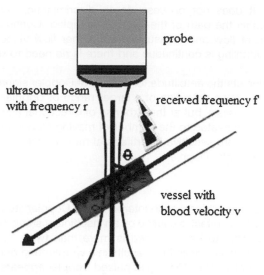

Fig. 11. Principles of Doppler imaging. The angle θ is the angle between the ultrasound beam and the longitudinal axis of the vessel. Its estimation is important in the calculation of the blood velocity. The Doppler shift frequency (Df) is the difference between transmitted (f) and received (f′) frequency: Df = f-f′.

the color red or blue, indicating flow toward and away from the transducer, respectively (**Fig. 12**).

Pulsed Doppler allows a sampling volume (or gate) to be positioned in a vessel visualized on the gray-scale image and displays a spectrum of the full range (as opposed to the mean velocity, as in color Doppler) of blood velocities within the gate plotted as a function of time. The amplitude of the signal is approximately proportional to the number of red blood cells and is indicated as a shade of gray.

Continuous wave Doppler uses a special transducer with two crystals. Sound is transmitted and received continuously by use of the separate transmitting and

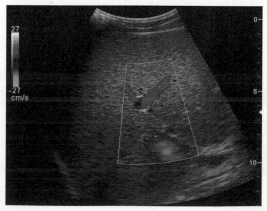

Fig. 12. Example of color Doppler image on hepatic vessels. The vessel in the near field (*red*) is a portal vessel; its flow is going toward the probe. The vessel in the far field (*blue*) is a hepatic vein; its flow is going away from the probe.

receiving crystals. It does not possess depth discrimination, which means that anything moving within the path of the beam is sampled. Continuous Doppler can determine direction of flow and measure much higher flow velocities than pulsed Doppler because sampling is continuous and there is no need to wait for echoes to return.

Power Doppler depicts the amplitude, or power, of Doppler signals rather than the frequency shift. This allows detection of a larger range of Doppler shifts and better visualization of small vessels, but at the expense of directional and velocity information. Color brightness is related to the number of moving blood cells. It is much less angle dependant but more sensitive to artifactual motion, and the frame rate tends to be slower than with color Doppler.

ALIASING ARTIFACT

Aliasing is one of the main artifacts encountered during Doppler studies and is the only one discussed here. This artifact is caused by an insufficient sampling rate and occurs when the frequency shift to be measured is more than twice the pulse repetition frequency (Nyquist frequency or limit). It results in a wraparound of the Doppler spectrum in pulsed or color Doppler. Aliasing at pulsed Doppler appears as the displaying of the spectrum of higher velocities lower in the scale. Aliasing at color Doppler manifests as a mixture of colors or as a focus of color in the vessel, which indicates an opposite direction than the normal flow. Aliasing can be reduced by increasing the pulse repetition frequency or using a lower frequency transducer, thus decreasing the Doppler shift.

PATIENT PREPARATION

For every transcutaneous ultrasonographic examination, the area has to be shaved and the skin cleaned with water or alcohol. Acoustic gel is then applied to improve the contact between the probe and the skin. Organs are scanned in sagittal and transverse plans with the goal of building a three-dimensional image in the examiner's mind, which is useful for distinguishing nodular from tubular structures. It is important to bear in mind that ultrasound is sensitive for evaluating tissue changes but is poorly specific. Sampling of the imaged lesion for cytologic study is often necessary to reach a final diagnosis.

SUMMARY

The acquisition of good quality ultrasound images depends on different factors, such as ultrasound equipment that is used, the technique of the operator, and his or her knowledge of the physical principles of this medical imaging technique. The most important acoustic artifacts need to be understood because they should not be over- or misinterpreted by the clinician in order to help in the diagnostic process.

REFERENCES

1. Fraser AF, Nagaratnam V, Callicott RB. The comprehensive use of Doppler ultrasound in farm animal reproduction. Vet Rec 1971;88(8):202–5.
2. Braun U. Atlas und lehrbuch der ultraschalldiagnostik beim rind [Atlas and textbook of ultrasonographic diagnosis in the cow]. Berlin: Parey Buchverlag; 1997. p. 279 [in German].
3. Herring DS, Bjornton G. Physics, facts, and artifacts of diagnostic ultrasound. Vet Clin North Am Small Anim Pract 1985;15(6):1107–21.

4. Nyland TG, Mattoon JS, Herrgesell EJ, et al. Physical principle, instrumentation, and safety of diagnostic ultrasound. In: Small animal diagnostic ultrasound. 2nd edition. Philadelphia: WB Saunders; 2002. p. 1–18.
5. Kremkau FW. Ultrasounds. In: Diagnostic ultrasound, principles and instruments. 7th edition. Philadelphia: WB Saunders; 2006. p. 17–53.
6. Penninck DG. Artifacts. In: Nyland TG, Mattoon JS, editors. Small animal diagnostic ultrasound. 2nd edition. Philadelphia: WB Saunders; 2002. p. 19–29.
7. Amory H, Jakovljevic S, Lekeux P. Quantitative M-mode and two-dimensional echocardiography in calves. Vet Rec 1991;128(2):25–31.
8. Pipers FS, Reef VB, Hamlin RL, et al. Echocardiography in the bovine animal. Bovine Pract 1978;30:114–8.

Ultrasonography of the Gastrointestinal Tract in Cattle

Ueli Braun, Prof Dr med vet, Dr med vet h c

KEYWORDS

- Cattle • Ultrasonography • Reticulum • Omasum
- Abomasum • Intestine

Ultrasonography is an ideal diagnostic tool for the investigation of bovine gastrointestinal disorders, the most common of which are traumatic reticuloperitonitis, left and right displacement of the abomasum, ileus of the small intestine, and dilatation and displacement of the cecum. An ultrasonographic examination is performed on non-sedated, standing cattle using a 3.5 MHz to 5.0 linear or convex transducer. When a tentative diagnosis has been made based on the clinical findings, often only the region in question is examined. For example, in cases with suspected traumatic reticuloperitonitis, the examination is performed in the sternal and parasternal regions, and in cattle suspected of having cholestasis, only the costal part of the abdominal wall on the right side is examined. Even experienced clinicians may not be able to pinpoint the organ affected and make a diagnosis in patients in which abdominal disease is suspected, however. In such cases, both sides of the abdomen are examined. Normally, the reticulum,[1,2] spleen,[1–4] rumen,[2] and parts of the abomasum[5,6] are seen on the left side, and the liver,[7–9] omasum,[10,11] parts of the abomasum,[5,6] small intestine,[12,13] large intestine,[14,15] and right kidney[16] are seen on the right. The uterus may be seen on either side depending on the stage of pregnancy.

This article describes the ultrasonographic techniques used for examination of the reticulum, rumen, omasum, abomasum, small intestine, and large intestine. The normal findings are presented followed by a description of the most important diseases of these organs.

RETICULUM/RUMEN

Ultrasonographic Examination of the Reticulum and Normal Findings

For ultrasonographic examination of the reticulum, the transducer is applied to the ventral aspect of the thorax on the left and right of the sternum and to the left and right lateral thorax up to the level of the elbow.[1,2,17,18] The reticulum is first examined from

Department of Farm Animals, University of Zurich, Winterthurerstrasse 260, CH-8057 Zürich, Switzerland
E-mail address: ubraun@vetclinics.uzh.ch

Vet Clin Food Anim 25 (2009) 567–590
doi:10.1016/j.cvfa.2009.07.004
0749-0720/09/$ – see front matter © 2009 Elsevier Inc. All rights reserved.

the left side and then the right. The normal reticulum appears as a half-moon-shaped structure with an even contour (**Fig. 1**). It contracts at regular intervals and when relaxed, it is situated immediately adjacent to the diaphragm and ventral portion of the abdominal wall. The different layers of the reticular wall usually cannot be imaged, and the honeycomb-like structure of the mucosa is not often seen clearly. In cattle with ascites, the tunica serosa of the reticulum appears as a narrow echogenic line, the tunica muscularis is seen as a hypoechogenic line, and the tunica mucosa is seen as a wider echogenic line (**Fig. 2**). Contents of the reticulum cannot be normally imaged because of their partly gaseous composition. Foreign bodies and magnets also cannot usually be seen in the reticulum because of the gas content of the reticulum. Radiography is the method of choice for identifying radiodense foreign bodies and magnets.[19]

The craniodorsal blind sac of the rumen and the transition to the ventral sac of the rumen can be seen caudal to the reticulum (**Fig. 3**). The abomasum is frequently seen between the craniodorsal blind sac of the rumen or rumen and ventral abdominal wall, immediately caudal to the reticulum. For assessment of reticular motility, the transducer is placed on the left ventral thoracic region. The reticulum is located and observed for 3 minutes without moving the transducer. The number, amplitude, and speed of reticular contractions and the duration of the interval of relaxation between two biphasic reticular contractions are assessed. The reticulum normally contracts once per minute in a biphasic manner, in which the first contraction is incomplete.[1,2] Thus, in the 3-minute observation period, the reticulum has three biphasic contractions. Contraction of the craniodorsal blind sac of the rumen is seen immediately after the second reticular contraction. Rumination is associated with an additional ruminal contraction, which occurs immediately before the biphasic contraction.

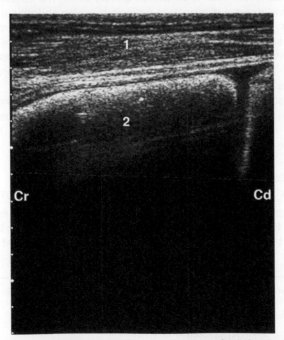

Fig. 1. Ultrasonogram of the normal reticulum imaged from the left sternal region. Ventral abdominal wall (1), reticulum (2). Cd, caudal; Cr, cranial.

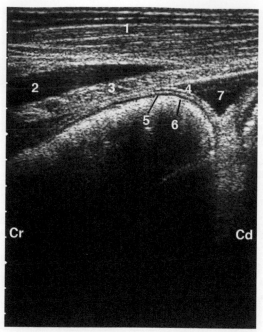

Fig. 2. Ultrasonogram of the normal reticulum in a cow with mild ascites imaged from the left sternal region. Ventral abdominal wall (1), musculophrenic vein (2), diaphragm (3), tunica serosa of the reticulum (4), tunica muscularis of the reticulum (5), tunica mucosa of the reticulum (6), mild ascites (7). Cd, caudal; Cr, cranial.

Control of Reticular Motility

Reticular motility is initiated and controlled by the vagus nerve, which in turn is under the influence of the gastric center in the medulla oblongata.[20] Several factors, including eating, rumination, and stress, affect reticular motility.[21,22] The number of reticular contractions is highest during eating (approximately 1.5/min) and lowest when the cow is stressed (a little less than 1/min).

In cattle with vagal indigestion, the number of reticular contractions may be reduced, normal, or increased.[21,23] In 144 cows with vagal indigestion, the number of contractions ranged from 0 to 12 per 3 minutes. Cows with reticulo-omasal stenosis had significantly more reticular contractions (4.6 contractions/3 min) than cows with functional stenosis of the pylorus (3.6 contraction/3 min). Reticular hypermotility also commonly occurs in cows with mechanical stenosis in the region of the reticulum;[24] two of three cows with reticulo-omasal stenosis caused by a rope foreign body had 6 contractions per 3 minutes. (For a discussion of reticular motility in traumatic reticuloperitonitis, see the section on traumatic reticuloperitonitis.)

Drugs also affect reticular motility. Atropine, scopolamine, and xylazine inhibit reticular motility.[25,26] Reticular atony occurred within 0 to 3 minutes of intravenous administration of these drugs and lasted 3 to 111 minutes. The drug dose was directly proportional to the onset and duration of atony.

Rumen

The rumen can be imaged in the region of the left costal part of the abdominal wall. From dorsal to ventral are the dorsal sac of the rumen, the longitudinal groove of

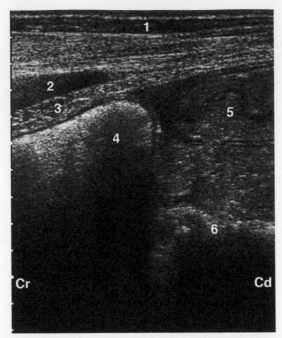

Fig. 3. Ultrasonogram of the reticulum, craniodorsal blind sac of the rumen, and abomasum imaged from the left sternal region. Ventral abdominal wall (1), musculophrenic vein (2), diaphragm (3), reticulum (4), abomasum (5), craniodorsal blind sac of the rumen (6). Cd, caudal; Cr, cranial.

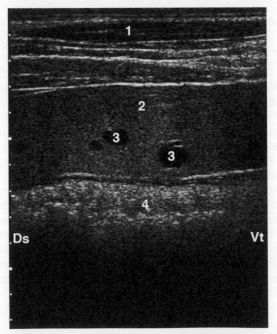

Fig. 4. Ultrasonogram of the normal spleen imaged from the distal portion of the sixth intercostal space. Lateral thoracic wall (1), spleen (2), spleen vessels (3), rumen (4). Ds, dorsal; Vt, ventral.

rumen, and the ventral sac of the rumen. The ruminal wall appears echogenic. Reverberation artifacts running parallel to the ruminal wall are seen in the region of the dorsal gas cap.[27] The ingesta are located in the middle of the rumen and appear echogenic with gaseous inclusions. The fluid in the ventral aspect of the rumen is hypoechogenic.[27]

Spleen

The spleen is located craniodorsally on the rumen. The spleen can be seen in the intercostal spaces 7 to 12.[3,4] It is 2 to 5 cm thick and tapered ventrally. The splenic capsule appears as an echogenic line. The splenic parenchyma consists of numerous small, regularly spaced echoes, and vessels within the parenchyma appear as anechoic round to oval or elongated images (**Fig. 4**). The long axis is oblique and runs from caudodorsal to cranioventral.

Traumatic Reticuloperitonitis

In cattle with traumatic reticuloperitonitis, ultrasonography can be used to identify morphologic changes in the region of the cranial, ventral, or caudal reticular wall.[28] The caudoventral reticular wall is the most frequently affected, often in association with the craniodorsal blind sac of the rumen. The changes in the contour of the reticulum depend on the severity of the inflammatory changes. Deposits of fibrinous tissue interspersed with fluid pockets are frequently seen on the reticular serosa and structures adjacent to the reticulum (**Figs. 5–8**). The extent of the inflammatory lesions

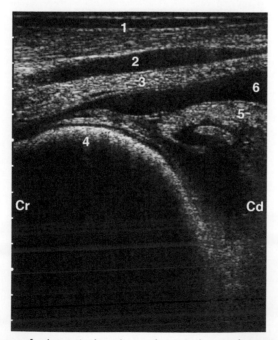

Fig. 5. Ultrasonogram of echogenic deposits on the reticulum and accumulation of fluid in a cow with traumatic reticuloperitonitis imaged from the left ventral thorax. Ventral abdominal wall (1), musculophrenic vein (2), diaphragm (3), reticulum (4), echogenic deposits of fibrin (5), accumulation of fluid (6). Cd, caudal; Cr, cranial.

varies greatly but may occasionally extend to the region of the flank fold. Remarkably, these inflammatory lesions can resolve within 6 months of effective treatment.[29] Ultrasonography revealed that 9 of 16 cows had no remaining adhesions 6 months after treatment and the adhesions in the other 7 cows had markedly regressed.[29]

Reticular abscesses have an echogenic capsule of varying thickness that surrounds a homogeneous hypoechogenic to moderately echogenic center (**Figs. 9** and **10**). The contents of an abscess are frequently partitioned by echogenic septa. Abscesses are usually caudoventral to the reticulum but may be cranial or lateral to the reticulum. Abscesses are often seen between the reticulum and spleen, reticulum and liver, or reticulum and omasum or abomasum. Reticular abscesses vary in diameter from a few centimeters to more than 15 cm. In certain cases, it is possible to drain abscesses through an ultrasound-guided transcutaneous incision.[30] The abscess must be immediately adjacent to and attached to the abdominal wall, however, and the intercostal space over the abscess must be large enough.

Reticular activity is almost always affected in cattle with traumatic reticuloperitonitis. The frequency, amplitude, or speed of contractions—singly or combined—may be abnormal. The frequency can be reduced from three to two, one or no contractions per 3 minutes. The reduction in the amplitude of contractions varies; when formation of adhesions is extensive, reticular contractions appear indistinct via ultrasonography. Although the pattern of biphasic contraction often is maintained, the reticulum contracts by only 1 to 3 cm. The speed of reticular contractions may be normal but can be markedly reduced.

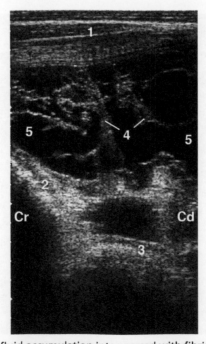

Fig. 6. Ultrasonogram of fluid accumulation interspersed with fibrin in a cow with traumatic reticuloperitonitis imaged from the left ventral thorax. Ventral abdominal wall (1), caudal wall of the reticulum (2), craniodorsal blind sac of the rumen (3), strands of fibrin (4), fluid accumulation (5). Cd, caudal; Cr, cranial.

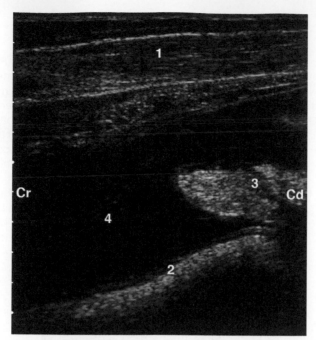

Fig. 7. Ultrasonogram of echogenic deposits on the reticulum and accumulation of fluid in a cow with traumatic reticuloperitonitis imaged from the left ventral thorax. Ventral abdominal wall (1), reticulum (2), echogenic deposits of fibrin (3), accumulation of fluid (4). Cd, caudal; Cr, cranial.

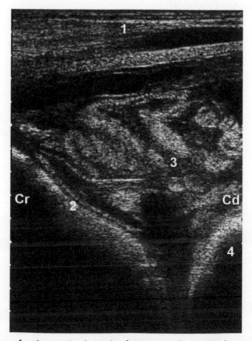

Fig. 8. Ultrasonogram of echogenic deposits between the reticulum and the craniodorsal blind sac of the rumen in a cow with traumatic reticuloperitonitis imaged from the left ventral thorax. Ventral abdominal wall (1), reticulum (2), echogenic deposits of fibrin(3), craniodorsal blind sac of the rumen (4). Cd, caudal; Cr, cranial.

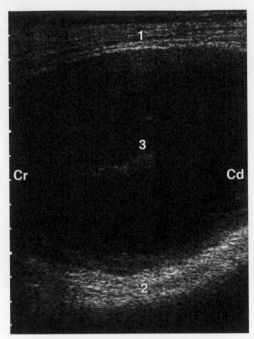

Fig. 9. Ultrasonogram of an abscess ventral to the reticulum of a cow with traumatic reticuloperitonitis imaged from the left ventral thorax. Ventral abdominal wall (1), reticulum (2), abscess (3). Cd, caudal; Cr, cranial.

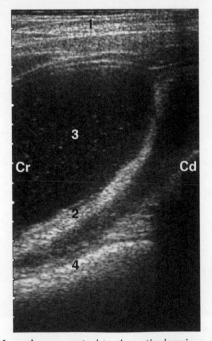

Fig. 10. Ultrasonogram of an abscess ventral to the reticulum in a cow with traumatic reticuloperitonitis imaged from the left ventral thorax. Ventral abdominal wall (1), abscess capsule (2), abscess lumen (3), reticulum (4). Cd, caudal; Cr, cranial.

An inflammatory effusion is often seen near the reticulum in cattle with traumatic reticuloperitonitis. Peritoneal effusion is visible ultrasonographically as an accumulation of fluid without an echogenic margin and restricted to the reticular area (**Fig. 11**). Depending on the fibrin and cell content, the fluid may be anechoic or hypoechogenic. Fibrinous deposits are easily identified in the fluid; sometimes, bands of fibrin are seen within the effusion. Occasionally, the peritoneal effusion is considerable and extends to the caudal abdomen (**Fig. 12**). The lesions may be within (omental bursitis) or outside the omentum (peritonitis). In such cases, the greater omentum is commonly seen as an echogenic structure surrounded by fluid.

The spleen, particularly its distal portion, is often affected in cattle with traumatic reticuloperitonitis. Fibrinous changes are frequently seen as echogenic deposits of varying thickness (**Fig. 13**), often surrounded by fluid, between the spleen and reticulum or rumen. The spleen may be covered with fibrinous deposits. Occasionally, one or more splenic abscesses are visible (**Fig. 14**), and the vasculature may be dilated, which indicates splenitis.

OMASUM

The omasum is visible in the sixth to eleventh intercostal spaces.[10,11] It has a crescent shape with only the wall closest to the transducer visible as a thick echogenic line (**Fig. 15**). The size of the omasum varies with the intercostal spaces from 16.3 ± 1.5 cm to 56.9 ± 10.0 cm. The size of the omasum is greatest in the ninth intercostal space

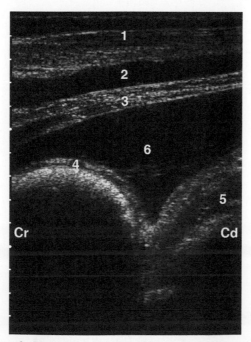

Fig. 11. Ultrasonogram of a small fluid accumulation caudal to the reticulum in a cow with traumatic reticuloperitonitis imaged from the sternal part of the ventral abdomen. Ventral abdominal wall (1), musculophrenic vein (2), diaphragm (3), reticulum (4), craniodorsal blind sac of the rumen with fibrin depositis (5), hypoechoic fluid accumulation (caused by inflammation) (6). Cd, caudal; Cr, cranial.

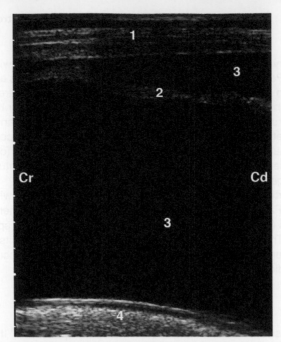

Fig. 12. Ultrasonogram of a large fluid accumulation caused by peritonitis in a cow with traumatic reticuloperitonitis. The rumen is imaged from the left side of the ventral abdomen. Ventral abdominal wall (1), omentum (2), fluid accumulation (3), rumen (4). Cd, caudal; Cr, cranial.

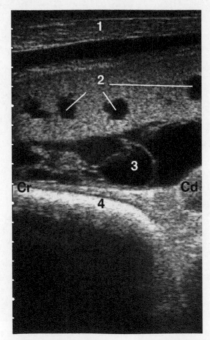

Fig. 13. Ultrasonogram of inflammatory changes between the reticulum and the spleen in a cow with traumatic reticuloperitonitis imaged from the left ventral thorax. Ventral abdominal wall (1), spleen with dilated vessels (2), fluid-containing fibrin between the reticulum and the spleen (3), reticulum (4). Cd, caudal; Cr, cranial.

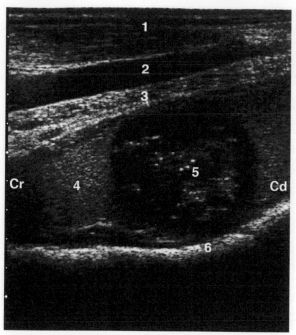

Fig. 14. Ultrasonogram of a large abscess in the spleen imaged from the left ventral thorax. Ventral thoracic wall (1), musculophrenic vein (2), diaphragm (3), spleen (4), abscess in the spleen (5), reticulum indented by the spleen (6). Cd, caudal; Cr, cranial.

and decreases cranially and caudally. The omasum is located closest to the right abdominal wall in the eighth and ninth intercostal spaces, and in many cows it is immediately adjacent to it in this region. Unlike the reticulum, the omasum of healthy cows does not have any apparent active motility of its own. The omasal laminae cannot be imaged in healthy cows because of intraluminal gas. Occasionally, the attachments of the omasal laminae are seen as short echogenic cone-shaped structures that protrude from the inner wall of the omasum. Occasionally the omasal laminae can be seen in ill cattle (**Fig. 16**) with an increased fluid content in the omasum, usually caused by abomasal reflux. The position and size of the omasum change in cattle with right and left displacement of the abomasum, abomasal volvulus, traumatic reticuloperitonitis, ileus and reticulo-omasal stenosis.[10,31] Omasal motility can be observed in rare cases of reticulo-omasal stenosis. Primary diseases of the omasum are rare; one publication described the ultrasonographic findings in a cow that had a leiomyoma in the omasum.[32]

ABOMASUM

Ultrasonography is a valuable technique for the assessment of the size, position, and content of the abomasum. The abomasum can be visualized approximately 10 cm caudal to the xyphoid process from the left and right paramedian regions and from the ventral midline.[5,6] The bulk of the abomasum is situated to the right of the ventral midline. The abomasum is frequently seen immediately caudal to the reticulum between the craniodorsal blind sac of the rumen, or the rumen, and the ventral abdominal wall

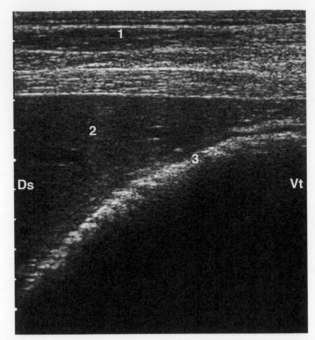

Fig. 15. Ultrasonogram of the normal omasum imaged from the eighth intercostal space of the right side. The wall of the omasum appears as a curved echogenic line. The liver is situated on the omasum dorsolaterally. Costal part of the abdominal wall (1), liver (2), omasal wall (3). Ds, dorsal; Vt, ventral.

(see **Fig. 3**). The wall of the abomasum appears at the most as a thin echogenic line. The abomasum is easily differentiated from neighboring organs by the ultrasonographic appearance of its contents, however, which are seen as a heterogeneous moderately echogenic mass with echogenic stippling. Parts of the abomasal folds occasionally can be seen as echogenic structures within the content of the abomasum. Passive and slow movements of the abomasal contents are frequently seen.

The position of the abomasum changes in late pregnancy because of the expanding uterus.[33–35] The abomasum changes from a more longitudinal to a transverse position but within 14 days of parturition resumes its normal longitudinal position.

Abomasocentesis

Percutaneous ultrasound-guided abomasocentesis can be performed to evaluate the nature and chemical composition of abomasal contents.[36] Centesis is performed at a site in which the abomasum appears large and in which no other organs are in the way. Abomasal fluid is assessed mainly for color, smell, and the presence of blood, and the pH is determined. Blood does not normally occur in abomasal fluid. In most cases, blood originates from an abomasal ulcer[36] and rarely from the rumen or small intestine.

Left Displacement of the Abomasum

An ultrasonographic examination is useful to confirm the diagnosis of left displacement of the abomasum in unclear cases.[37] The last three intercostal spaces on the

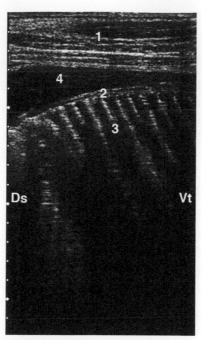

Fig. 16. Ultrasonogram of the omasum of a cow with abomasal volvulus imaged from the tenth intercostal space. The omasal laminae appear as thin echogenic lines. Costal part of the abdominal wall (1), omasal wall (2), omasal laminae (3), greater omentum (4). Ds, dorsal; Vt, ventral.

left side are examined ventrally to dorsally with the transducer held parallel to the ribs. Normally, the rumen is immediately adjacent to the left abdominal wall. On ultrasonograms, the ruminal wall is medial to the abdominal wall and from ventral to dorsal appears as a smooth, thick, echogenic line, which is indented at the left longitudinal sulcus. With left displacement of the abomasum, the wall of the rumen often is still immediately adjacent to the abdominal wall in the ventral region. When the transducer is moved dorsally, it becomes apparent that the wall of the rumen is pushed medially and then can no longer be imaged ultrasonographically. Instead the abomasum is seen—located between the abdominal wall and rumen. Moving the transducer further dorsally, the abomasum disappears and the rumen reappears on the screen.

The abomasal contents do not appear uniform because ventrally there are fluid ingesta and dorsally there is a gas cap that varies in extent. The ingesta visible ventrally in the abomasum appear hypoechogenic (**Fig. 17**). Occasionally, the abomasal folds are visible among the ingesta and appear as elongated, echogenic, sickle-shaped structures. The ruminal wall often can be seen medial to the ingesta. The abomasal gas cap, seen further dorsally, is characterized by reverberation artifacts (**Fig. 18**) similar to those observed during the ultrasonographic examination of lung.

Right Displacement of the Abomasum and Abomasal Volvulus

Ultrasonography also is a useful diagnostic tool in doubtful cases of right displacement of the abomasum and abomasal volvulus. The area immediately caudal to the last rib and the caudal three to four intercostal spaces on the right side are examined

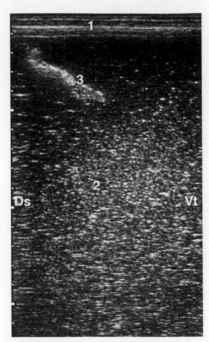

Fig. 17. Ultrasonogram of left displacement of the abomasum imaged from the ventral region of the twelfth intercostal space. Abdominal wall (1), abomasum with hypoechogenic ingesta (2), abomasal fold (3). Ds, dorsal; Vt, ventral.

from ventral to dorsal with the transducer held parallel to the ribs.[18,38,39] Normally, loops of small intestine are imaged in cross-section and, less commonly, longitudinally in the ventral abdomen. Further dorsally, the liver is seen immediately adjacent to the right abdominal wall. In animals with right displacement of the abomasum or abomasal volvulus, the liver is displaced from the abdominal wall. The abomasum is seen where the liver would normally be, immediately adjacent to the right abdominal wall. Its ultrasonographic appearance is the same as that described previously for left displacement.

The ultrasonographic appearance of right displacement of the abomasum cannot be differentiated from abomasal volvulus.[38,39] In both disorders, the liver, omasum, and small and large intestine may be displaced, depending on the size of the abomasum.[38,40] In contrast to healthy cows, in which the liver always can be imaged on the right side, there is a significant decrease in the frequency with which the liver is seen from the different intercostal spaces in cows with abomasal displacement or volvulus. In fact, sometimes the liver cannot be imaged on the right side at all because it is displaced from the abdominal wall by the abomasum. The omasum and small and large intestine are also less frequently seen in cows with right displacement of the abomasum and abomasal volvulus compared with healthy cows.

Defects in Abomasal Emptying

Defects in emptying of the abomasum occur with functional or mechanical pyloric stenosis. Abomasal emptying can also be impaired secondary to intestinal ileus. With all these disorders, the abomasum is dilated but not displaced dorsally or torsed. Depending on its degree of fill, the dilated abomasum can be imaged on the right side

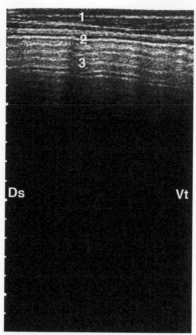

Fig. 18. Ultrasonogram of left displacement of the abomasum imaged from the dorsal region of the twelfth intercostal space. The abomasal gas cap is not visible because of reverberation artifacts at the abomasal surface. Abdominal wall (1), abomasal wall (2), reverberation artifacts (3). Ds, dorsal; Vt, ventral.

from the ventral region of intercostal spaces 8 to 12 or even from the ventral abdomen caudal to the ribs. In contrast to left or right displacement, there is no accumulation of gas in the non-displaced, dilated abomasum. The abomasal contents appear predominantly hypoechogenic and homogeneous and, because of sequestration of hypochloric acid, are frequently fluid in nature. This often allows for good visualization of the abomasal folds, which appear as thin, echogenic, wavy structures (**Fig. 19**). In animals with ileus, the loops of intestine are dilated and clearly visible. With pyloric stenosis, the small intestine is empty.

Abomasitis/Abomasal Ulcers

Discrete lesions of the abomasal mucosa, such as chronic abomasitis, parasitic nodules, erosions, and type 1 ulcers, cannot be imaged ultrasonographically using a 3.5- or 5.0-MHz transducer. Type 3 abomasal ulcers produce abdominal changes similar to those of fibrinous traumatic reticuloperitonitis with abscessation. Type 4 abomasal ulcers produce signs of generalized peritonitis with ascites, fibrinous adhesions, and thickening of the intestinal wall. Abomasal ulcers have never been imaged with ultrasound.

INTESTINE
Normal Small Intestine

For ultrasonography of the small intestine in cattle, the area from the tuber coxae to the eighth intercostal space and from the transverse processes of the vertebrae to the linea alba on the right side is examined.[12,13] The appearance of loops of small intestine

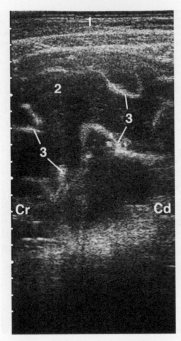

Fig. 19. Ultrasonogram of the abomasum dilated secondary to ileus of the jejunum imaged from the right paramedian region. The abomasal contents appear hypoechogenic and the abomasal folds are clearly visible as thin, echogenic wavy structures. Abdominal wall (1), abomasum (2), abomasal folds (3). Cd, caudal; Cr, cranial.

and their diameter, contents, and motility are assessed. The wall of the normal small intestine is 2 to 3 mm thick and its luminal diameter is 2 to 4 cm.[13] Evaluation of the contents of the small intestine in cattle is usually straightforward because there is generally no gas. Unlike small animals and humans, ruminants digest carbohydrates principally in the forestomachs, from which the gas is eructated.[41] The ultrasonographic appearance of the contents of the small intestine varies. Most commonly, the intestine contains mucus or feed, which appears hyperechogenic. In these cases, not only the intestinal wall closest to the transducer but also the intestinal contents and the wall furthest from the transducer can be visualized. This is also true for intestine filled with fluid, which is hypoechogenic. In rare cases with gaseous intestinal contents, the intestinal wall closest to the transducer appears as a hyperechogenic line adjacent to an acoustic shadow. Because of reflection of the ultrasound waves at the soft tissue–air interface, the intestinal contents and the intestinal wall furthest from the transducer cannot be visualized. In contrast with results in dogs, there is no difference between the diameter of most of the small intestine before and after feeding in cattle.[42] This uniformity is probably because the forestomachs constitute a feed reservoir and ingesta pass along the intestine continuously, independent of feed intake, and without changes in the diameter of the intestinal lumen, which would be measurable by ultrasonography.

The cranial part of the duodenum is relatively easy to identify because it originates from the abomasum and is in close proximity to the liver and gallbladder. It is seen in cross-section or longitudinally medial or ventral to the gallbladder and almost always from the tenth or eleventh intercostal space. The diameter of the cranial part of the duodenum ranges from 0.9 to 5.5 cm.[13] The descending duodenum also is easily imaged in most cattle. From the tenth, eleventh, or twelfth intercostal space and from the dorsal region of the right flank, it is observed in cross-section or longitudinally. The following characteristics allow accurate identification of the descending duodenum. It is situated immediately adjacent to the abdominal wall and runs horizontally and caudally between the serosal lamellae of the omentum, which appears as an echogenic envelope around the descending duodenum. It then courses caudally to form the caudal duodenal flexure at the level of the tuber coxae. After this, it runs medially and cranially to form the ascending duodenum. The diameter of the descending duodenum varies from 1.5 to 3.5 cm. The ascending duodenum is situated more than 20 cm from the right abdominal wall and cannot be imaged via ultrasonography.

The jejunum and ileum form the longest part of the small intestine and cannot be differentiated from one another ultrasonographically. It is typical to see more than ten loops of jejunum and ileum immediately adjacent to one another from the flank and lateral abdominal wall and from intercostal spaces 9 to 12.[13] The loops of small intestine are usually seen in cross-section and occasionally longitudinally. They can be differentiated from the descending duodenum because they are not surrounded by omentum and because they are constantly in motion (**Fig. 20**). Loops of jejunum and ileum are seen from the tenth intercostal space in approximately 70% of cows and from the ninth intercostal space in approximately 10% of cows. The diameter of the jejunum and ileum ranges from 2 to 4 cm. The number of loops of jejunum and ileum visible longitudinally and in cross-section is approximately the same when imaged from the flank and the twelfth intercostal space, but it decreases when imaged from the successive intercostal spaces.

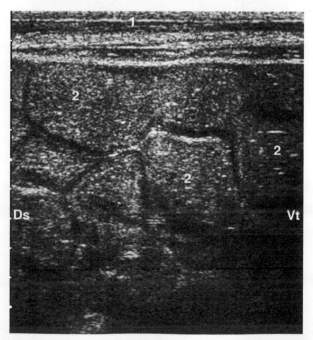

Fig. 20. Ultrasonogram of cross-sections through loops of the jejunum imaged from the right flank. Several loops of jejunum, seen in cross-section, are situated immediately adjacent to one another. Abdominal wall (1), loops of jejunum (2). Ds, dorsal; Vt, ventral.

Ileus of the Small Intestine

When ileus of the small intestine is suspected, an ultrasonographic examination should evaluate the diameter, motility, and anatomic arrangement of the small intestine, evidence of peritonitis, and the possible cause of the ileus.[18,43] The most important parameters are diameter and motility of the small intestine; identification of the cause of ileus via ultrasonography is rarely possible. In cattle with ileus, the small intestine is dilated in at least one area and has a diameter of more than 3.5 cm.[43] The motility of the small intestine is usually reduced or absent. Sometimes, hypoechogenic fluid, which is attributable to transudation, is visible between the dilated loops of intestine. Independent of the localization of ileus and its cause, the loops of small intestine are most commonly imaged in cross-section (**Fig. 21**), often in cross-section and longitudinally (**Fig. 22**) but rarely only longitudinally.

The site of ileus markedly affects the number of dilated loops of intestine seen in cross-section and longitudinally from either the flank or each intercostal space. When only one or a few usually markedly dilated loops of small intestine are seen (**Fig. 23**), ileus of the duodenum is most likely.[43,44] More than five loops of small intestine seen in one area usually indicates ileus of the jejunum or ileum. Rarely, when the ileus is localized in the proximal jejunum, only one or two dilated loops of small intestine are imaged. The number of dilated loops of small intestine increases if the localization of the ileus is more distal. Conversely, in the eighth and ninth intercostal spaces, the number of dilated loops of small intestine generally decreases.

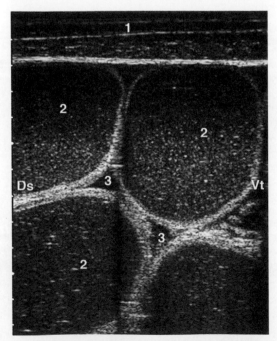

Fig. 21. Ultrasonogram of cross-sections through dilated loops of the jejunum in a cow with ileus imaged from the twelfth intercostal space. The contents of the loops appear echogenic. There is anechoic fluid between the loops. Abdominal wall (1), dilated loops of the jejunum (2), anechoic fluid between the loops of the jejunum (3). Ds, dorsal; Vt, ventral.

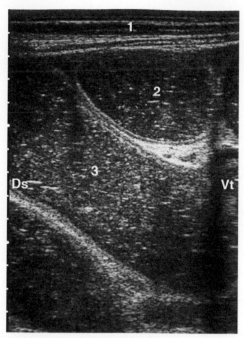

Fig. 22. Ultrasonogram of cross- and longitudinal sections through dilated loops of the jejunum in a cow with ileus imaged from the twelfth intercostal space. The contents of the loops appear echogenic. Abdominal wall (1), loop of jejunum in cross-section (2), loop of jejunum in longitudinal section (3). Ds Dorsal, Vt Ventral.

The loops become more dilated with ileus of the proximal small intestine. The largest diameter of intestine measured from the twelfth intercostal space varied from 6.5 to 9.9 cm (7.7 ± 1.9) in animals with ileus of the duodenum, from 3.5 to 9.8 cm (5.5 ± 1.7) in animals with ileus of the jejunum, and from 4.4 to 5.5 cm (5.0 ± 0.4 cm) in animals with ileus of the ileum.[43] When interpreting the diameter of the intestine, it is important to remember that in healthy cows, in which the intestine is full of ingesta, all parts of the intestine have a similar diameter. By contrast, in animals with ileus, in addition to the extremely dilated loops of intestine proximal to the ileus, there are usually empty loops of intestine distal to the ileus. The intestinal lumen of a healthy cow is constantly changing, whereas the increased intestinal diameter of a cow with ileus remains unchanged because the intestinal motility is markedly reduced or absent.

The contents of the small intestine appear predominantly echogenic and rarely anechoic. Different parts of the intestine of the same animal may be echogenic or an-echoic. Intraluminal gas, which is associated with reverberation artifacts, is rarely observed. In most cows with ileus of the small intestine, intestinal motility is markedly reduced or absent. Movement of intestinal contents often is apparent, however, although no intestinal contractions are visible. This flowing movement is presumably caused by the passive movement of the intestine by respiratory activity and possibly by the movement of adjacent organs, such as the rumen or abomasum.

The cause of ileus seldom can be determined ultrasonographically, often because the cause of ileus is further from the abdominal wall than the penetration capacity of the transducer. A common cause of ileus is intussusception, the ultrasonographic

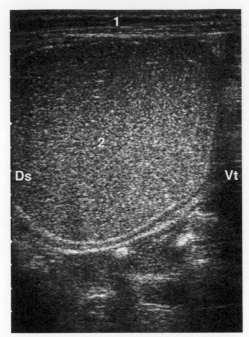

Fig. 23. Ultrasonogram of a cross-section through the dilated duodenum of a cow with duodenal ileus imaged from the tenth intercostal space. Abdominal wall (1), dilated duodenum in cross-section (2). Ds, dorsal; Vt, ventral.

appearance of which in cross-section has been described as bowel within bowel, bull's eye lesion, target pattern, or multiple layered, onion ring–type mass with varying echogenicities. Typically, the invaginated intestinal wall is swollen. Depending on the severity of edema and the imaging plane, the affected area of intestine may appear hyperechogenic or hypoechogenic. Viewed longitudinally, the typical lumen-within-a-lumen appearance can be clearly identified and has been described as a "sandwich" configuration. In rare cases, compression of the small intestine by abscesses in the region of the liver or compression of the duodenum between the liver and gallbladder can be identified. Ileus also can be caused by generalized peritonitis with fibrinous adhesions involving the small intestine. In such cases, thickening of the intestinal wall, fibrinous deposits, and accumulation of intra-abdominal fluid are usually seen. In cattle with hemorrhagic bowel syndrome, the blood clots occasionally can be imaged as an echogenic masses in the lumen of the small intestine (**Fig. 24**).[45] In a heifer with duodenal ileus, ultrasonography showed that the gallbladder was not in its normal position, and exploratory laparotomy revealed that the displaced gallbladder was causing obstruction of the duodenum.[46]

Failure of ingesta to pass through the small intestine results in delayed passage of ingesta through the abomasum, omasum and rumen, which consequently become dilated (see the section on defects in abomasal emptying).

Incomplete perforation of the intestine usually leads to chronic peritonitis. Ultrasonographically, this is seen as intra-abdominal fluid with bands of fibrin, which may have a spiderweb-type of appearance among the loops of intestine and organs. Free intra-abdominal gas with its associated reverberation artifacts may be seen if intestinal gas has leaked through the perforation.

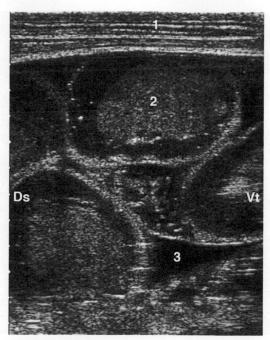

Fig. 24. Ultrasonogram of the jejunum in a cow with hemorrhagic bowel syndrome imaged from the right lateral abdominal wall. The blood clots have the appearance of echogenic masses in the lumen of the small intestine. Abdominal wall (1), blood clots in the lumen of the small intestine (2), fluid between the intestinal loops (3). Ds, dorsal; Vt, ventral.

Normal Large Intestine

Carbohydrates remaining in the ingesta after their passage through the forestomachs are fermented in the large intestine, and the gas produced makes it more difficult to image this section of the bowel.[12] The large intestine is always visible from the flank and is situated medial to the descending duodenum, whereby the colon is more dorsal and the proximal loop of the colon and cecum are more ventral. The large intestine is usually easy to differentiate from the small intestine based on its marked gas content.[12,14,15] Because of the gas, only the wall of the large intestine closest to the transducer can be imaged and appears as a thick echogenic line. Reverberation artifacts that originate from the tissue-gas interphase may become superimposed on the image of the wall and obscure it, however. The wall of the large intestine furthest from the transducer cannot be imaged. Usually, the proximal loop of the large colon, the cecum, and the colon can be visualized. The proximal loop of the large colon and the cecum appears as thick, echogenic, continuous and slightly curved lines. The spiral loop of the colon has the appearance of a garland with several echogenic arched lines next to each other. In contrast to the small intestine, which has vigorous peristaltic activity and segmental contractions, few contractions are observed in the large intestine.

Cecal Dilatation

Diagnosis of cecal dilatation usually is straightforward but may be difficult when the dilatation is complicated by retroflexion of the cecum. In that case, either no abnormal

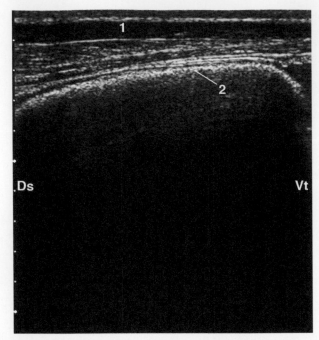

Fig. 25. Ultrasonogram of a dilated cecum of a cow with cecal dilatation and torsion imaged from the right flank. The cecal wall closest to the transducer appears as a curved echogenic line. The cecal contents and wall furthest from the transducer are not visible. Lateral abdominal wall (1), cecal wall (2). Ds, dorsal; Vt, ventral.

transrectal findings can be palpated or a distended viscus can be palpated only with the tips of the fingers. The differential diagnoses must include ileus of the small intestine and right displacement of the abomasum, respectively. A diagnosis by clinical examination alone may not be possible, but ultrasonography allows the differentiation of right displacement of the abomasum, ileus of the small intestine, and cecal dilatation. A dilated cecum always can be imaged from the lateral abdominal wall;[14,47] in some cases, it may be seen from the twelfth, eleventh, and tenth intercostal spaces. The dilated cecum and the proximal loop of the colon are almost always immediately adjacent to the abdominal wall. Because of the gaseous contents, only the wall of the dilated cecum and proximal loop of the colon closest to the transducer are seen ultrasonographically. They appear as thick, echogenic, semicircular lines (**Fig. 25**). In cases that involve fluid ingesta instead of gaseous contents in the cecum and proximal loop of the colon, the lumen appears moderately echogenic. Differentiation of cecum and proximal loop of the colon may be difficult ultrasonographically unless the ileocecal fold of the peritoneum between the two can be identified.

REFERENCES

1. Götz M. Sonographische untersuchungen an der haube des rindes [dissertation]. Zurich: Faculty of Veterinary Medicine, University of Zurich; 1992.
2. Braun U, Götz M. Ultrasonography of the reticulum in cows. Am J Vet Res 1994; 55(3):325–32.
3. Sicher D. Sonographische untersuchungen an lunge, mediastinum und milz des rindes [dissertation]. Zurich: Vetsuisse Faculty, University of Zurich; 1995.

4. Braun U, Sicher D. Ultrasonography of the spleen in 50 healthy cows. Vet J 2006; 171(3):513–8.
5. Wild K. Sonographische untersuchungen am labmagen des rindes [dissertation]. Zurich: Vetsuisse Faculty, University of Zurich; 1995.
6. Braun U, Wild K, Guscetti F. Ultrasonographic examination of the abomasum of 50 cows. Vet Rec 1997;140(4):93–8.
7. Braun U. Ultrasonographic examination of the liver in cows. Am J Vet Res 1990; 51(10):1522–6.
8. Gerber D. Sonographische befunde an der leber des rindes [dissertation]. Zurich: Vetsuisse Faculty, University of Zurich; 1993.
9. Braun U, Gerber D. Influence of age, breed, and stage of pregnancy on hepatic ultrasonographic findings in cows. Am J Vet Res 1994;55(9):1201–5.
10. Blessing S. Sonographische untersuchungen am psalter des rindes [dissertation]. Zurich: Vetsuisse Faculty, University of Zurich; 2003.
11. Braun U, Blessing S. Ultrasonographic examination of the omasum in 30 healthy cows. Vet Rec 2006;159(24):812–5.
12. Marmier O. Sonographische untersuchungen am darm des rindes [dissertation]. Zurich: Vetsuisse Faculty, University of Zurich; 1993.
13. Braun U, Marmier O. Ultrasonographic examination of the small intestine of cows. Vet Rec 1995;136(10):239–44.
14. Amrein EM. Ultraschalluntersuchungen bei kühen mit blinddarmdilatation [dissertation]. Zurich: Faculty of Veterinary Medicine, University of Zurich; 1999.
15. Braun U, Amrein E. Ultrasonographic examination of the caecum and proximal and spiral ansa of the colon of cattle. Vet Rec 2001;149(2):45–8.
16. Braun U. Ultrasonographic examination of the right kidney in cows. Am J Vet Res 1991;52(12):1933–9.
17. Kaske M, Midasch A, Rehage J. Sonographic investigation of reticular contractions in healthy sheep, cows and goats and in cows with traumatic reticulo-peritonitis. Journal of Veterinary Medicine 1994;41(10):748–56.
18. Braun U. Atlas und lehrbuch der ultraschalldiagnostik beim rind [Atlas and textbook of ultrasonography in cattle]. Berlin: Parey Buchverlag; 1997.
19. Braun U, Flückiger M, Nägeli F. Radiography as an aid in the diagnosis of traumatic reticuloperitonitis in cattle. Vet Rec 1993;132(5):103–9.
20. Constable PD, Hoffsis GF, Rings DM. The reticulorumen: normal and abnormal motor function. Part I. Primary contraction cycle. Comp Cont Educ Pract Vet 1990;12(7):1008–15.
21. Rauch S. Haubenmotorik bei gesunden kühen und bei kühen mit Hoflund-syndrom [dissertation]. Zurich: Vetsuisse Faculty, University of Zurich; 2007.
22. Braun U, Rauch S. Ultrasonographic evaluation of reticular motility during rest, eating, rumination and stress in 30 healthy cows. Vet Rec 2008;163(19): 571–4.
23. Braun U, Rauch S, Haessig M. Ultrasonographic evaluation of reticular motility in 144 cattle with vagal indigestion. Vet Rec 2009;164(1):11–3.
24. Braun U, Schweizer G, Flückiger M. Radiographic and ultrasonographic findings in three cows with reticulo-omasal obstruction due to a foreign body. Vet Rec 2002;150(18):580–1.
25. Gansohr B Untersuchungen zur eingabe von fremdkörpernacktmagneten beim rind [dissertation]. Zurich: Vetsuisse Faculty, University of Zurich; 2001.
26. Braun U, Gansohr B, Haessig M. Ultrasonographic evaluation of reticular motility in cows after administration of atropine, scopolamine and xylazine. J Vet Med A 2002;49(6):299–302.

27. Tschuor A, Clauss M. Investigations on the stratification of forestomach contents in ruminants: an ultrasonographic approach. Eur J Wildl Res 2008;54:627–33.

28. Braun U, Götz M, Marmier O. Ultrasonographic findings in cows with traumatic reticuloperitonitis. Vet Rec 1993;133(17):416–22.

29. Herzog K, Kaske M, Bischoff C, et al. Post surgical development of inflammatory adhesions and reticular function in cows suffering from traumatic reticuloperitonitis. Dtsch Tieräztl Wochenschr 2004;111(2):57–62.

30. Braun U, Iselin U, Lischer C, et al. Ultrasonographic findings in five cows before and after treatment of reticular abscesses. Vet Rec 1998;142(8):184–9.

31. Braun U, Blessing S, Lejeune B, et al. Ultrasonography of the omasum in cows with various gastrointestinal diseases. Vet Rec 2007;160(25):865–9.

32. Mohamed T, Oikawa S, Koiwa K, et al. Ultrasonographic diagnosis of omasal leiomyoma in a cow. Vet Rec 2004;155(17):530–1.

33. Van Winden SC, Brattinga CR, Müller KE, et al. Position of the abomasum in dairy cows during the first six weeks after calving. Vet Rec 2002;151(15):446–9.

34. Sendag S, Seeger T, Wehrend A. Sonographische untersuchung über die lageänderungen des labmagens bei kühen im peripartalen zeitraum. Dtsch Tierärztl Wochenschr 2005;112(9):351–4.

35. Wittek T, Constable PD, Morin DE. Ultrasonographic assessment of change in abomasal position during the last three months of gestation and first three months of lactation in Holstein-Friesian cows. J Am Vet Med Assoc 2005;227(9):1469–75.

36. Braun U, Wild K, Merz M, et al. Percutaneous ultrasound-guided abomasocentesis in cows. Vet Rec 1997;140(23):599–602.

37. Braun U, Pusterla N, Schönmann M. Ultrasonographic findings in cows with left displacement of the abomasum. Vet Rec 1997;141(13):331–5.

38. Feller B. Sonographische untersuchungen bei kühen mit rechtsseitiger labmagenverlagerung mit und ohne torsion [dissertation]. Zurich: Vetsuisse Faculty, University of Zurich; 2006.

39. Braun U, Feller B. Ultrasonographic findings in cows with right displacement of the abomasum and abomasal volvulus. Vet Rec 2008;162(10):311–5.

40. Braun U, Feller B, Haessig M, et al. Ultrasonographic examination of the omasum, liver and small and large intestines in cows with right displacement of the abomasum and abomasal volvulus. Am J Vet Res 2008;69(6):774–84.

41. Gürtler H. Die physiologie der verdauung und absorption. In: Kolb E, editor. Lehrbuch der physiologie der haustiere. Stuttgart: VEB Gustav Fischer; 1980. p. 177–339.

42. Penninck DG, Nyland TG, Fisher PE, et al. Ultrasonography of the normal canine gastrointestinal tract. Vet Radiol 1989;30(6):272–6.

43. Braun U, Marmier O, Pusterla N. Ultrasonographic examination of the small intestine of cows with ileus of the duodenum, jejunum or ileum. Vet Rec 1995;137(9):209–15.

44. Lejeune B, Lorenz I. Ultrasonographic findings in 2 cows with duodenal obstruction. Can Vet J 2008;49(4):386–8.

45. Dennison AC, VanMetre DC, Callan RJ, et al. Hemorrhagic bowel syndrome in dairy cattle: 22 cases (1997–2000). J Am Vet Med Assoc 2002;221(5):686–9.

46. Boerboom D, Mulon PY, Desrochers A. Duodenal obstruction caused by malposition of the gallbladder in a heifer. J Am Vet Med Assoc 2003;223(10):1475–7.

47. Braun U, Amrein E, Koller U, et al. Ultrasonographic findings in cows with dilatation, torsion and retroflexion of the caecum. Vet Rec 2002;150(3):75–9.

Ultrasonography of the Liver in Cattle

Ueli Braun, Prof Dr med vet, Dr med vet h c

KEYWORDS

- Cattle • Ultrasonography • Liver • Gallbladder
- Cholecystocentesis

Hepatic diseases are of great importance in cattle. Fascioliasis, hepatic abscesses, hepatic neoplasia, metabolic disturbances (eg, fatty liver disease) and diseases of major vessels (eg, thrombosis of the caudal vena cava) caused by hepatic abscesses that have broken into the vein are some examples. Until recently, diagnosis of many hepatic diseases was difficult because signs may be nonspecific. In many cases, diagnostic methods such as hepatospecific enzyme tests are insufficient. A complete ultrasonographic examination of the liver should give detailed information about the size, position, and ultrasonographic parenchymal pattern of the liver, the size and position of the gallbladder and the intra- and extrahepatic bile ducts, and the topography of the major vessels. Ultrasound-guided collection of hepatic biopsy samples, centesis and aspiration of abscesses, and cholecystocentesis and aspiration of bile samples (for examination for fluke eggs and determination of bile acids concentration) can be performed safely. In the first part of this article, the methods of ultrasonographic examination of the liver and the ultrasonographic appearance of the normal liver are discussed, followed in the second part by a description of specific liver diseases.

ULTRASONOGRAPHIC EXAMINATION OF THE LIVER AND NORMAL FINDINGS

The bovine liver is situated immediately adjacent and medial to the right body wall; its cranial aspect is hidden by the lung. The ultrasonographic examination is performed on the right side of the standing animal. The liver is examined ultrasonographically from caudal to cranial, beginning caudal to the last rib and ending at the fifth intercostal space and from dorsal to ventral in every intercostal space using a real-time 3.5- to 5.0-MHz linear or convex transducer.[1–4] First, the various hepatic structures are assessed subjectively; then the exact size of some of them is determined. Depending on the patient, cholecystocentesis and aspiration of a bile sample for microscopic examination, collection of a liver biopsy sample, or aspiration of an abscess may be performed.

Department of Farm Animals, University of Zurich, Winterthurerstrasse 260, CH-8057 Zürich, Switzerland
E-mail address: ubraun@vetclinics.uzh.ch

Vet Clin Food Anim 25 (2009) 591–609
doi:10.1016/j.cvfa.2009.07.003
0749-0720/09/$ – see front matter

Subjective Assessment of Hepatic Structure

Subjective assessment of hepatic structure includes assessment of the hepatic parenchyma, the position of the liver, the diaphragmatic and visceral surfaces, the angle of the liver, the caudal vena cava, the hepatic veins, the portal vein and its branches in the hepatic parenchyma, the gallbladder, and the biliary system. Dorsally, the liver can be imaged to the ventral acute margin of the lung. Parts of the liver beneath the lungs cannot be visualized via ultrasonography. The reticulum is seen adjacent to the liver in the sixth and seventh intercostal spaces. It appears as a half-moon–shaped structure and is characterized by regular biphasic contractions.[5,6] In the eighth to tenth intercostal spaces, the liver is adjacent to the omasum, the wall of which is clearly recognizable as a thick echogenic line.[7,8] Loops of intestine are situated adjacent to the liver in the eleventh and twelfth intercostal spaces.[9,10] In most cases, the right kidney can be imaged high dorsally in the twelfth intercostal space, where the so-called "hepatic window" is created at the site of the impressio renalis of the liver.[11]

The measurable size of the liver is largest in the intercostal spaces 10 to 12 and becomes progressively smaller cranially because of superimposition of the lungs. The parenchymal pattern of the normal liver consists of numerous weak echoes homogeneously distributed over the entire liver. The portal and hepatic veins can be seen within the liver, and their diameter increases toward the portal vein and the caudal vena cava. The lumen of these vessels appears anechoic. In contrast to the hepatic veins, the wall of the portal veins is characterized by an echogenic border that facilitates its identification. The portal veins can be clearly differentiated from the hepatic vein only in the area of the stellate ramifications of the portal vein. The intrahepatic bile ducts are only visible when they are calcified or when bile stasis is present.

The caudal vena cava is always situated more dorsally and medially than the portal vein and usually can be visualized in the twelfth and eleventh intercostal spaces (**Fig. 1**). It is rarely visualized in the tenth intercostal space and never in the more cranial intercostal spaces, because it is hidden by the lungs. The caudal vena cava has a characteristic triangular shape on cross-section because it is embedded in the sulcus of the vena cava in the liver. The diameter of the caudal vena cava does not change from the twelfth intercostal space to the tenth intercostal space and measures from 1.8 to 5 cm (**Table 1**).[1] Toward the liver, hepatic veins are seen joining the caudal vena cava. The common trunk of the left gastric vein and the splenic vein or individual splenic and gastric veins are observed in cross-section before they unite, medial to the caudal vena cava and outside of the hepatic parenchyma. These veins are usually circular on cross-section.

The portal vein is always situated ventrally and laterally to the caudal vena cava and is usually visible in the twelfth to eighth intercostal spaces (**Fig. 2**). The portal vein is circular on cross-section and has stellate ramifications into the hepatic parenchyma. The diameter of the portal vein in the twelfth and eleventh intercostal spaces is between 2.9 and 5.3 cm and decreases cranially. In contrast to the hepatic veins, the walls of the portal veins are easier to identify because they are characterized by an echogenic border. Differentiation of hepatic and portal veins is only possible in the area of the stellate branching of the portal vein.

The gallbladder is situated between the ninth and eleventh intercostal spaces. It is usually visible in one, sometimes in two, and rarely in three intercostal spaces. The normal gallbladder is a pear-shaped cystic structure of variable size and is easy to recognize (**Fig. 3**). Ultrasonographically, the gallbladder has an image typical of a fluid-filled vesicle and on ultrasonograms appears almost anechoic

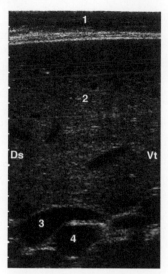

Fig. 1. Ultrasonogram of normal liver and caudal vena cava imaged from the eleventh inter-costal space. The abdominal wall (1), liver (2), caudal vena cava (3), common trunk of the splenic vein and the left gastric vein (4) are shown before the entry into the portal vein. Ds, dorsal; Vt, ventral.

surrounded by a thin white rim. The gallbladder is situated on the visceral surface of the liver. Depending on the degree of fullness, the gallbladder extends beyond the ventral liver margin such that it becomes situated directly adjacent to the abdominal wall. The size of the gallbladder varies greatly. By following the neck of the gall-bladder and the cystic duct, one usually can identify the common hepatic duct. The common bile duct cannot always be visualized. It originates from the cystic duct several centimeters away from the neck of the gallbladder. It sometimes can be seen at this point in cross-section, where it appears as a circular structure, with a diameter of approximately 0.3 cm. Normally, the course of the common bile duct to the duodenal papilla cannot be imaged.

Table 1
Results of ultrasonographic examination of the caudal vena cava and the portal vein of 186 cows

Variable	ICS (No. of Cows)	Mean	SD	Normal Range (mean ± 2 SD)
Caudal vena cava				
Diameter (cm)	12 (174)	3.6	0.6	2.2–5.0
	11 (179)	3.7	0.7	2.3–5.1
	10 (40)	3.4	0.8	1.8–5.0
Portal vein				
Diameter (cm)	12 (157)	4.3	0.5	3.2–5.3
	11 (186)	4.0	0.5	2.9–5.1
	10 (186)	3.4	0.6	2.3–4.5
	9 (165)	2.6	0.5	1.7–3.6
	8 (79)	2.0	0.4	1.1–2.8

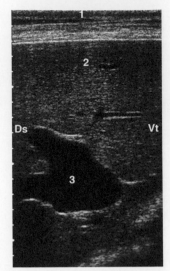

Fig. 2. Ultrasonogram of the liver and portal vein imaged from the tenth intercostal space. The abdominal wall (1), liver (2), and portal vein (3) are shown. Ds, dorsal; Vt, ventral.

Assessment of Position and Size of the Liver and its Vessels

To quantitate findings that were obtained by subjective assessment, the position and size of the liver and its vessels can be determined by measuring various structures in individual intercostal spaces. Examples are the determination of the dorsal and ventral margins of the liver and the size of the liver in different intercostal spaces and the diameters of the caudal vena cava and the portal vein and the thickness of the liver over these vessels. The method of measurement has been described in detail.[1–4] The

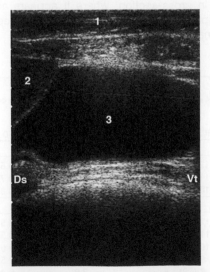

Fig. 3. Ultrasonogram of liver and gallbladder imaged from the ninth intercostal space. Abdominal wall (1), liver (2), gallbladder (3). Ds, dorsal; Vt, ventral.

dorsal and ventral margins of the liver are measured in relation to the midline of the back. For example, the dorsal margin is determined by measuring the distance between the dorsal margin of the liver and the midline of the back using a tape measure. Determination of the ventral margin of the liver is analogous. The visible size of the liver in a given intercostal space is determined by subtracting the distance between the dorsal liver margin and midline of the back from the distance between ventral liver margin and midline of the back.[1,2,4] For determination of the diameter of the caudal vena cava and the portal vein and the thickness of the liver over these vessels, the ultrasonographic image is electronically stored at maximal inspiration of the cow. The appropriate measurements are then made electronically on the ultrasonogram by means of the two cursors. The means and ranges determined from a study involving 186 cows were reported.[2–4] The results indicate that breed and age do not influence the different variables. There are significant correlations between body size, height at the withers, and milk production and several of the variables determined by ultrasonography. There is also a correlation between the stage of pregnancy and variables determined by ultrasonography. The diameter of the caudal vena cava increases with advancing pregnancy; in contrast, the diameter of the portal vein decreases.

Ultrasound-Guided Cholecystocentesis

Cholecystocentesis always should be performed in cows with suspected hepatic disease, especially if fascioliasis is a possibility. Microscopic examination of bile for liver fluke eggs is the most reliable method of diagnosing fascioliasis.[12–14] In cows with chronic fascioliasis and negative fecal findings, cholecystocentesis and microscopic examination of bile is the best diagnostic method. Bacteriologic and cytologic examination of bile is important in cows with suspected cholecystitis or pyocholecystitis. Inflammatory changes and bacteria such as *Fusobacterium necrophorum* have been detected in the bile of cows with cholestasis.[15] The risk of bile peritonitis is low when percutaneous ultrasound-guided cholecystocentesis is performed carefully. Complications related to cholecystocentesis did not occur in short- and long-term studies in cows.[3]

In cows, the gallbladder is readily accessible for ultrasonographic examination and centesis. The dorsal area of the gallbladder is accessible only transhepatically because it is situated on the visceral surface of the liver. Depending on the amount of bile, the gallbladder may extend beyond the ventral margin of the liver so that it lies adjacent to the abdominal wall, where it can be reached transperitoneally. The gallbladder can be reached transhepatically or transperitoneally. In humans, the transhepatic approach to the gallbladder is considered the safest because the liver acts to seal off the site of centesis, which reduces the risk of bile peritonitis caused by leakage of bile into the abdomen.[16]

In our experience involving more than 1000 cows, transperitoneal cholecystocentesis seems to be as safe as transhepatic cholecystocentesis. Percutaneous cholecystocentesis is performed at the location where the gallbladder is best visualized via ultrasonography. This is usually in the tenth or eleventh intercostal space. A spinal needle (20 gauge × 3.5 in) with stylet is introduced and guided by ultrasonography through the skin and abdominal wall toward the gallbladder (**Fig. 4**). Depending on the position of the gallbladder, the needle is advanced transhepatically or transperitoneally to the wall of the gallbladder and, with a slight thrust, is pushed through. The end of the needle within the gallbladder is usually visible in ultrasonograms. The stylet is removed, and using a syringe, 10 mL of bile is aspirated. The bile sample can be used for the bacteriologic and cytologic examination or for the determination of bile

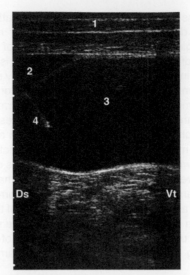

Fig. 4. Ultrasonogram of transhepatic cholecystocentesis of the gallbladder under ultrasonographic control imaged from the tenth intercostal space. Abdominal wall (1), liver (2), gallbladder (3), spinal needle (4) penetrating the abdominal wall, the liver, and the gallbladder. Ds, dorsal; Vt, ventral.

acids. It is not suitable for the microscopic detection of liver fluke eggs, however, because the latter are not evenly distributed within the bile but rather sediment to the lowest point in the gallbladder. To stir up liver fluke eggs, 10 mL of isotonic NaCl solution is infused in the gallbladder. Immediately afterward, 10 mL of diluted bile is aspirated for examination for liver fluke eggs. Bile is poured into a centrifuge tube and placed in a refrigerator overnight. Then the sediment is aspirated by use of a Pasteur pipette, placed on a glass slide, and examined microscopically.

HEPATIC ABSCESS

The ultrasonographic examination is of substantial importance in the diagnosis of hepatic abscesses in cows. The ultrasonographic appearance of hepatic abscesses has been described in feedlot cattle,[17–21] cows,[22,23] and a breeding bull.[24] In cattle with experimentally induced hepatic abscesses, the portal vein was inoculated with *F necrophorum* under ultrasonographic guidance.[17,19] The develop and ultrasonographic appearance of the hepatic abscesses were then recorded via regular ultrasonographic examinations, and it was shown that the ultrasonographic appearance changed during the course of disease.

Abscesses result in circumscribed structural changes in the hepatic parenchyma (**Fig. 5**). The ultrasonographic appearance of hepatic abscesses in cattle is variable. The content of the abscess appears anechogenic to hyperechogenic. Abscesses may appear homogeneous or heterogeneous. A heterogeneous ultrasonogram with single or multiple hyperechogenic foci and no evidence of a capsule indicates an early stage in the development of the abscess. Homogeneous content, capsule formation, and substantial size (**Fig. 6**) indicate that the abscess is longstanding. The abscess may be divided into several chambers by septa, which indicates partial destruction of the liver. The individual compartments may become confluent during the course

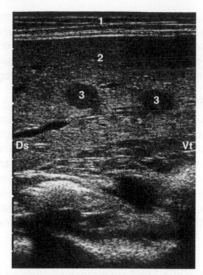

Fig. 5. Ultrasonogram from a cow with multiple abscesses in the liver imaged from the eleventh intercostal space. Abdominal wall (1), liver (2), hepatic abscesses (3). Ds, dorsal; Vt, ventral.

of the disease. The diameter of an abscess ranges from 3 to 20 cm, and the abscess may extend across one to five intercostal spaces.[22]

Aspiration of Hepatic Abscesses

A diagnosis of hepatic abscess often cannot be made based solely on its ultrasonographic appearance because the appearance of hepatic abscesses varies greatly and may change with time. The differential diagnosis of circumscribed changes in the liver must include neoplasia and cysts. Ultrasound-guided centesis of such changes

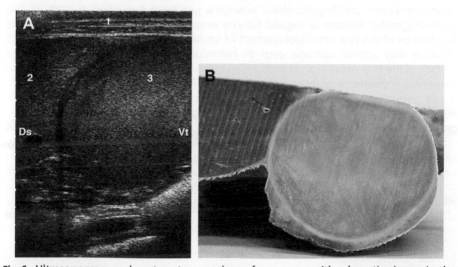

Fig. 6. Ultrasonogram and postmortem specimen from a cow with a hepatic abscess in the right lobe of the liver. The liver was frozen before cutting. Abdominal wall (1), liver (2), liver abscess (3). Ds, dorsal; Vt, ventral.

should be performed to confirm the diagnosis.[22] It is important that the needle (20 gauge × 3.5 in, 0.90 × 90 mm) used for centesis is closed with a stylet during introduction into and withdrawal from the lesion. A definitive diagnosis of hepatic abscess can be made in nearly all cases based on the macroscopic nature of the aspirated material. When in doubt, the latter can be examined bacteriologically and cytologically.

Treatment of Liver Abscesses

In the author's experience, multiple small abscesses with a diameter of less than 3 cm often can be treated effectively with a broad-spectrum antibiotic (eg, amoxicillin) over 14 days. Percutaneous ultrasound-guided lancing and draining can be attempted to treat larger solitary abscesses provided that they are situated immediately adjacent to the abdominal wall. It may be possible to drain abscesses located farther away from the abdominal wall via laparotomy[25] or through the reticulum.[26] Cattle often have multiple abscesses, however, (eg, in the caudal vena cava or lungs), and treatment is not indicated in these patients. It is critical that other organs be examined.

HEPATIC TUMORS

Hepatic tumors are rare in cattle. Most are metastastic tumors that reach the liver from the gastrointestinal tract via the portal vein or from the lungs via the hepatic artery. In rare cases the tumor may originate in the liver. Hepatic tumors are divided into hepatocellular and cholangiocellular adenoma and carcinoma.[27] Hepatocellular carcinoma is usually solitary and may be surrounded by intrahepatic metastases. Occasionally, the tumor may penetrate through the capsule and attach itself to the peritoneum. It is characteristic for a hepatocellular carcinoma to rupture into the large hepatic veins and caudal vena cava.[27] The tumors also may extend to the portal vein, spleen, and stomach, which may result in portal hypertension. Cholangiocellular carcinomas are usually multifocal or diffuse; rarely are they solitary tumors. The liver of animals with this type of tumor is otherwise usually normal.

Ultrasonographically, hepatic tumors are characteristically single or multiple circumscribed structures.[28] The ultrasonographic appearance of bile duct carcinoma, adenocarcinoma, and hepatocellular adenoma has been described in cattle.[28] The ultrasonographic features of hepatic tumors essentially reflect changes in the shape and texture of the liver and displacement of vessels and bile ducts.[29] The neoplastic changes may appear homogeneous or heterogeneous.[28] Tumors situated on the surface of the liver result in a circumscribed bulge in the hepatic contour. The ultrasonographic appearance of most metastases is different from that of the liver (**Fig. 7**). Some metastases also have the same echogenicity as the liver; they are recognized as bulges in the contour of the liver. The echogenic pattern of metastases varies greatly and depends on its vascularity and rate of growth. Rapidly growing metastases that are composed of predominantly tumor cells are hypoechogenic, because they have few acoustic surfaces. In contrast, slowly growing metastases usually contain vascular and connective tissue and appear more echogenic. In cases with rupture of a tumor into a vessel, echogenic thrombi may be seen. Occasionally the portal vein becomes congested when there is a decrease in liver perfusion.[28] Percutaneous ultrasound-guided liver biopsy is recommended to confirm a tentative diagnosis of neoplasia and in most cases can be used to determine the type of tumor.

DIFFUSE HEPATIC DISEASE

Many diseases result in diffuse hepatic damage with nonspecific ultrasonographic features; the echogenicity may be increased or decreased. In contrast to

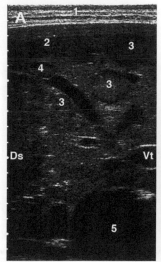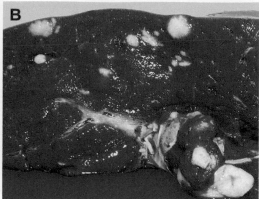

Fig. 7. Ultrasonogram and postmortem specimen of the liver in a cow with lymphosarcoma imaged from the eleventh intercostal space. Abdominal wall (1), liver (2), tumor nodules (3), tumor invaded into a hepatic vein (4), portal vein (5). Ds, dorsal; Vt, ventral.

circumscribed structural changes, the liver is uniformly affected. Fatty liver degeneration is the most common hepatic disease with a diffuse distribution of lesions. Hepatic cirrhosis and congestion are seen less often.

Diffuse hepatic damage is often observed on ultrasonograms, but its ultrasonographic features are not specific.[29] A liver biopsy sample is usually obtained to aid in the diagnosis. Diffuse hepatic disease is often accompanied by enlargement of and an increase in the weight of the liver. Estimating the weight of the liver using ultrasonographic measurements may aid in diagnosing diffuse hepatic disease. The most reliable criterion is the thickness of the liver as measured over the caudal vena cava and over the portal vein.[2] The weight of the liver (y) (kg) can be estimated using the formula y = -3.97 + 1.036 × thickness of liver (cm) measured in the eleventh intercostal space (r = 0.76, $P < .01$). Other indications of enlargement of the liver are rounding and blunting of the margins of the liver and an increase in the ventral angle of the liver.

FATTY LIVER DISEASE

In animals with diffuse fatty liver disease, the number and intensity of the internal echoes increase as the severity of the disease increases.[30–32] In advanced stages of the disease, the liver appears white on ultrasonograms and is difficult to differentiate from surrounding tissue. In severe fatty liver disease, weakening of the echoes occurs as the distance from the abdominal wall increases because the fat-containing hepatocytes enhance the acoustic impedance. The result is that the region near the abdominal wall is hyperechogenic, whereas areas more distant are hypoechoegenic or cannot be imaged at all (**Fig. 8**).

The contrast between the liver and vessels is also decreased. Often only large vessels are seen; small vessels may be poorly imaged or not seen at all. This is because the small vessels are compressed by swollen hepatic tissue.[29] In the hyperechogenic areas of the diseased liver there is an increase in scattered echoes, which

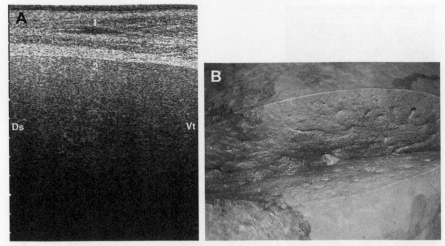

Fig. 8. Ultrasonogram and postmortem specimen of the liver of a cow with severe fatty liver degeneration. The liver is hyperechoic near the abdominal wall and cannot be visualized far from the abdominal wall. Abdominal wall (1), liver (2). Ds, dorsal; Vt, ventral.

project onto the vessels and result in deterioration of the contrast between the hepatic parenchyma and hepatic vessels. Several authors have tried with moderate success to determine the fat content of the liver using its ultrasonographic echogenicity.[30–33] A more promising method seems to be calibrated, computer-aided B-mode ultrasonography.[34] The mean transcutaneous liver tissue echo level correlates well with liver fat score (r = 0.80). The most reliable method of determining the fat content of the liver is histologic evaluation of a liver biopsy sample. In rare cases, multifocal areas of fat deposition can be recognized in the liver (**Fig. 9**).[35] These fatty areas are intensely echogenic and contrast the rest of the hepatic parenchyma.

CONGESTION OF THE LIVER

As a result of an increased fluid content with systemic congestion, the liver becomes enlarged and has noticeably fewer parenchymal echoes. Chronic liver congestion eventually leads to an increase in the amount of connective tissue in the liver. The ultrasonographic appearance then changes from that of acute liver congestion to one similar to that seen with liver cirrhosis, in which the parenchyma appears heterogeneous and hyperechogenic with strong individual echoes.

SENECIOSIS

Diseases caused by the ingestion of poisonous plants of the *Senecio* species are common and have the greatest economic impact of all plant poisonings. Plants of the *Senecio spp* contain toxic substances termed pyrrolizidine alkaloids,[27,36] which constitute cumulative hepatotoxins after transformation in the liver to pyrrole metabolites. They inhibit mitosis of hepatocytes and cause megalocytosis. Proliferation of the endothelium of the centrilobular and hepatic veins results in the occlusion of these vessels and veno-occlusive fibrosis. Other hepatic changes are generalized fibrosis and hyperplasia of bile ducts, which lead to impaired hepatic perfusion and portal hypertension with ascites. Ultrasonographic evaluation of patients with seneciosis reveals an enlarged and heterogeneous liver with echogenic nodular lesions

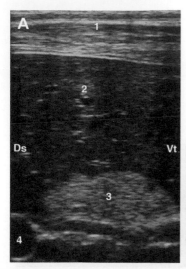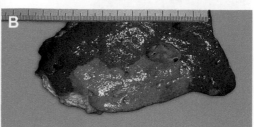

Fig. 9. Ultrasonogram and postmortem specimen of focal fatty liver disease imaged from the tenth intercostal space. Abdominal wall (1), liver (2), focal fatty liver degeneration (3), portal vein (4). Ds, dorsal; Vt, ventral.

(Fig. 10).[37] Endothelial proliferation in the centrolobular veins and veno-occlusive fibrosis result in decreased blood flow from the hepatic veins into the caudal vena cava. The lumina of the hepatic veins and caudal vena cava are distinctly smaller than normal on ultrasonograms. There is concurrent congestion in the portal vein, which leads to intrahepatic portal hypertension and an increase in the diameter of the portal vein. The results can be imaged via ultrasonography and include ascites and edema of the omentum, mesentery, gastrointestinal tract, and gallbladder wall.[37] In advanced stages of the disease, histologic evaluation of a liver biopsy sample reveals severe liver fibrosis, which alerts the clinician to the possibility of seneciosis.

BILE DUCTS AND GALLBLADDER
Calcification of the Bile Ducts

The most common cause of bile duct calcification is chronic fascioliasis. Calcified bile ducts result in discrete sonographic changes in the liver parenchyma. They are intensely hyperechogenic and accompanied by an acoustic shadow distally. In cross-section, calcified bile ducts appear as ring-like (**Fig. 11**); in longitudinal section, they appear as tube-like hyperechogenic structures.

Cholestasis

In obstructive cholestasis, the flow of bile is mechanically impaired. The most common causes of biliary obstruction in cattle are fascioliasis, fibrinous or purulent products, and solid deposits; other less common causes include gall stones and tissue proliferation.[38] Inflammatory products that result from cholangitis also may impair the flow of bile. In rare cases, the flow of bile may be obstructed by compression of the major bile ducts by tumors, abscesses, or peritoneal changes. In cows with suspected cholestasis, the diagnostic examination should include the determination of the activities of hepatic enzymes, ultrasonographic examination of the liver, histologic examination

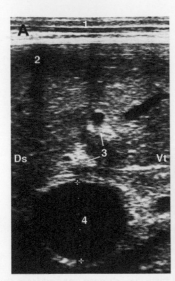
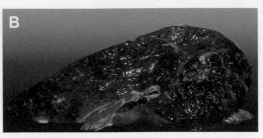

Fig. 10. Ultrasonogram and postmortem specimen of the liver of a cow with seneciosis imaged from the eleventh intercostal space. There are multiple hyperechogenic nodules, and the portal vein is dilated because of intrahepatic portal hypertension. Abdominal wall (1), liver (2), hyperechoic nodular alterations (3), dilated portal vein (4). Ds, dorsal; Vt, ventral. The postmortem specimen shows a cross-section through the enlarged liver. The liver parenchyma consists of small (1–2 cm) and large nodules (2–4 cm). Histopathologically there were multifocal nodules of regenerative hyperplasia with varying numbers of megalocytic hepatocytes throughout the parenchyma. Approximately two thirds of portal triads and bile ducts had distinct fibroplasia and proliferation, respectively.

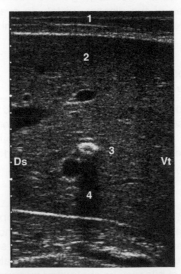

Fig. 11. Ultrasonogram of a calcified bile duct (in cross-section) in a cow with fascioliasis. The calcified bile duct appears as a ring-shaped echogenic structure and is accompanied by an acoustic shadow. Abdominal wall (1), liver (2), calcified bile duct (3), acoustic shadow (4). Ds, dorsal; Vt, ventral.

of a liver biopsy specimen, and ultrasound-guided cholecystocentesis with examination of a bile sample.[39]

Obstructive cholestasis almost always can be diagnosed on the basis of the observation of dilated bile ducts. Ultrasonographic assessment of the dilatory pattern of the intra- and extrahepatic bile ducts and gallbladder may reveal the location of the obstruction and other abnormalities, such as a hepatic abscess. A proximal obstruction, which occurs in the area of the hepatic hilus, can be differentiated from a distal obstruction, which occurs in the region of the duodenal papilla. With a proximal obstruction, only the intrahepatic bile ducts are dilated. With a distal obstruction, there is dilatation of the common bile duct and the gallbladder, which may be associated with dilatation of the intrahepatic bile ducts. Normally, the intrahepatic bile ducts, which run parallel to the branches of the portal vein, are not visible ultrasonographically; however, when they are dilated they become visible (**Fig. 12**). Severe congestion results in lacunar dilatation of the bile ducts (**Fig. 13**).

Dilatation of the gallbladder alone is not an indication of cholestasis. In many anorexic cows, there is no reflex stimulus for emptying of the gallbladder, and its volume increases without any impairment of the flow of bile. Thickening of the wall of the gallbladder because of inflammation suggests disease, however. Abnormal gallbladder content, such as sediment or concretion, without thickening of the wall of the gallbladder also can be observed in anorexic cows with various problems not specific to the liver. The content of the gallbladder can appear homogeneous or heterogeneous. Homogeneous content usually appears echogenic, and heterogeneous content consists of an echogenic sediment and a hypoechogenic supernatant (**Fig. 14**). Thickening of the wall of the gallbladder without other signs of cholestasis suggests edematous rather than inflammatory changes. Edema of the wall of the gallbladder occurs in patients with right-sided cardiac insufficiency, thrombosis of the caudal vena cava, and hypoproteinemia. In cattle suspected of having cholestasis, ultrasound-guided cholecystocentesis is indicated (see the section on

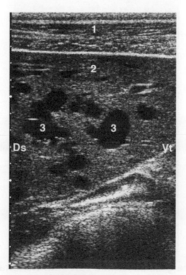

Fig. 12. Ultrasonogram of dilated bile ducts in the liver of a cow with cholestasis imaged from the tenth intercostal space. Abdominal wall (1), liver (2), dilated bile ducts (3). Ds, dorsal; Vt, ventral.

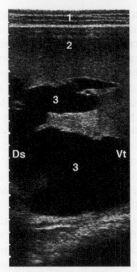

Fig. 13. Ultrasonogram of dilated bile ducts in the liver of a cow with cholestasis imaged from the tenth intercostal space. Abdominal wall (1), liver (2), dilated bile ducts (3). Ds, dorsal; Vt, ventral.

cholecystocentesis). A sample of bile is then examined microscopically and bacteriologically and undergoes testing for liver fluke eggs.

Without resolution of obstructive cholestasis, rupture of the gallbladder may ensue with subsequent generalized peritonitis or intra-abdominal hemorrhage. In three cows with rupture of the gallbladder, the lead ultrasonographic findings were generalized peritonitis with ascites and fibrin deposition.[40] In only one cow with characteristic

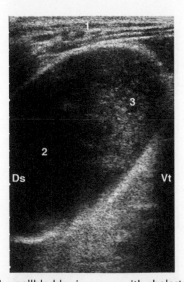

Fig. 14. Ultrasonogram of the gallbladder in a cow with cholestasis imaged from the ninth intercostal space. The gallbladder contains an echogenic sediment and an anechoic supernatant. Abdominal wall (1), anechoic supernatant in the gallbladder (2), sediment in the gallbladder (3). Ds, dorsal; Vt, ventral.

signs of cholestasis, which included icterus, bilirubinuria, and elevated liver enzyme activity, a rupture of the gallbladder could be tentatively diagnosed intra vitam.[38,40] The ultrasonographic findings included thickening of the gallbladder wall, which was poorly demarcated, and dilatation of intrahepatic and extrahepatic bile ducts. Abdominocentesis yielded bile-containing fluid.

Pneumobilia

Pneumobilia or aerobilia refers to air or gas accumulation in the bile ducts and may be the result of various causes.[41] Pneumobilia may be the result of gas-producing bacteria in suppurative cholangitis. Pneumobilia of individual bile ducts attributable to suppurative cholangitis has been described in cattle.[39] On ultrasonograms, pneumobilia appears as hyperechogenic structures that reflect the branching of the bile ducts from central to peripheral. Depending on the position of the transducer, these echoes may be band-shaped or miliary structures that are accompanied by reverberations or a distal acoustic shadow.

CAUDAL VENA CAVA

The lumen of the caudal vena cava may be dilated or narrowed. Congestion in the systemic circulatory system results in dilatation of the caudal vena cava. Causes include right-sided cardiac insufficiency, thrombosis of the caudal vena cava, and compression of the caudal vena cava in the thorax or subphrenic region by space-occupying lesions. The ultrasonographic appearance of the caudal vena cava is a substantial aid in diagnosing congestion in the systemic circulation. In cases with congestion of the caudal vena cava, a change in the cross-sectional shape of the vein is important for making a reliable diagnosis.[42–46] The caudal vena cava loses its normal triangular shape when congested and becomes round to oval (**Fig. 15**) on ultrasonograms. At the same time, the diameter of the vein increases.

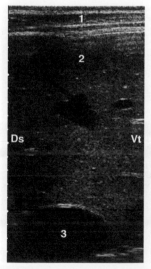

Fig. 15. Ultrasonogram of the caudal vena cava in a cow with thrombosis of the caudal vena cava imaged from the twelfth intercostal space. The caudal vena cava has an oval shape and an enlarged diameter because of congestion. Abdominal wall (1), liver (2), caudal vena cava (3). Ds, dorsal; Vt, ventral.

Congestion of the caudal vena cava also results in marked dilatation of the hepatic veins that empty into it (**Fig. 16**) and other signs of liver congestion (see the section on liver congestion), including an edematous gallbladder wall. Occasionally ascites can be seen. In animals with congestion of the caudal vena cava, dilatation of the jugular veins indicates right-sided cardiac insufficiency, whereas normal jugular veins indicate obstruction or compression of the caudal vena cava between the liver and the heart. In cattle with thrombosis of the caudal vena cava, the thrombus is rarely seen; ultrasonographic identification of a thrombus has been reported in only one cow[44] and one heifer;[47] in the latter a thrombus was also seen in the right hepatic vein. Imaging a thrombus is difficult because it is situated cranially in the caudal vena cava, where it is obscured from view by the lungs. It may be possible to see a liver abscess in cattle with thrombosis of the caudal vena cava, however. A further report describes the antemortem diagnosis of caudal vena cava thrombosis by intraoperative ultrasonography in two cows.[48]

The caudal vena cava also can have a narrow lumen, the most common cause of which is compression by an enlarged rumen. Impairment of the venous circulation of the liver because of severe hepatic cirrhosis, for example, also may result in narrowing of the lumen of the caudal vena cava when the venous blood flow is severely decreased.[37] In such cases, the portal vein is dilated because of congestion.

PORTAL VEIN

In portal hypertension, there is dilatation of the portal vein with an increase in its diameter. Causes include prehepatic portal hypertension caused by thrombosis of the portal vein, intrahepatic portal hypertension caused by hepatic cirrhosis, tumors, and abscesses, and posthepatic portal hypertension attributable to right-sided cardiac insufficiency or thrombosis or compression of the caudal vena cava. In such cases, the lumen of the portal vein is abnormally large and has a diameter that exceeds 5.5 cm in the twelfth intercostal space. There often is dilatation of the stellate

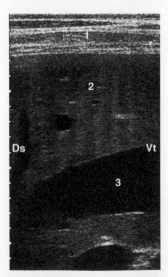

Fig. 16. Ultrasonogram of the right hepatic vein in a cow with thrombosis of the caudal vena cava imaged from the eleventh intercostal space. The right hepatic vein is markedly dilated because of congestion. Abdominal wall (1), liver (2), right hepatic vein (3). Ds, dorsal; Vt, ventral.

ramifications of the portal vein and the intrahepatic portal veins. The portal vein was not visible via ultrasonography in the region of the hepatic portal in a 10-week-old Holstein-Friesian calf with an elevated concentration of serum ammonia caused by a portosystemic shunt.[49] Instead, the cranial mesenteric vein was prominent, and the portocaval shunt was identified using color Doppler sonography.

Centesis and Catheterization of the Portal Vein

Percutaneous ultrasound-guided centesis and catheterization of the portal vein are procedures that can be performed for various experimental reasons.[19,50–54]

SUMMARY

Ultrasonography is a valuable tool for the diagnosis of liver disease. Discrete or diffuse lesions can be imaged, aspirated, and biopsied under visual guidance. This imaging modality also can be used to aspirate bile from the gallbladder for the diagnosis of liver flukes. Ultrasonography cannot be used to evaluate liver regions obscured by the lungs, however.

REFERENCES

1. Braun U. Ultrasonographic examination of the liver in cows. Am J Vet Res 1990; 51(10):1522–6.
2. Gerber D. Sonographische befunde an der leber des rindes [dissertation]. Vetsuisse faculty, University of Zurich, 1993.
3. Braun U, Gerber D. Percutaneous ultrasound-guided cholecystocentesis in cows. Am J Vet Res 1992;53(7):1079–84.
4. Braun U. Ultrasonographic examination of the liver and gallbladder in cows: normal findings. Compendium on Continuing Education for the Practicing Veterinarian 1996;18(2):S61–72.
5. Götz M. Sonographische untersuchungen an der haube des rindes [dissertation]. Faculty of veterinary medicine, University of Zurich, 1992.
6. Braun U, Götz M. Ultrasonography of the reticulum in cows. Am J Vet Res 1994; 55(3):325–32.
7. Blessing S. Sonographische untersuchungen am psalter des rindes [dissertation]. Vetsuisse faculty, University of Zurich, 2003.
8. Braun U, Blessing S. Ultrasonographic examination of the omasum in 30 healthy cows. Vet Rec 2006;159(24):812–5.
9. Marmier O. Sonographische untersuchungen am darm des rindes [dissertation]. Vetsuisse faculty, University of Zurich, 1993.
10. Braun U, Marmier O. Ultrasonographic examination of the small intestine of cows. Vet Rec 1995;136(10):239–44.
11. Braun U. Ultrasonographic examination of the right kidney in cows. Am J Vet Res 1991;52(12):1933–9.
12. Wolfensberger R. Vergleichende untersuchungen auf fasziolose und dikrozöliose in galle, kot und leber beim rind [dissertation]. Vetsuisse faculty, University of Zurich, 1993.
13. Braun U, Wolfensberger R, Hertzberg H. Diagnosis of liver flukes in cows: a comparison of the findings in the liver, in the feces, and in the bile. Schweiz Arch Tierheilk 1995;137(9):438–44.
14. Rapsch C, Schweizer G, Grimm F, et al. Estimating the true prevalence of *Fasciola hepatica* in cattle slaughtered in Switzerland in the absence of an absolute diagnostic test. Int J Parasitol 2006;36(10–11):1153–8.

15. Braun U, Götz M, Guscetti F. Ultrasonographic findings in a cow with extra-hepatic cholestasis and cholangitis. Schweiz Arch Tierheilkd 1994;136(8):275–9.
16. Martin EC, Getrajdman GI. Does the gallbladder have a future? Radiology 1989; 170(3):969–73.
17. Itabisashi T, Yamamoto R, Satoh M. Ultrasonogram of hepatic abscess in cattle inoculated with Fusobacterium necrophorum. Jpn J Vet Sci 1987;49(4):585–92.
18. Jönsson G, Bergsten C, Carlsten J, et al. Ultrasonic diagnosis of liver abscesses in intensively fed beef cattle. In: Proceedings of the 15th World Congress on Cattle Diseases. Palma de Mallorca;1988. p. 1428–30.
19. Lechtenberg KF, Nagaraja TG. Hepatic ultrasonography and blood changes in cattle with experimentally induced hepatic abscesses. Am J Vet Res 1991;52(6):803–9.
20. Liberg P, Jönsson G. Ultrasonography and determination of proteins and enzymes in blood for the diagnosis of liver abscesses in intensively fed beef cattle. Acta Vet Scand 1993;34(1):21–8.
21. Tan ZL, Lechtenberg KF, Nagaraja TG, et al. Serum neutralizing antibodies against Fusobacterium necrophorum leukotoxin in cattle experimentally induced or naturally developed hepatic abscesses. J Anim Sci 1994;72(2):502–8.
22. Braun U, Pusterla N, Wild K. Ultrasonographic findings in 11 cows with a hepatic abscess. Vet Rec 1995;137(12):284–90.
23. Doré E, Fecteau G, Hélie P, et al. Liver abscesses in Holstein dairy cattle: 18 cases (1992–2003). J Vet Intern Med 2007;21(4):853–6.
24. Tromp JF, Loeb E, Kuiper R. Een geval van leverabcessen bij een stier [A case of liver abscesses in a bull]. Tijdschr Diergeneeskd. 2005;130(24):758–61.
25. Fubini SL, Ducharme NG, Murphy JP, et al. Vagus indigestion syndrome resulting from a liver abscess in dairy cows. J Am Vet Med Assoc 1985;186(12):1297–300.
26. Dirksen G. Bakteriell bedingte lebernekrosen und -abszesse. In: Dirksen G, Gründer HD, Stöber M, editors. Innere medizin und chirurgie des rindes. 4th edition. Berlin: Parey Buchverlag; 2002. p. 631–4.
27. Stalker MJ, Hayes MA. Liver and biliary system. In: Grant Maxie M, editor. Jubb, Kennedy, and Palmer's pathology of domestic animals. 5th edition. Edinburgh: Saunders Elsevier; 2007. p. 297–388.
28. Braun U, Nuss K, Soldati G, et al. Clinical and ultrasonographic findings in four cows with liver tumours. Vet Rec 2005;157(16):482–4.
29. Kremer H, Dobrinski W, Schreiber MA. Leber. In: Kremer H, Dobrinski W, editors. Sonographische diagnostik, innere medizin und angrenzende gebiete. 4th edition. München: Urban & Schwarzenberg; 1993. p. 63–88.
30. Grote D. Sonographische untersuchungen zur leberdiagnostik beim rind unter besonderer berücksichtigung des fettlebersyndroms [dissertation]. Hannover, Germany: University of Veterinary Medicine; 1992.
31. Lauener JW. Zweidimensionale sonographie in der fettleberdiagnostik bei milch-kühen: untersuchungen zur diagnostischen sensitivität und spezifität [disserta-tion]. Hannover, Germany: University of Veterinary Medicine; 1993.
32. Acorda JA, Yamada H, Ghamsari SM. Ultrasonographic features of diffuse hepa-tocellular disorders in dairy cattle. Vet Radiol Ultrasound 1994;35(3):196–200.
33. Delling U. Intraoperative ultraschalluntersuchung der leber und der gallenblase des rindes [dissertation]. Leipzig, Germany: University of Leipzig; 2000.
34. Thijssen JM, Starke A, Weijers G, et al. Computer-aided B-mode ultrasound diag-nosis of hepatic steatosis: a feasibility study. IEEE Trans Ultrason Ferroelectr Freq Control 2008;55(6):1343–54.
35. Mohamed T, Oikawa S, Kurosawa T, et al. Focal fatty liver in a heifer: utility of ultra-sonography in diagnosis. J Vet Med Sci 2004;66(3):341–4.

36. Radostits OM, Gay CC, Hinchcliff KW, et al. Pyrrolizidine alkaloid poisoning. In: Radostits OM, Gay CC, Hinchcliff KW, et al, editors. Veterinary medicine: a textbook of the diseases of cattle, horses, sheep, pigs, and goats. 10th edition. Philadelphia: WB Saunders; 2007. p. 1878–81.
37. Braun U, Linggi T, Pospischil A. Ultrasonographic findings in three cows with chronic ragwort (Senecio alpinus) poisoning. Vet Rec 1999;144(5):122–6.
38. Dirksen G. Gallengangs- und gallenblasenentzündung. In: Dirksen G, Gründer HD, Stöber M, editors. Innere medizin und chirurgie des rindes. 4th edition. Berlin: Parey Buchverlag; 2002. p. 634–9.
39. Braun U, Pospischil A, Pusterla N, et al. Ultrasonographic findings in cows with cholestasis. Vet Rec 1995;137(21):537–43.
40. Braun U, Schweizer G, Pospischil A. Clinical and ultrasonographic findings in three cows with ruptured gallbladders. Vet Rec 2005;156(11):351–3.
41. Banholzer P, Weigold B. Gallenwege. In: Kremer H, Dobrinski W, editors. Sonographische diagnostik, innere medizin und angrenzende gebiete. 4th edition. München: Urban & Schwarzenberg; 1993. p. 113–21.
42. Braun U, Schefer U, Gerber D, et al. Ultrasonographic findings in a cow with ascites due to thrombosis of the caudal vena cava. Schweiz Arch Tierheilkd 1992;134(5):235–41.
43. Braun U, Flückiger M, Feige K, et al. Diagnosis by ultrasonography of congestion of the caudal vena cava secondary to thrombosis in 12 cows. Vet Rec 2002; 150(7):209–13.
44. Braun U, Salis F, Gerspach C. Sonographischer nachweis eines echogenen thrombus in der vena cava caudalis bei einer kuh [Diagnosis by ultrasonography of a thrombus in the caudal vena cava of a cow]. Schweiz Arch Tierheilkd 2003; 145(7):340–1.
45. Braun U, Schweizer G, Wehbrink D, et al. Ultraschallbefunde bei einem rind mit aszites infolge thrombose der vena cava caudalis [Ultrasonographic findings in a heifer with ascites due to thrombosis of the caudal vena cava]. Tierarztl Prax 2005;33G(6):389–94.
46. Braun U. Clinical findings and diagnosis of thrombosis of the caudal vena cava in cattle. Vet J 2008;175(1):118–25.
47. Mohamed T, Sato H, Kurosawa T, et al. Ultrasonographic localisation of thrombi in the caudal vena cava and hepatic veins in a heifer. Vet J 2004;168(1):103–6.
48. Sigrist I, Francoz D, Leclère M, et al. Antemortem diagnosis of caudal vena cava thrombosis in 2 cows. J Vet Intern Med 2008;22(3):684–6.
49. Buczinski S, Duval J, D'Anjou MA, et al. Portacaval shunt in a calf: clinical, pathologic, and ultrasonographic findings. Can Vet J 2007;48(4):407–10.
50. Braun U, Koller-Wild K, Bettschart-Wolfensberger R. Ultrasound-guided percutaneous portocentesis in 21 cows. Vet Rec 2000;147(22):623–6.
51. Mohamed T, Sato H, Kurosawa T, et al. Bile acid extraction rate in the liver of cows fed high-fat diet and lipid profiles in the portal and hepatic veins. Journal of Veterinary Medicine A 2002;49(3):151–6.
52. Mohamed T, Sato H, Kurosawa T, et al. Echo-guided studies on portal and hepatic blood in cattle. J Vet Med Sci 2002;64(1):23–8.
53. Braun U, Camenzind D, Ossent P. Ultrasound-guided catheterization of the portal vein in 11 cows using the Seldinger technique. J Vet Med Series A 2003;50:1–7.
54. Braun U, Camenzind D, Wanner M, et al. The influence of a fermentation-resistant glucose diet on the glucose concentration and other metabolites in portal and jugular blood in 15 cows. J Vet Med Series A 2003;50(1):8–13.

Cardiovascular Ultrasonography in Cattle

Sébastien Buczinski, Dr Vét, DÉS, MSc

KEYWORDS

- Echocardiography • Pericarditis • Endocarditis
- Ventricular septal defects • Vascular ultrasound

Diagnosing heart disease in cattle is challenging because clinical signs can be hidden until signs of congestive heart failure occur. An early diagnosis is of primary importance because the prognosis of the most common heart disorders ranges from guarded to poor.[1] Ancillary tests, such as complete cell blood count and serum biochemistry panel, may lack the sensitivity or specificity to detect heart disease.[1,2] By contrast, the main diseases of superficial vessels may be detected with a precautionary clinical examination; however, a precise diagnosis requires medical imaging to observe the suspected vessel and its content.[3] Medical imaging is also required for the assessment of deep vessels that cannot be clinically assessed. For all these reasons, cardiovascular ultrasonography may be valuable in the management of suspected cardiovascular disease. With the improvement of ultrasound equipment quality and portability, this ancillary test can be used in a farm setting or in hospital. This article reviews the diagnostic and prognostic applications of ultrasound concerning bovine heart disease and vascular disease.

ULTRASONOGRAPHY OF THE HEART: TECHNIQUE AND NORMAL FINDINGS

Echocardiography can be performed in the field as well as in hospital. The equipment required consists of a low-frequency probe (2.5–3.5 MHz) in adults[4–7] or a higher-frequency probe (3.75–5 MHz) in calves.[8–10] The narrow intercostal space, the cranial position of the heart in the chest, and the shape of the probe may be limiting factors for performing all the scanning views of the heart. A small, phased array (pencil-like) probe is preferred, if available (**Fig. 1**). However, a large sectorial probe may be sufficient to allow the diagnosis of bacterial endocarditis, pericarditis, and ventricular septal defects, the most common cardiac diseases in cattle.[1,11]

Echocardiograms are usually performed on standing animals.[4–11] For calves, the examination can also be performed with the animal restrained in right lateral

Clinique Ambulatoire Bovine/Bovine Ambulatory Clinic, Département des Sciences Cliniques, Faculté de Médecine Vétérinaire, Université de Montréal, Saint-Hyacinthe, QC, J2S 7C6, Canada
E-mail address: s.buczinski@umontreal.ca

Vet Clin Food Anim 25 (2009) 611–632
doi:10.1016/j.cvfa.2009.07.010
0749-0720/09/$ – see front matter © 2009 Elsevier Inc. All rights reserved.

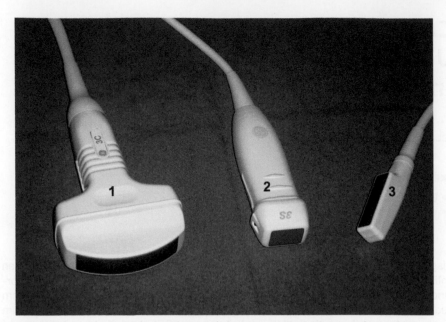

Fig. 1. Different probes may be used to perform echocardiography. Low-frequency probes, such as sectorial probes used to monitor pregnancy in small ruminants, (1) or, if available, a small, phased array probe (2), can be used in cattle. High-frequency linear probes (3) used in reproductive monitoring do not allow good penetration for adults but can sometimes be used in calves. The linear probes' major inconvenience is lack of dexterity in the intercostal space.

recumbency on a table with the standard imaging opening for small animals.[12] The area from the third to the fifth intercostal space in the cardiac region is clipped on both sides of the thorax. The skin is then rinsed with warm water or alcohol, and transmission gel is applied. The thoracic limbs can be moved cranially (**Fig. 2**)[11] or gently abducted[7] to facilitate better contact between the probe and the intercostal space.

Right Parasternal Ultrasonograms

The echocardiogram performed in the right side of the thorax allows to distinguish three long-axis and one short-axis view of the heart.[6,7,11] When the probe is applied parallel to the fourth intercostal space, the long-axis four-chambers view of the ventricles, atria, and the interventricular septum is observed (**Fig. 3**). The operator needs to remember that the moderator band (trabeculae septomarginalis) that connects the anterior and posterior walls of the right ventricle, frequently observed with this view (see **Fig. 3**), is thick in cattle and should not be misinterpreted as mural endocarditis. Placing the probe slightly more cranially with a slight clockwise rotation, the left ventricular outflow tract (LVOT) is observed—the left ventricle, left atria, aortic valve, and the aortic root (**Fig. 4**). The right ventricle and right atria are also observed with this view. A slight clockwise rotation in the same intercostal space or probe placement in the third intercostal space allows the visualization of the right ventricular outflow tract (RVOT) in which the right ventricle and atrium and the pulmonary valve and pulmonary trunk are observed (**Fig. 5**). The short-axis view of the heart is obtained by placing the probe perpendicular to the ribs in the fourth intercostal space to observe a transverse section of both ventricles (**Fig. 6**). The short-axis view may be

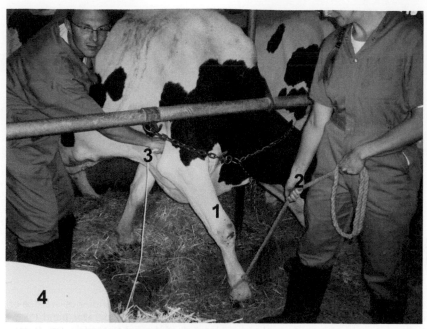

Fig. 2. Practical realization of echocardiography via the right side of the thorax in an on-farm setting. If needed, the right forelimb (1) can be moved cranially by a helper (2) so that the region of interest (3) can be examined. The ultrasound device is placed in a safe location (4) to avoid problems with other herdmates.

difficult to obtain because of symmetric images and interferences with the pleural surface.[7] As in small animals, other views may be obtained from the right side of the thorax;[12,13] however, their usefulness in clinical situations remains to be determined.

Left Parasternal Ultrasonograms

Echocardiography on the left side is especially useful when suspecting left heart disease. Preparation for an ultrasonographic examination of the cow is the same as for the right thorax. The caudal long-axis view of the heart is obtained by placing the probe on the fourth or the fifth intercostal space dorsally to the level of the olecranum directed slightly caudodorsally, allowing a view of the ventricles, atria, and the atrioventricular valves (**Fig. 7**). The probe is then turned slightly more cranially and rotated slightly counterclockwise to observe the LVOT (**Fig. 8**). The left parasternal cranial long-axis view of the RVOT (**Fig. 9**) is seen from the third[6,7] or fourth intercostal space.[7] Different echocardiographic measurements have been made in adult cows[5,7] or calves.[8–10] However, the usefulness of measured echocardiographic parameters in cattle in a clinical setting remains to be determined. The cardiac chamber dimensions may be an objective tool when suspecting heart dilation secondary to heart disease.[12,14] The left ventricular fractional shortening (FS) can also be measured using M-mode analysis of the right parasternal short- or long-axis view.[12,14,15] The FS represents the percentage of change of the left ventricular diameter between the diastole (end diastolic diameter of the left ventricle [LVd]) and the systole (end systolic diameter of the left ventricle [LVs]) by the formula FS (%)=100×(LVd−LVs)/LVd. In healthy

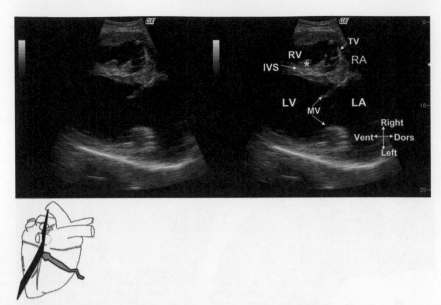

Fig. 3. Right long-axis view of the heart (four-chambers view). The tendinous chordae of the tricuspid valve are also seen as echoic lines (*arrowhead*). The moderator band (*) is also partially observed emerging from the posterior wall of the right ventricle. Ds, dorsal; IVS, interventricular septum; LA, left atrium; MV, mitral valve; RA, right atrium; RV, right ventricle; TV, tricuspid valve; Vt, ventral.

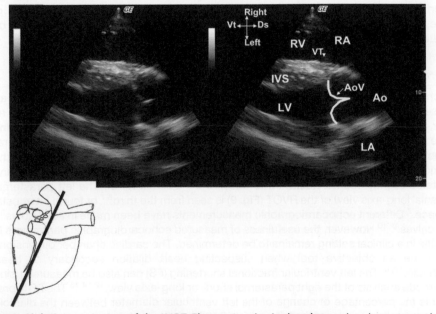

Fig. 4. Right long-axis view of the LVOT. The aortic valve is also observed and represented as a yellow line. Ao, aorta; AoV, aortic valve.

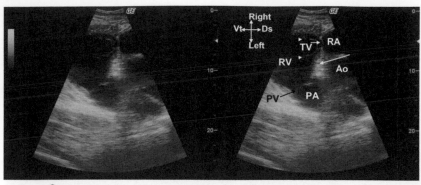

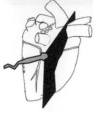

Fig. 5. Right parasternal cranial long-axis view of the right ventricular outflow on the third intercostal space. A small anechoic circular structure (*yellow arrow*), which is the coronary artery, is observed between the aorta and the right ventricle. The tendinous chordae of the tricuspid valve are also observed (*arrowheads*). Ao, aorta; Ds, dorsal; PA, pulmonary artery; PV, pulmonary valve; RA, right atrium; RV, right ventricle; TV, tricuspid valve; Vt, ventral.

Holstein and Jersey cows, the normal FS range varies between 28% and 55%.[7] In other species, the FS can be used as a rough method for assessing the global inotropism and the left systolic function that can be affected by various cardiac or noncardiac diseases.[12,14–16] This calculation is useful when suspecting myocardial disease in horses.[3,14] The main echocardiographic measurements of other cardiac structures are indicated in **Table 1**.[5,7] To date, the data are currently lacking in cattle concerning the prognostic values of echocardiographic measurements or calculated parameters.

PRACTICAL APPLICATION OF ECHOCARDIOGRAPHY IN BOVINE MEDICINE

Although the clinical manifestations of heart disease may be indicative of most cardiac disorders,[1] the definitive diagnosis requires ancillary tests, such as serum biochemistry panel, complete cell blood count, blood culture, pericardiocentesis, electrocardiography, and echocardiography.[1–3] Echocardiography is a noninvasive diagnostic imaging technique that permits cowside diagnosis, which can be useful in a field setting when clinical signs are not obvious or with commercial animals to allow rapid culling or euthanasia if the diagnosis and the associated prognosis are not compatible with financial restraints or animal welfare.

The echocardiographic findings in cases of suspected heart disease include specific cardiac findings and nonspecific findings that appear secondary to congestive heart failure (eg, pleural effusion, compression of the lung).[17] The most common cardiac diseases—pericarditis, infectious endocarditis, and ventricular septal defects[1]—can be suspected on the basis of clinical findings and echocardiographic findings.

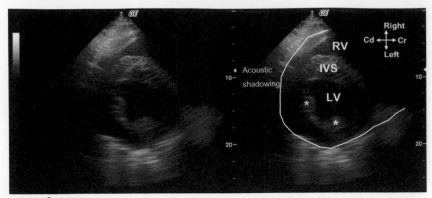

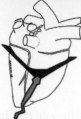

Fig. 6. Right short-axis view of the cardiac ventricles. Both ventricles are seen in transversal section. The papillary muscles of the left ventricle are observed (*), revealing the mushroom shape of the left ventricular lumen. Cd, caudal; Cr, cranial; IVS, interventricular septum; LV, left ventricle; RV, right ventricle.

Pericarditis and Pericardial Effusions

Pericarditis is the most common pericardial disorder in cattle.[1,17] Pericardial effusion is often secondary to hardware diseases and consists of a purulent effusion with varying amounts of fibrin clots.[11,17,18] Recently, idiopathic hemorrhagic pericarditis (IHP) has been mentioned as an uncommon cause of pericardial effusion with a good prognosis in cattle.[19,20] Echocardiography may help distinguish traumatic pericarditis, which has a poor prognosis, from IHP, which can be successfully treated with pericardial drainage.[17,19,20] Pericardial effusion should not be confused with bilateral pleuritis in which anomalies of the pleural space and the lung parenchyma can also be found.[14]

The main ultrasonographic finding of traumatic pericarditis is pericardial effusion, which is normally hypoechogenic to echogenic.[17] Some echoic fibrin clots can also be seen.[11,17,18,21,22] The pericardial layer, which is not seen in healthy animals, is typically seen as a thick echoic membrane surrounding the heart in cases of pericarditis (**Fig. 10**).[17] Hyperechoic points associated with a reverberation artifact can also be observed when free gas is present with septic pericardial effusion. The echocardiographic findings in cases of IHP consist of anechoic[19] to hypoechogenic[20] pericardial effusion with or without echogenic strands of fibrin.[19,20] Therefore, ultrasonographic findings may be useful in the diagnosis of idiopathic pericarditis when anechoic pericardial fluids with no echogenic fibrin clots are observed (**Fig. 11**). However, because IHP and septic pericarditis may have the same ultrasonographic aspects (ie, hypoechogenic fluid and echoic fibrin clots), the definitive diagnosis concerning the origin of pericardial effusion still needs to be confirmed by pericardiocentesis and examination of the pericardial fluid.[2,17–20]

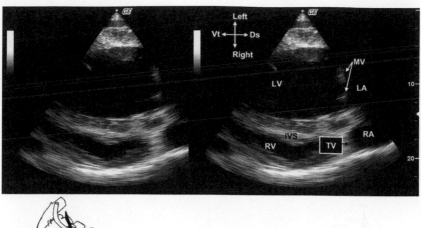

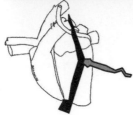

Fig. 7. Left caudal long-axis view of the heart. In this view, the four cardiac chambers are observed as well as the atrioventricular valves. Note that the tricuspid valve falsely appears thickened because the ultrasound beam crosses the valve near its attachment to the myocardium. Ds, dorsal; IVS, interventricular septum; LA, left atrium; LV, left ventricle; MV, mitral valve; RA, right atrium; RV, right ventricle; TV, tricuspid valve; Vt, ventral.

In horses, depending on the clinical and echocardiographic findings, three forms of pericarditis have been described: the effusive form (leading to cardiac tamponade caused by pericardial effusion), the fibrinous form (with accumulation of fibrin in the pericardium), and the constrictive form, in which pericardial thickening reduces the diastolic filling of the heart.[23] In cattle, this classification does not exist. Pericardial effusion typically compresses the right ventricle and atrium[17,20] and the left ventricle.[17,19] This compression is particularly visible during cardiac diastole when measuring the cardiac chamber dimensions. The end diastolic ventricular volume is reduced secondary to the increased pericardial pressure, which leads to a decrease in heart preload and a decreased cardiac output partially compensated by an increased heart rate at rest.[24] Epicardial deposits of echogenic fibrin may also be a limiting factor for ventricular diastole as found in cases of effusive-constrictive pericarditis syndrome in humans.[24]

Pericardial effusion may also be observed with the occurrence of other cardiac and noncardiac diseases.[14] Various heart neoplasms can lead to an anechoic pericardial effusion, discussed below. Anechogenic pericardial effusion can also be seen in cases of hypoproteinemia, right heart failure, or viral disease in horses.[23]

Evidence-based medicine concerning the clinical impact of echocardiographic findings in cattle with pericardial effusion is still lacking. Case series demonstrated that, as in horse,[23] echocardiography can be used to observe the beneficial effects of pericardial drainage and the progression of pericardial fluid accumulation.[19,20] However, for the moment, there are no prognostic echocardiographic factors that can be used by the bovine practitioner. Echocardiography is useful to confirm the suspicion of pericardial effusion, to observe the impact of pericardial effusion on the cardiac chambers or

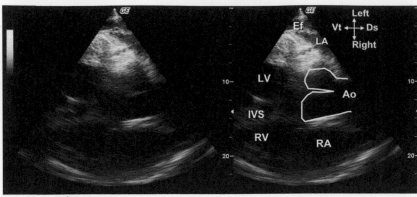

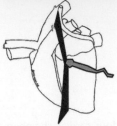

Fig. 8. Left parasternal long-axis view of the LVOT. The left atrium, left ventricle, and aorta are observed. The transversal view of the aortic valve is recognized as a thin echoic line. A small quantity of pleural effusion is also seen. Ao, aorta; Ds, dorsal; Ef, pleural effusion; IVS, interventricular septum; LA, left atrium; LV, left ventricle; RA, right atrium; RV, right ventricle; Vt, ventral.

function, to differentiate pericardial and pleural effusion, and to help the clinician choose the optimal site of the pericardiocentesis.[11]

Bacterial Endocarditis and Endocardial Diseases

Bacterial endocarditis is the most common endocardial disease in cattle.[1,25,26] The infection most frequently involves the valvular endocardium, leading to a thickened endocardium and valvular insufficiency.[27] Clinical diagnosis of bacterial endocarditis may be difficult in the absence of heart murmur and clinical signs of heart failure.[25,26] Cardiac auscultation reveals a murmur secondary to valvular insufficiency in 50%[25] to 80%[1] of cases. Clinical signs of heart failure are not definitive in cattle.[25] The auscultation of a cardiac murmur may be heard in cases of congenital heart disease[1,28] and even in healthy cows,[29] in addition to cases of bacterial endocarditis.

Echocardiography is a sensitive diagnostic tool for cases of bovine endocarditis in studies in a hospital setting.[25,26,30,31] The sensitivity for detecting valvular thickening or vegetation in cases of bacterial endocarditis has been reported to be 75% (4 of 6 cases),[26] 95% (21 of 22 cases),[25] and 100% (in 5 cases).[31] The tricuspid valve is the valve most frequently affected by bacterial endocarditis.[25,30] The infection of more than one valve may occur in 13%[25] to 53%[30] of cases. The mural endocardium may rarely be affected.[11,25] A recent German study showed that the sensitivity of echocardiography for detecting bacterial endocarditis depended on the site of the infection.[30] Tricuspid lesions were detected in 13 of 13 cases, mitral lesions in 7 of 8 cases, pulmonary lesions in 6 of 7 cases, and aortic lesions in 2 of 4 cases.[30]

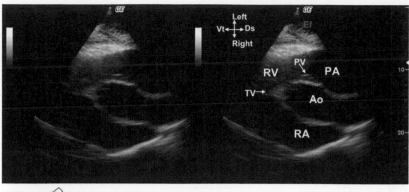

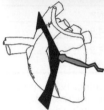

Fig. 9. Left view of the RVOT in a cow. Some pleural effusion is also seen on the left side of the thorax in this case of unilateral pleuritis. Ao, aorta; Ds, dorsal; Ef, pleural effusion; PA, pulmonary artery; PV, pulmonary valve; RA, right atrium; RV, right ventricle; TV, tricuspid valve; Vt, ventral.

However, at least one abnormal valve could be diagnosed in all 15 presented cases. The specificity of echocardiographic findings for bacterial endocarditis has not been determined in cattle. This specificity should be good to excellent because of the low incidence of noninfectious valvular anomalies in cattle [32–34] and the clinical presentation of most affected patients in advanced stage of the disease with obvious changes of the affected endocardium.

Typical echocardiographic findings in cases of bacterial endocarditis include a marked irregular thickening of the affected valvular leaflet or of the mural endocardium that can confer a vegetation or a "shaggy" appearance (**Fig. 12**).[21,25,30,35,36] All heart valves should be properly imaged (**Fig. 13**). The infected endocardium is more frequently echogenic[11,21,31,35] than hyperechoic with gaseous content.[11,31] A previous study by Yamaga and Too[31] stated that valvular vegetation with a diameter of less than 5 mm could be missed by echocardiography. Valvular thickening can also occur with ruptured chordae tendineae or flail valvular leaflets in horses,[14] but such conditions are rare in cattle.[3] Valvular blood and serous cysts, which are common in bovine atrioventricular valves,[37] could also theoretically (although not reported) cause a valvular thickening; however, the cysts are small (mean diameter of 2 mm).[37]

For these reasons, when valvular thickening is observed, bacterial endocarditis should be the first diagnosis on the differential list. Secondary to the valvular deformation, regurgitant lesions leading to cardiac chamber dilation may also occur.[11,14,31] The right atrium and right ventricle may enlarge secondary to tricuspid endocarditis (see **Fig. 12**).[31]

Although information is still lacking in cattle, echocardiography has been mentioned as an beneficial ancillary tool to monitor the valvular healing of equine endocarditis.[14,38] During the healing process, the lesions tend to be smaller, smoother, and

Table 1
Echocardiographic dimensions in healthy adult cattle

Parameter	Jersey Cows (n = 10)[7] Mean ±SD	Holstein Cows (n = 12)[7] Mean ±SD	Swiss Braunvieh (n = 25), Simmental (n = 21), and Holstein Cows (n = 5), Total of 51 cows[5] Mean ±SD
RVd (cm)	2.45±0.53	2.27±0.76	4.1±1.02
RVs (cm)	1.32±0.63	1.14±0.43	3.6±0.98
IVSd (cm)	2±0.4	2.2±0.51	2.4±0.33
IVSs (cm)	3.6±0.5	3.4±0.5	3.1±0.38
LVd (cm)	7.7±0.7	8.7±1.0	7.0±0.73
LVs (cm)	4.2±0.53	4.2±0.8	4.5±0.69
LAD (cm)	10.9±0.5	12±1.2	NP
Ao (cm)	5±0.26	6.4±0.62	4.9±0.92
PA (cm)	4.2±0.27	5.5±0.8	5.6±0.82
FS (%)	44.7±8.3	46.5±9.5	43.4±9.33

Ao, end-diastolic aortic diameter; FS, left ventricular fractional shortening; IVSd, end-diastolic interventricular septal thickness; IVSs, end-systolic interventricular septal thickness; LAD, left atrial diameter; LVd, end-diastolic left ventricle diameter; LVs, end-systolic left ventricle diameter; NP, not performed; PA, pulmonary artery diameter in diastole; RVd, end-diastolic right ventricle diameter; RVs, end-systolic right ventricle diameter.

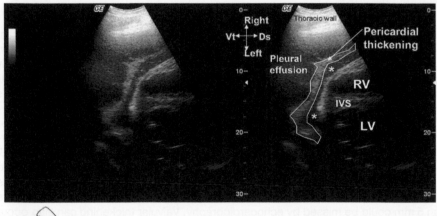

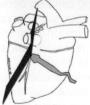

Fig. 10. Right long-axis view of the ventral part of the heart of a cow with pericarditis and pleuritis secondary to hardware disease. Pleural effusion displaced the heart dorsally. A small amount of hypoechoic pericardial effusion is observed (*). Pericardial thickening is demonstrated as an echoic line surrounding the cardiac silhouette. Ds, dorsal; IVS, interventricular septum; LV, left ventricle; RV, right ventricle; Vt, ventral.

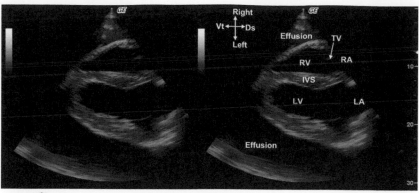

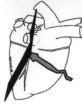

Fig. 11. Right four-chambers long-axis view of a bovine heart with anechoic pericardial effusion. An idiopathic hemorrhagic pericarditis was diagnosed after pericardial fluid analysis, the most important differential diagnosis in an anechoic pericardial effusion secondary to cardiac manifestation of a lymphoma. Ds, dorsal; IVS, interventricular septum; LA, left atrium; RA, right atrium; RV, right ventricle; TV, tricuspid valve; Vt, ventral.

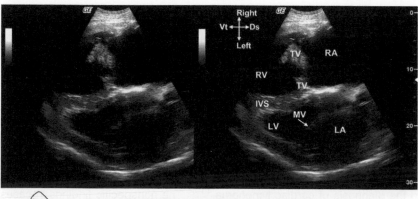

Fig. 12. Right four-chambers long-axis view of a tricuspid endocarditis in a cow. The affected valve is markedly thickened and has a "shaggy" appearance. Tricuspid regurgitation caused by valvular insufficiency led to a secondary right atrial dilation. Ds, dorsal; IVS, interventricular septum; LA, left atrium; LV, left ventricle; MV, mitral valve; RA, right atrium; RV, right ventricle; TV, tricuspid valve; Vt, ventral.

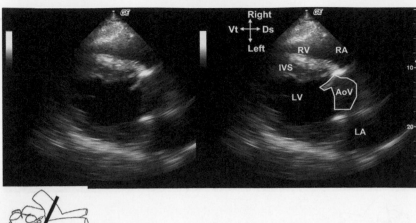

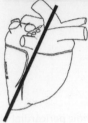

Fig.13. Right long-axis view of the LVOT of a cow with aortic endocarditis. The aortic trunk is totally obstructed by an echogenic heterogenous mass that represents the infectious vegetation. AoV, aortic valve; Ds, dorsal; IVS, interventricular septum; LA, left atrium; LV, left ventricle; RA, right atrium; RV, right ventricle; Vt, ventral.

more echoic.[38] Echocardiography could potentially be useful in bovine cases in which therapy is attempted.

Finally, thickening and increased echogenicity of the valves has also been found in cattle as a result of experimental intoxication with *Trisetum flavescens* silage.[39] The echocardiographic findings in these cases had a specificity of 100% for detecting valvular calcifications when compared with histology.

Cardiac Neoplasms

The most common cardiac neoplasm in cattle is cardiac lymphoma in areas where the bovine leukosis virus infection has not been eradicated.[3] The typical signs of enzootic lymphoma (eg, polyadenomegaly, exophthalmos) may [40,41] or may not [42,43] be present concomitant to clinical signs of heart failure. Echocardiographic findings may be helpful in the diagnosis of cardiac lymphoma.[40–44] The nonspecific findings in cases of cardiac lymphoma include varying quantities of anechoic pericardial effusion [40,42,43] with small amounts of echoic fibrin strands.[40,41] The most striking abnormal findings are located in the right atrium, which, as in humans [44] is the most common cardiac site of primary tumor involvement.[40–43] A right atrial dilation can be observed [40,41] or masked by echocardiographic signs of cardiac tamponade due to pericardial effusion.[42] The infiltrated atrial wall, epicardium, or endocardium appears thickened.[40,42] This infiltration may lead to the observation of a luminal echogenic mass with multiple hypoechoic foci.[40,42] Still, the definitive diagnosis must be supported by isolation of neoplastic cells.[3]

Echocardiographic data concerning other types of cardiac neoplasms are scant in ruminants. An echogenic mass at the base of the heart was the main echocardiographic finding in two cows that each had a tumor of the mediastinal fusiform cells.[26] An echogenic round mass that partially obstructed the right atrium was also found in a case of ovine cardiac fibrosarcoma.[45] In both cases, however, the final diagnosis required histologic analysis of the abnormal mass.[26,45]

Congenital Heart Disease

Congenital heart disease has been estimated to represent 2.7% of congenital problems in calves.[46] The most common bovine congenital heart disease is ventricular septal defect (VSD).[28,47] The echocardiographic findings are compatible with a septal defect in the membranous part of the interventricular septum.[28,48] As in horses, the right long-axis view of the LVOT is best for observing the defect (**Fig. 14**).[14] In cases of a subpulmonic location of the defect, the short-axis view of the interventricular septum between the LVOT and RVOT may also be helpful.[3] Although the size of the defect ($\leq$2.5 cm) and the peak velocity of shunt flow ($\geq$4 m/s) through the VSD (assessed by Doppler ultrasound) have been mentioned as positive prognostic factors in horses with VSD,[49] this information is still lacking in cattle.[28,32] However, the direction of blood flow across the defect is important for suspecting an inversion of the shunt associated with pulmonary hypertension, also called Eisenmenger's complex, which has a poor prognosis.[28,50] The direction of the blood across the defect can be assessed by Doppler ultrasound or by the bubble test.[3,51] The bubble test is simple contrast echocardiography that allows a view of the repartition of a bolus of agitated sterile saline solution injected via the jugular vein during the cardiac cycle.[51] The injected solution increases the echogenicity of the blood in the right heart, which helps to see if the blood in the right heart can be found in the left heart chambers (ie, if an

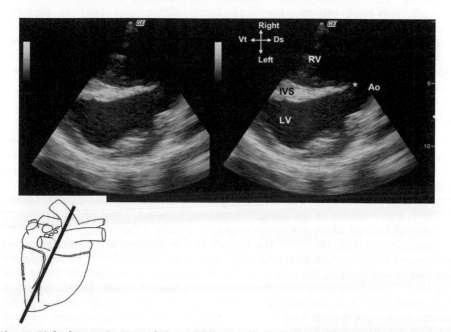

Fig. 14. Right long-axis view of the LVOT in a calf presenting with a pansystolic murmur heard maximally on the right side of the thorax. The membranous part of the interventricular septum is lacking (*), which is diagnostic of VSD. Ao, aorta; Ds, dorsal; IVS, interventricular septum; LV, left ventricle; RV, right ventricle; Vt, ventral.

intracardiac right-to-left shunt is present). Other echocardiographic findings in cases of VSD consist of left atrial, left ventricular, and right ventricular enlargement, and pulmonary artery dilation.[3,28]

Other congenital anomalies have also been diagnosed by echocardiography.[32,34,52–58] The tetralogy of Fallot found in a VSD—dextroposition of the aorta, right ventricular hypertrophy, and pulmonary stenosis—can be imaged with cardiac ultrasonography.[32,52–54] The other, rarer congenital heart diseases may also be imaged; however, their diagnosis may be difficult if not performed by a specialist in echocardiography.[52,55–58]

Cor Pulmonale

Cor pulmonale is represented by right ventricular hypertrophy or right heart failure secondary to pulmonary hypertension that can be caused by high altitude or chronic lung disease.[3,59,60] Echocardiographic findings in two cows were nonspecific.[59] The pulmonary artery was enlarged when compared with the aorta in equine cases of cor pulmonale.[61,62] A pulmonary insufficiency was also noted with Doppler ultrasound.[61,62] Right ventricular and atrial dilation may also be observed, leading to a tricuspid insufficiency.[62] However, information is still lacking concerning the real clinical use of echocardiography in detecting this disease in cattle.

Other Cardiac Diseases

Myocarditis and cardiomyopathy can also be encountered in cattle.[3] However, the data are scant concerning their echocardiographic manifestations.[21,41,50,63,64] The echocardiographic findings in cases of dilated cardiomyopathy include a reduced[21,41] to normal[63] FS. The right cardiac chambers are classically enlarged with [41,63] or without[21] left heart dilation. The right heart dilation may lead to tricuspid regurgitation.[63]

The echocardiographic findings in cases of bovine myocarditis have been limited to abscessation of the myocardium.[64] The abscesses were observed as anechoic lesions in the myocardium.[64] The localization of the abscess in the heart is important because they can be missed when performing standard echocardiograms.[50]

PRACTICAL ULTRASONOGRAPHY OF THE VASCULAR SYSTEM

Vascular ultrasonography can be helpful in the noninvasive diagnosis of vascular disease when clinical signs are insufficient to make a diagnosis and also for deep vessel assessment.[3,14,65] The technique for the ultrasonographic examination of the main vessels in cattle has been described, including the jugular,[66,67] mammary,[68] tarsal,[69] caudal vena cava,[70] ovarian and vaginal,[71] and musculophrenic veins.[72] Information is also available for the aorta,[39,73] carotid,[66] uterine,[74] and caudal arteries.[75] The normal findings of venous ultrasonography include a thin echogenic wall with anechoic content (**Fig. 15**).[11,65,66] The superficial vein diameter and appearance can be affected by how much pressure is applied to the probe.[11,65,66] Venous valves can also be observed as thin echoic to hyperechoic lines in the vascular lumen (see **Fig. 15**).[65,68] The ultrasonographic appearance of arteries is grossly the same except for a small variation in diameter between the systolic and diastolic phases of the cardiac cycle—the arterial wall is thicker than the venous wall, arteries are less deformable than the superficial veins, and no valvulae are observed in their lumen.[14,65] If the Doppler function is available, blood flow can be assessed when performing ultrasonography (see **Fig. 15**). The main vascular diseases in cattle include inflammation of the vessel wall, thrombosis, and aneurysm.[3,11,14]

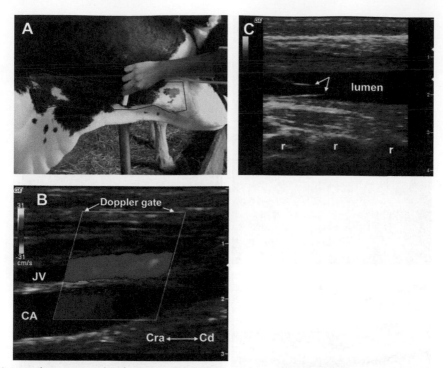

Fig. 15. Ultrasonographic findings of the jugular vein and the carotid artery region in cows. The cow is restrained with a lateral extension of the neck to perform the examination (*A*). If this procedure is performed in a calf, the examination can be performed with the animal in lateral recumbency. Normal findings (*B*) include visualization of the superficial jugular vein and the carotid artery. The jugular vein is a compressible tubular structure with a thin echoic wall and anechoic content; thin echoic lines can be observed in the lumen of the vessel and are compatible with venous valves (*C; yellow arrows*). When the color flow Doppler is available (*B*), it shows the opposite laminar blood flow direction in both vessels. CA, carotid artery; Cd, caudal; Cra, cranial; JV, jugular vein, r, tracheal ring.

Phlebitis and Thrombophlebitis

The ultrasonographic appearance of periphlebitis, phlebitis, and thrombophlebitis of the jugular [67,76–78] and limb [69,79,80] vessels have been described in cows. Periphlebitis (inflammation of perivenous tissues) is accompanied by multiple hypoechoic areas compatible with interstitial fluid and necrotic content (**Fig. 16**).[76] In cases of phlebitis, the venous wall is thickened and the echoic intima is difficult to observe. Phlebitis and periphlebitis are often observed together as a consequence of irritant perivascular injections (see **Fig. 16**).[11,14] Thrombosis and thrombophlebitis are characterized by the observation of a luminal hypoechoic to echoic mass that totally or partially occludes the affected vessel (**Fig. 17**). Although most of time the thrombus has a homogeneous echogenicity,[67,77] some anechoic areas can also be seen within the thrombosed area, especially in mature thrombus.[80] A cavitating lesion with anechoic content is a frequent finding in septic thrombophlebitis in horses,[81] but has not been reported in cattle.[67,77,79,80] Transcutaneous ultrasound is a reliable tool to assess the precise extent of the thrombus[69,79,80] as well as recanalization in the healing thrombosed area if Doppler ultrasound is available (see **Fig. 17**).[81] Ultrasound-guided puncture biopsy of the thrombus can also be safely done for diagnostic

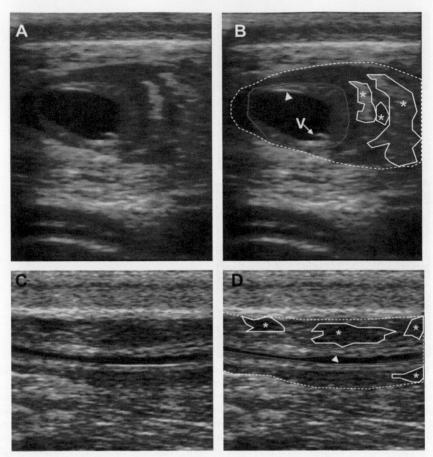

Fig.16. Transverse (*A*, *B*) and longitudinal (*C*, *D*) ultrasonograms of the jugular vein of a cow with periphlebitis and phlebitis secondary to perivascular dextrose injection by the owner. The anechoic venous lumen is observed with (*A*, *B*) or without (*C*, *D*) distal manual compression. The vascular wall is thickened (*continuous red line*). The thin echoic intima (*arrowhead*) is discontinued. Anechoic or hyperechoic areas (*) are observed in the swollen perivascular tissues (*dotted line*). A venous valve (V) is also observed.

or therapeutic purposes.[81] Thrombi have also been observed in the ovarian and vaginal veins, and in the caudal vena cava[82–84] and the hepatic vein.[84] To date, no information is available concerning the use of ultrasonography other than for diagnostic purposes.

Arterial Thrombosis

Arterial thrombosis is a rare event that can occur as a result of various inflammatory processes (**Fig. 18**).[3] Ultrasonographic findings of arterial thrombosis have been described in distal aortic thrombosis in calves.[73] They are the same as for venous thrombosis, including a hypoechoic to echoic area that partially to totally obstructs blood flow. Ultrasonography can be an interesting tool in monitoring thrombus size reduction.[73] The color-flow Doppler is also an interesting tool for assessing blood flow across the thrombosed area.[73]

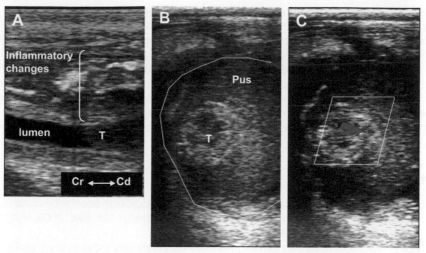

Fig. 17. Ultrasonographic appearance of chronic jugular thrombophlebitis in an adult Holstein cow. (*A*) The longitudinal view of the jugular vein shows a hypoechoic thrombus (T) that totally obstructs the venous lumen. The peripheral venous tissues are swollen with echoic to hyperechoic content. (*B*) As the beam is relocated from the mandible to the thorax and rotated perpendicular to the vessel, a cavitary lesion (*dotted line*) is observed in periphery of the vein. This cavitary lesion has heterogenic content that is similar to pus. (*C*) Doppler interrogation of the thrombosed area shows laminar flow throughout the thrombus (*red area*) compatible with recanalization of the thrombosed area by new vessels.

Other Vascular Diseases

The ultrasonographic findings of other vascular diseases have been described in cases of portacaval shunt in calves,[85] calcification of blood vessels secondary to experimental *Trisetum flavescens* silage feeding in cows,[39] patent ductus venosus,[86] and aneurysm of the ductus arteriosus in a heifer.[87] Although the data are limited to case reports or case-series concerning the use of ultrasonography in cattle, the

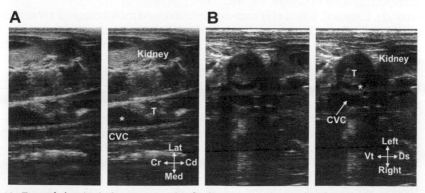

Fig. 18. Transabdominal ultrasonographic findings in a calf with distal aortic thrombosis. The calf was placed in right lateral recumbency. The thrombus is seen in longitudinal (*A*) and transversal (*B*) views and almost totally occupies the aortic lumen (*) near the left kidney. The caudal vena cava is also observed. Cd, caudal; Cr, cranial; CVC, caudal vena cava; Ds, dorsal ; Lat, lateral; Med, medial; T, thrombus; Vt, ventral.

vascular ultrasonography potentially may help in the diagnosis and management of many vascular diseases.[14,65] The Doppler vascular assessment, which is not discussed in this review, has shown promising results in cattle, especially for the genital tract.[74,88–90]

In conclusion, ultrasonography can be of tremendous help in the management of cardiovascular disease in cattle. In most cases, cardiovascular ultrasonography permits an antemortem diagnosis that can be especially useful in cases with a poor prognosis to avoid ineffective treatment. This early diagnosis can also be helpful in highly valuable animals by allowing an earlier therapeutic attempt and for monitoring the healing process.

REFERENCES

1. Bexiga R, Mateus A, Philbey AW, et al. Clinicopathological presentation of cardiac diseases in cattle and its impact on decision making. Vet Rec 2008;162(18): 575–80.
2. Buczinski S. Les maladies cardiaques bovines: revue des moyens diagnostiques disponibles et de leur intérêt [Bovine heart diseases: a review of the ancillary tests and their clinical values]. Ann Med Vet 2007;151(1):15–23 [in French].
3. Reef VB, McGuirk SM. Diseases of the cardiovascular system. In: Smith BP, editor. Large animal internal medicine. 3rd edition. St. Louis (MO): Mosby; 2002. p. 443–78.
4. Pipers FS, Reef VB, Hamlin RL, et al. Echocardiography in the bovine animal. Bov Pract 1978;30:114–8.
5. Braun U, Schweizer T. Bestimmung der Herzdimensionen beim rind mit hilfe der 2-D-mode-echocardiographie [Assessment of heart dimension in the cow with the help of 2-D-mode echocardiography]. Berl Munch Tierarztl Wschr 2001;114(1–2): 46–50 [in German].
6. Braun U, Schweizer T, Pusterla N. Echocardiography of the normal bovine heart: technique and ultrasonographic appearance. Vet Rec 2001;148(2):47–51.
7. Hallowell G, Potter TJ, Bowen IM. Methods and normal values for echocardiography in adult dairy cattle. J Vet Cardiol 2007;9(2):91–8.
8. Amory H, Jakovljevic S, Lekeux P. Quantitative M-mode and two-dimensional echocardiography in calves. Vet Rec 1991;128(2):25–31.
9. Amory H, Lekeux P. Effect of growth on functional and morphological echocardiographic variables in Friesian calves. Vet Rec 1991;128(15):349–54.
10. Amory H, Kafidi N, Lekeux P. Echocardiographic evaluation of cardiac morphologic and functional variables in double-muscled calves. Am J Vet Res 1992; 53(9):1540–7.
11. Buczinski S. L'examen échographique de l'appareil cardiovasculaire et lymphatique. In: Buczinski S, editor. Echographie des bovins. Rueil-Malmaison, France: Point-vétérinaire Wolter-Kluwer; 2009. p. 47–67 [in Spanish].
12. Buczinski S. L'examen échographique de l'appareil cardiovasculaire et lymphatique [Ultrasonography of the cardiovascular and lymphatic system]. In: Buczinski S, editor. Echographie des bovins. [Bovine ultrasonography]. Rueil-Malmaison, France: Point-vétérinaire, Wolter-Kluwer; 2009. p. 47–67 [in French].
13. Thomas WP, Gaber CE, Jacobs GJ, et al. Recommendations for standards in transthoracic two-dimensional echocardiography in the dog and cat. J Vet Intern Med 1993;7(4):247–52.
14. Reef VB. Cardiovascular ultrasonography. In: Reef VB, editor. Equine diagnostic ultrasound. Philadelphia: Saunders; 1997. p. 215–72.

15. Slama M, Maizel J. Echocardiographic measurement of ventricular function. Curr Opin Critical Care 2006;12(3):241–8.
16. Young LE, Rogers K, Wood JLN. Left ventricular size and systolic function in thoroughbred racehorses and their relationships to race performance. J Appl Physiol 2005;99(4):1278–85.
17. Braun U. Traumatic pericarditis in cattle: clinical, radiographic and ultrasonographic findings. Vet J, in press.
18. Braun U, Lejeune B, Rauch S, et al. Sonographische Befunde bei 22 Rindern mit Pericarditis traumatica [Ultrasonographic findings in 22 cows with traumatic pericarditis]. Schweiz Arch Tierheilkd 2008;150(6):281–6 [In German].
19. Jesty SA, Sweeney RW, Dolente BA, et al. Idiopathic pericarditis and cardiac tamponade in two cows. J Am Vet Med Assoc 2005;226(9):1555–8.
20. Firshman AM, Sage AM, Valberg SJ, et al. Idiopathic hemorrhagic pericardial effusion in cows. J Vet Intern Med 2006;20(6):1499–502.
21. Schweizer T, Sydler T, Braun U. Kardiomyopathie, Endokarditis valvularis thromboticans und Perikarditis traumatica beim Rind – Klinische und echokardiographische Befunde an drei Fallberichten [Cardiomyopathy, valvular thombotic endocarditis and traumatic pericarditis in cows—clinical and echocardiographic findings on 3 case reports]. Schweiz Archiv Tierheilkd 2003;145(9):425–30 [In German].
22. Sojka JE, White MR, Widmer WR, et al. An unusual case of traumatic pericarditis in a cow. J Vet Diag Invest 1990;2(2):139–42.
23. Worth LT, Reef VB. Pericarditis in horses: 18 cases (1986–1995). J Am Vet Med Assoc 1998;212(2):248–53.
24. LeWinter MM, Kabbani S. Pericardial diseases. In: Zipes DP, Libby P, Bonow RO, Braunwald E, editors. Braunwald's heart disease: a textbook of cardiovascular medicine. 7th edition. Philadelphia: Elsevier Saunders; 2005. p. 1757–79.
25. Healy AM. Endocarditis in cattle: a review of 22 cases. Irish Vet J 1996;49(1): 43–8.
26. Buczinski S, Francoz D, Fecteau G. Congestive heart failure in cattle: 59 cases (1990–2005). Nice, France: 24th World Buiatric Congress; 2006. p. OS18–1.
27. Kasari TR, Roussel AJ. Bacterial endocarditis. Part I. Pathophysiologic, diagnostic, and therapeutic considerations. Compendium Contin Educ Pract Vet 1989;11(5):655–9.
28. Buczinski S, Fecteau G, DiFruscia R. Ventricular septal defects in cattle: 25 cases. Can Vet J 2006;47(3):246–52.
29. Rezakhani A, Zarifi M. Auscultatory findings of cardiac murmurs in clinically healthy cattle. Online J Vet Res 2007;11:62–6.
30. Starke A, Hollenberg C, Strattner, et al. Sonographische Untersuchungen zur Endocarditis des Rindes. Lovran, Croatia. In: IVth Central European Buiatric Congress. p. 349–57 [In German].
31. Yamaga Y, Too K. Diagnostic ultrasound imaging of vegetative valvular endocarditis in cattle. Jpn J Vet Res 1987;35(1):49–63.
32. Buczinski S, Fecteau G, Francoz D, et al. Les affections cardiaques congénitales du veau: une approche clinique diagnostique simple [Congenital heart disease in calves: a simple and practical approach]. Med Vet Quebec 2005;35(2):79–85 [in French].
33. Gopal T, Leipold HW, Dennis SM. Congenital cardiac defects in calves. Am J Vet Res 1986;47(5):1120–1.
34. Watson TDG, Marr CM, McCandlish IAP. Aortic valvular dysplasia in a calf. Vet Rec 1991;129(17):380–2.

35. Estepa JC, Mayer-Valor R, Lopez I, et al. What is your diagnosis? J Am Vet Med Assoc 2006;228(1):37–8.
36. Ware WA, Bonagura JD, Rings DM. Echocardiographic diagnosis of pulmonary valve vegetation endocarditis in a cow. J Am Vet Med Assoc 1986; 188(2):185–7.
37. Shekarforoush SS, Rezakhani A, Katannejad A. The prevalence of blood and serous cysts in the atrioventricular valves of the heart of cattle. Revue Med Vet 2006;157(10):477–80.
38. Maxson AD, Reef VB. Bacterial endocarditis in horses: ten cases (1984–1995). Equine Vet J 1997;29(5):394–9.
39. Franz S, Gasteiner J, Schilcher F, et al. Use of ultrasonography to detect calcifications in cattle and sheep fed Trisetum flavescens silage. Vet Rec 2007;161(22): 751–4.
40. Schmitz DG, Seahorn TL. Use of echocardiography to detect tumors in the heart of a bull with bovine leukosis. J Am Vet Med Assoc 1991;205(11):1590–2.
41. Yamaga Y, Too K. Echocardiographic detection of bovine cardiac diseases. Jpn J Vet Res 1986;34(3–4):251–67.
42. Van Biervliet J, Kraus M, Woodie B, et al. Thoracoscopic pericardiotomy as a palliative treatment in a cow with pericardial lymphoma. J Vet Cardiol 2006;8(1): 69–73.
43. Ivany JM, Illanes OG. Congestive heart failure due to epicardial lymphosarcoma in a Holstein cow. Can Vet J 1999;40(11):819–20.
44. Faganello G, Belham M, Thaman R, et al. A case of primary cardiac lymphoma: analysis of the role of echocardiography in early diagnosis. Echocardiography 2007;24(8):889–92.
45. Braun U, Hagen A, Pusterla N, et al. Echocardiographic diagnosis of a cardiac fibrosarcoma in the right atrium of a sheep. Schweiz Arch Tierheilk 1995; 137(5):187–92.
46. Leipold HW, Dennis SM, Huston K. Congenital defects in cattle: nature, cause and effect. Adv Vet Sci Comp Med 1972;16:103–50.
47. Ohwada K, Murakami T. Morphologies of 469 cases of congenital heart diseases in cattle. J Jpn Vet Med Assoc 2000;53:205–9.
48. Pipers FS, Reef V, Wilson J. Echocardiographic detection of ventricular septal defects in calves. J Am Vet Med Assoc 1985;187(8):810–6.
49. Reef VB. Evaluation of ventricular septal defects in horses using two-dimensional and Doppler echocardiography. Eq Vet J 1995;19(Suppl):86–96.
50. Gavaghan BJ, Kittleson MD, Decock H. Eisenmenger's complex in a Holstein-Friesian cow. Aust Vet J 2001;79(1):37–40.
51. Bonagura JD, Pipers FS. Diagnosis of cardiac lesions by contrast echocardiography. J Am Vet Med Assoc 1983;182(4):396–402.
52. Hagio M, Murakami T, Otsuka H. Two dimensional echocardiographic diagnosis of bovine congenital heart disease: echocardiographic and anatomic correlation. Jpn J Vet Sci 1987;49(5):883–97.
53. Mohamed T, Sato H, Kurosawa T, et al. Tetralogy of Fallot in a calf: clinical, ultrasonographic, laboratory and postmortem findings. J Vet Med Sci 2004;66(1): 73–6.
54. Nakade T, Uchida Y, Otomo K. Three cases of bovine extreme tetralogy of Fallot. J Vet Med Sci 1993;55(1):161–7.
55. Schwarzwald C, Gerspach C, Glaus T, et al. Persistent truncus arteriosus and patent foramen ovale in a Simmentaler × Braunvieh calf. Vet Rec 2003;152(11): 329–33.

56. Prosek R, Oyama MA, Church WM, et al. Double-outlet right ventricle in an Angus calf. J Vet Intern Med 2005;19(2):262–7.
57. Zulauf M, Tschudi T, Meylan M. Double outlet right ventricle (DORV) bei einem 15 Monate alten rind. Schweiz Arch Tierheilkd 2001;143(3):149–54.
58. Prescott JRR, Slater JD, Jackson PGG. Patent ductus arteriosus in an 11-month-old heifer. Vet Rec 1997;140(16):430–1.
59. Angel KL, Tyler JW. Pulmonary hypertension and cardiac insufficiency in three cows with primary lung disease. J Vet Intern Med 1992;6(4):214–9.
60. Rhodes J. Comparative physiology of hypoxic pulmonary hypertension: historical clues from brisket disease. J Appl Physiol 2005;98(3):1092–100.
61. Sage AM, Valberg S, Hayden DW, et al. Echocardiography in a horse with cor pulmonale from recurrent airway obstruction. J Vet Intern Med 2006;20(3):694–6.
62. Schwarzwald CC, Stewart AJ, Morrison CD, et al. Cor pulmonale in a horse with granulomatous pneumonia. Equine Vet Educ 2006;18(4):182–7.
63. Guglielmini C. Echocardiographic and Doppler echocardiographic findings of dilated cardiomyopathy in a heifer. Vet Rec 2003;153(17):535–6.
64. Reef VB, Hattel AL. Echocardiographic detection of tetralogy of Fallot and myocardial abscesses in a calf. Cornell Vet 1984;74(2):81–95.
65. Trush A, Hartshorne T. Peripheral vascular ultrasound: how, why and when. 2nd edition. Edinburgh, UK: Elsevier; 2005. p. 235.
66. Braun U, Föhn J, Pusterla N. Ultrasonographic examination of the ventral neck region in cows. Am J Vet Res 1994;55(1):14–21.
67. Pusterla N, Braun U. Ultrasonographic evaluation of the jugular vein of cows with catheter-related thrombophlebitis. Vet Rec 1995;137(17):431–4.
68. Braun U, Hoegger R. B-mode and colour Doppler ultrasonography of the milk vein in 29 healthy Swiss Braunvieh cows. Vet Rec 2008;163(2):47–9.
69. Kofler J, Buchner A, Sendhofer A. Application of real-time ultrasonography for the detection of tarsal vein thrombosis in cattle. Vet Rec 1996;138(2):34–8.
70. Braun U. Ultrasonographic examination of the liver in cows. Am J Vet Res 1990; 51(10):1522–6.
71. Bleul U, Hagedorn A, Kähn W. Thrombosis of the ovarian and vaginal veins after caesarean section in a cow. Vet Rec 2005;156(24):780–2.
72. Braun U, Hoegger R, Haessig M. Colour Doppler sonography of the musculo-phrenic vein in cows. Vet J 2009;179:451–4.
73. Buczinski S, Francoz D, Mulon PY. Ultrasonographic diagnosis of distal aortic thrombosis in two calves. J Vet Intern Med 2007;21(2):348–51.
74. Bollwein H, Meyer HH, Maierl J, et al. Transrectal Doppler sonography of uterine blood flow. Therio 2000;53(8):1541–52.
75. Aiken GE, Kirsh BH, Strickland JR, et al. Hemodynamic responses of the caudal artery to toxic tall fescue in beef heifers. J Anim Sci 2007;85(9):2337–45.
76. Pusterla N, Braun U. Sonographische Bild perivaskülarer Jugularvenenerkran-kungen beim Rind [Ultrasonographic findings of the jugular perivenous diseases in cattle]. Tierärztl Prax 1995;23(4):360–2 [In German].
77. Pusterla N, Braun U. Prophylaxis of intravenous catheter-related thrombophlebitis in cattle. Vet Rec 1996;139(12):287–9.
78. Rouleau G, Babkine M, Dubreuil P. Factors influencing the development of jugular thrombophlebitis in cattle and comparison of 2 types of catheter. Can Vet J 2003; 44(5):399–404.
79. Kofler J, Martinek B, Kübber-Heiss A, et al. Generalised distal limb vessel thrombosis in two cows with digital and inner organ infections. Vet J 2004;167(1): 107–10.

80. Kofler J, Kübber-Heiss A. Long-term ultrasonographic and venographic study of the development of tarsal vein thrombosis in a cow. Vet Rec 1997;140(26):676–8.
81. Gardner SY, Reef VB, Spencer PA. Ultrasonographic evaluation of horses with thrombophlebitis of the jugular vein: 46 cases (1985–1988). J Am Vet Med Assoc 1991;199(3):370–3.
82. Sigrist I, Francoz D, Leclère M, et al. Antemortem diagnosis of caudal vena cava thrombosis in 2 cows. J Vet Intern Med 2008;22(3):684–6.
83. Braun U, Salis F, Gerspach C. Sonographic detection of an echogenic thrombus in the vena cava caudalis in a cow. Schweiz Arch Tierheilkd 2003;145(7):340–1.
84. Mohamed T, Sato H, Kurosawa T, et al. Ultrasonographic localisation of thrombi in the caudal vena cava and hepatic veins in a heifer. Vet J 2004;168(1):103–6.
85. Buczinski S, Duval J, d'Anjou MA, et al. Portacaval shunt in a calf: clinical, pathologic and ultrasonographic findings. Can Vet J 2007;48(4):407–10.
86. Reimer JM, Donawick WJ, Reef VB, et al. Diagnosis and surgical correction of patent ductus venosus in a calf. J Am Vet Med Assoc 1988;193(12):1539–41.
87. Pravettoni D, Re M, Riccaboni P, et al. Aneurysm of the ductus arteriosus in a heifer. Vet Rec 2005;156(24):783–5.
88. Matsui M, Miyamoto A. Evaluation of ovarian blood flow by colour Doppler ultrasound: practical use for reproductive management in the cow. Vet J 2009;181: 232–40.
89. Honnens A, Voss C, Herzog K, et al. Uterine blood flow during the first 3 weeks of pregnancy in dairy cows. Therio 2008;70(7):1048–56.
90. Herzog K, Bollwein H. Application of Doppler ultrasonography in cattle reproduction. Reprod Domest Anim 2007;42(2):51–8.

Ultrasonography of the Bovine Respiratory System and Its Practical Application

Marie Babkine, DMV, MSc[a],*, Laurent Blond, DrVét, MSc[b]

KEYWORDS

- Ultrasonography • Bovine • Respiratory system
- Pleura • Lung

Numerous diagnostic methods are used to evaluate diseases that affect the bovine respiratory system, including auscultation, percussion, bloodwork, radiography, ultrasonography, and more invasive procedures such as aspirations and biopsies.[1,2] Ultrasonography is a noninvasive diagnostic tool that has been used for the past several years in veterinary and human medicine to assess the lungs, the pleura, and the mediastinum. Ultrasonography of the upper respiratory system has been the subject of several publications in equine medicine, particularly the normal appearance of the larynx.[3] In cattle, ultrasonography of the upper respiratory system is less frequent[4] because of the use of endoscopy; however, ultrasonography may be useful in the evaluation of masses such as abscesses in the soft tissue surrounding the larynx and trachea (**Fig. 1**).

Ultrasonography of the larynx gives valuable information complementary to the endoscopic examination, specifically for imaging the arytenoid cartilages. Abnormalities such as abscesses can be visible during the ultrasonographic examination. In **Fig. 2**, right and left arytenoid cartilages of the same animal are present. The right arytenoid cartilage appears enlarged and heterogenous, which is indicative of arytenoid abscessation. This lesion was confirmed at surgery. Such types of images may help clinicians make decisions between surgical or medical therapy.[3]

In human medicine, ultrasonography of the lungs is one of the important tools in the management of critical patients and urgent cases, not only for the detection of pleural effusion but also for the identification of pneumothorax, alveolar consolidation, and

[a] Centre Hospitalier Universitaire Vétérinaire, Faculté de Médecine Vétérinaire, Université de Montréal, Saint-Hyacinthe, Québec, J2S 7C6, Canada
[b] Département des Sciences Cliniques, Faculté de Médecine Vétérinaire, Université de Montréal, CP 5000, Saint-Hyacinthe, Québec J2S 6K9, Canada
* Corresponding author.
E-mail address: marie.babkine@umontreal.ca (M. Babkine).

Vet Clin Food Anim 25 (2009) 633–649
doi:10.1016/j.cvfa.2009.07.001
0749-0720/09/$ – see front matter © 2009 Published by Elsevier Inc.

vetfood.theclinics.com

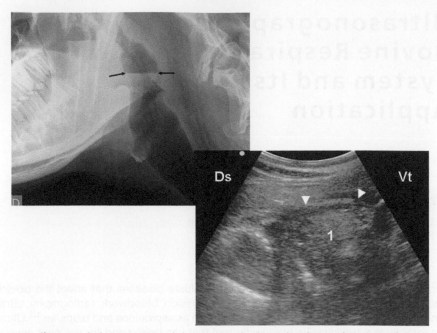

Fig. 1. Perilaryngeal abscess in an adult cow. On the lateral radiographic view of the skull, the presence of an irregularity of the soft tissue in the region of the larynx is visible, indicative of an abscess (*arrows*). An ultrasound of the region caudal to the left mandible showed the presence of a mass of medium echogenicity surrounded by a capsule (*arrowhead*). The content of the mass (1) is heterogeneous. On the dorsal side of the mass there is presence of gas. These images are compatible with an abscess. Ultrasound-guided puncture of this mass is possible. Ds, dorsal; Vt, ventral.

interstitial syndromes.[5] In cattle, ultrasonongraphy of the lungs and pleura has been the subject of several research projects and publications.[6–10] It is particularly useful for detection and characterization of pleural effusion, especially small amounts, the detection of superficial pulmonary lesions or consolidation, pulmonary atelectasia, and pneumothorax. In some cases, an ultrasonographic examination brings further precision to a radiographic examination.[11] This is particularly true regarding the cranioventral part of the thorax, because radiographs of this region are more difficult to analyze because of overlap of the soft tissue, bone, and the cardiac silhouette.

ULTRASOUND OF THE LOWER RESPIRATORY SYSTEM: TECHNIQUE AND NORMAL APPEARANCE

The ultrasound examination is performed using either a linear or sectorial probe with a frequency of 7.5 to 3.5 MHz, depending on the depth of the lesion observed using an intercostal approach (**Fig. 3**). A thoracic inlet approach similar to the one described in small animals[12] is also possible in some cases for examination of the more cranial regions of the thorax but is more restricted and more difficult (**Fig. 4**). The area between the fifth and twelfth intercostal spaces is shaved on the right and left sides in the shape of a triangle that spans the caudal edge of the thoracic limb, the transverse vertebral processes, and a line stretching from the elbow to the dorsal corner of the thirteenth rib and following the diaphragm (see **Fig. 3**). Each intercostal space

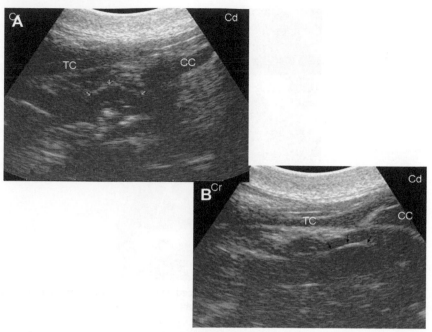

Fig. 2. Ultrasound image of the larynx of a calf that presented with upper airway obstruction. An abscess of the right arytenoid cartilage was confirmed in surgery. (*A*) Right lateral view of the larynx. The right arytenoid cartilage (*white arrows*) appears heterogenous. (*B*) left lateral view of the larynx of the same calf. The left arytenoid cartilage (*black arrows*) appears normal. CC, cricoid cartilage; Cd, caudal; Cr, cranial; TC, thyroid cartilage.

is examined after the application of acoustic gel and the probe is placed parallel to the ribs.

Normally, the visceral pleura and the lung surface form a hyperechogenic line known as the pleural line. The parietal pleura can only be differentiated from the visceral pleura during a real-time examination, during which the gliding sign, which is the

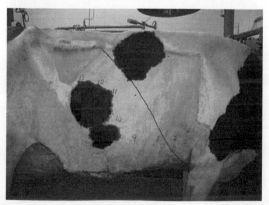

Fig. 3. Intercostal approach used during an ultrasound of the thorax. The examination area is delimited caudally by the black line, dorsally at the level of the transverse process of the thoracic vertebra, and cranially at the caudal edge of the thoracic limb.

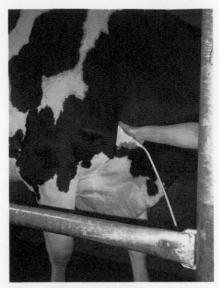

Fig. 4. Thoracic inlet approach. The probe is placed medially to the shoulder to make adequate contact with the cranial part of the thorax.

sliding movement of the lung during respiration, can be observed. Air contained in the lung tissue blocks the progression of the ultrasound waves, which causes reverberation artifacts (**Fig. 5**). As a result, normal air-filled pulmonary tissue cannot be imaged. Comet-tail artifact is a particular form of reverberation that represents a series of closely spaced, discrete echoes indicating the focal accumulation of a small amount of highly reflective material, often gas bubbles.

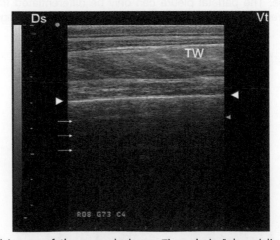

Fig. 5. Ultrasound image of the normal pleura. The echoic "pleural line" (*arrowhead*) is caused by the total reflection of the ultrasonic beam at the transition to the normally aerated lung. The reverberation artifacts (*arrows*) resulted from reflection of the ultrasound waves by air in the lung. Ds, dorsal; TW, thoracic wall; Vt, ventral.

ULTRASONOGRAPHIC APPEARANCE OF THE MOST FREQUENTLY OBSERVED THORACIC PATHOLOGIES

Lesions of the Thoracic Wall

Trauma is the most common cause of thoracic wall disease, with neoplasms being less frequent. In cattle, rib fractures are likely the most common thoracic wall lesion. Radiography is a noninvasive and nonpainful tool that may allow observation of this type of lesion, but the limited number of possible projections, overlap between various structures, and the lack of radiographic equipment in private practice can make the diagnosis difficult. A fractured rib is easily visible with ultrasound, however. A discontinuity in the alignment of the cortex of the rib bone and a change in the echogenicity of the surrounding soft tissue caused by inflammation or hemorrhage are observed (**Fig. 6**).

Pleural Lesions

Pleural effusion is defined by the accumulation of fluid between the parietal and the visceral pleura,[13] and it is caused by a pathology of the pleura itself or a condition affecting the surrounding tissues. If pleural effusion is present, the two pleura separate from one another (**Fig. 7**), and there is a liquid-like content that can range from anechoic to more or less echoic, depending on its particular or cellular content. The effusion is usually located in the ventral part of the thorax but can be located around a pulmonary lesion. In this case the accumulation is mild with a separation of the two pleura over a few millimeters (**Fig. 8**). Generally, a transudate, such as that observed in the case of cardiac insufficiency (see **Fig. 7**) is anechoic. In the case of an exudate, the content is more echoic with the presence of cellular material or strands of fibrin (**Figs. 9** and **10**). The exact nature of an exudate can only be determined by analysis of the liquid, however.

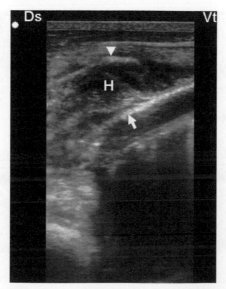

Fig. 6. Rib fracture in a 3-day-old calf. Ultrasound image of the fifth rib. A discontinuity in cortex alignment is observed. The proximal fragment (*arrowhead*) is separated from the distal fragment (*arrow*) by a heterogeneous tissue of medium echogenicity compatible with a hematoma (H).

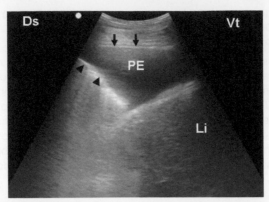

Fig. 7. Pleural effusion (PE). The parietal pleura (*black arrow*) and the visceral pleura (*black arrowheads*) are separated by the presence of an anechoic liquid. Ds, dorsal; Li, liver; Vt, ventral.

Compared with radiography, ultrasonography allows pleural effusion to be visualized in a much more definitive manner and qualifies the nature and the extent of the effusion.[11] In practice, ultrasonography is mostly used for diagnostic purposes in the case of pleural effusion. The images are often characteristic, and ultrasound-guided aspiration provides a safe way to obtain liquid for analysis. Another use for such technology is the identification of the area to be drained so as to provide relief to the patient. It is also an objective tool for monitoring patients secondary to therapy.

Irregular or thickened pleura
The pleura can have an irregular or fragmented appearance (**Fig. 11**) and be thickened. These images become objective when pathologic regions are compared with the

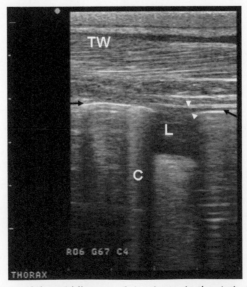

Fig. 8. Ultrasound image of the middle part of the thorax in the sixth right intercostal space of a cow with bronchopneumonia. Mild pleural effusion is observed (*between arrowheads*) associated with a focal pulmonary lesion (L). The visceral pleura (*black arrow*) is interrupted at the site of the pulmonary lesion. C, comet-tail artifact; TW, thoracic wall.

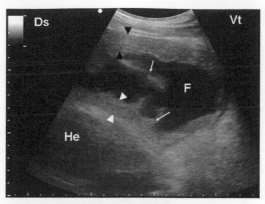

Fig. 9. Ultrasound image of the ventral part of the left thorax at the fifth intercostal space of a cow with cranioventral peritonitis and fibrinous pleuresia. The heart (He) is visible; the pericardium is also covered by a thick layer of fibrin (*white arrowhead*). Strands of fibrin (*white arrow*) are floating in an anechogenic liquid (F). A thick layer of fibrin (*black arrowhead*) is also covering the parietal pleura. Ds, dorsal; Vt, ventral.

corresponding areas on the opposite side, which is presumed to be healthy. It is possible to determine which of the two pleura is affected by observing their movement, because it is always the visceral pleura that moves.

Pneumothorax
A pneumothorax is the result of an accumulation of free air between the visceral and parietal pleura. Normally, breathing allows the operator to observe the sliding movement of one pleura along the other. The two pleura are not distinguishable during an ultrasound examination other than by their movement. When a pneumothorax is present, air infiltrates between the two pleura and the sliding movement is no longer visible. The obtained image is just immobile artifacts of reverberation (**Fig. 12**). An

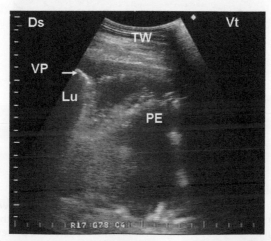

Fig. 10. Ultrasound image of the ventral part of the thorax in the sixth left intercostal space of a cow with septic pleuresia. The visceral pleura (VP) is separated from the parietal pleura. The lung (lu) is displaced dorsally by an important amount of pleural effusion (PE) that is anechoic with dispersed echoic material. Ds, dorsal; TW, thoracic wall; Vt, ventral.

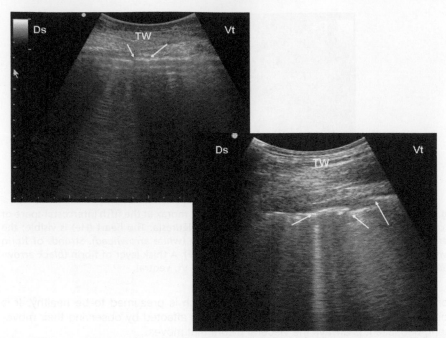

Fig. 11. Ultrasound image of an irregular, fragmented pleura (*white arrow*). Ds, dorsal; TW, thoracic wall; Vt, ventral.

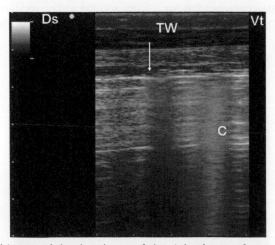

Fig. 12. Ultrasound image of the dorsal part of the right thorax of a cow with a pneumothorax. In movement, in the dorsal part of the thorax, to the left of the separating line (*white arrow*), the gliding sign is no longer visible. This indicates the presence of a pneumothorax. In the more ventral portion of the thorax (*to the right of the demarcation line*), the gliding sign is present, indicating the movement of the pleura against one another. In this region, the presence of comet tails, which begin at the visceral pleura, is also noted (C). Ds, dorsal; TW, thoracic wall; Vt, ventral.

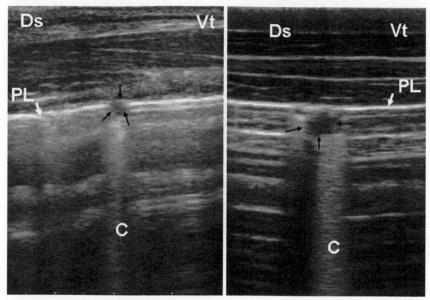

Fig. 13. Ultrasound image of the thorax of a cow with bronchopneumonia. The small circular hypoechogenic area (*surrounded by black arrows*) at the lung surface (0.5 cm in diameter on the left, 1 cm in diameter on the right) represents a superficial fluid alveologram with a comet-tail artifact (C). C, comet-tail artifact; Ds, dorsal; PL, pleural line; Vt, ventral.

ultrasonographic examination of the thorax allows assessment of the extent of the pneumothorax and facilitates the installation of a thoracic drain as a way of providing relief to the patient.

Pulmonary Lesions

Only pulmonary lesions next to the visceral pleura are visible using ultrasonography.

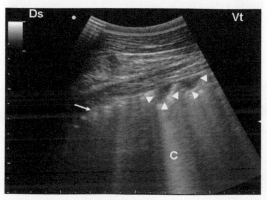

Fig. 14. Ultrasound image of the middle part of the thorax in the eighth intercostal space of a cow with pulmonary metastases of a hemangiosarcoma in the muscles of the left thigh. The presence of several more or less circular hypoechoic zones is scattered throughout the superficial part of the lungs. On this figure, two lesions are visible (*surrounded by white arrowheads*), with the presence of comet-tail artifacts (C). The pleural line (*white arrow*) is also irregular. C, comet-tail artifact; Ds, dorsal; Vt, ventral.

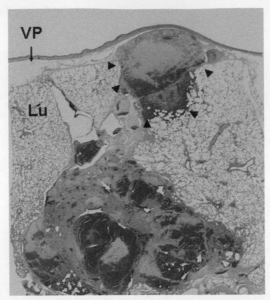

Fig. 15. Histology slide of pulmonary metastases. Under the visceral pleura (VP), the presence of metastases is noted (*surrounded by black arrowheads*). Normal lung tissue is also visible (Lu). Upon ultrasonographic examination, this circular area appears hypoechoic, as presented in **Fig. 13**. The tissues surrounding this zone are not visible because they are filled with air.

Masses or nodules

Small pulmonary nodules that measure approximately 1 cm in diameter are sometimes encountered in the case of bronchopneumonia in cattle.[9] These lesions correspond to alveoli that are filled with either liquid or a more cellular material or consolidated pulmonary lobules. They are known as alveolograms and are characterized by circular lesions of various sizes that are either hypoechoic or anechoic

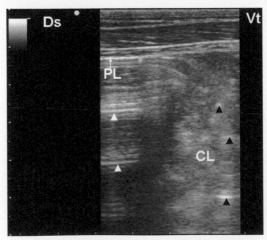

Fig. 16. Ultrasound image of the cranioventral region of the thorax of a calf with pneumonia. Dorsally, the pleural line (PL) is visible with reverberation artifacts (*white arrowhead*). This normal area is distinctly different from the ventral portion of the lung that contains hypoechoic tissues with small hyperechoic spots. This part of the lung is visible and consolidated (CL). The hyperechoic spots are bronchoaerograms (*black arrowhead*). Ds, dorsal; Vt, ventral.

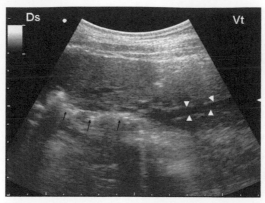

Fig. 17. Ultrasound image of the ventral thorax in the sixth right intercostal space of a cow with bronchopneumonia. The pulmonary tissue appears hypoechoic and contains ramified fluid bronchograms (*surrounded by white arrowheads*). The hyperechoic zones around the bronchi correspond to inclusions of air (*black arrow*). Ds, dorsal; Vt, ventral.

(**Fig. 13**). These small nodules might be small abscesses, inflamed or necrotic areas, or metastases (**Figs. 14** and **15**). They can be aspirated using ultrasonography as a guide for diagnostic purposes.

In cattle, the masses or cavitary lesions that are observed in pulmonary tissue are most commonly abscesses,[14] although neoplasms and hematomas are possible.[15,16] An abscess is characterized by a well-defined circular region with a content of variable echogenicity. It is possible to observe these abscesses only if they are located against the visceral pleura. An ultrasound-guided aspiration allows analysis of the contents for diagnostic purpose. Transthoracic drainage using a trochar is only possible if the two pleura are affected by adherences, which is demonstrated by the absence of movement between the two pleura, or "gliding sign."

Pulmonary consolidation
When pulmonary consolidation is present, the lung tissue appears hypoechoic and its echo texture may look like liver parenchyma. It is possible to observe

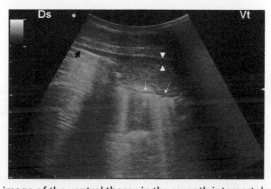

Fig. 18. Ultrasound image of the ventral thorax in the seventh intercostal space of a cow with a fibrinous pleuresia and cranioventral peritonitis. On the left side, a normal pleural line (*black arrow*) is observed with reverberation artifacts. Ventrally (*on the right side of the image*), the lung is consolidated and separated from the costal wall by a small amount of pleural effusion (*white arrowhead*). In the consolidated lung tissue a ramified fluid bronchogram is visible (*white arrows*). Ds, dorsal; Vt, ventral.

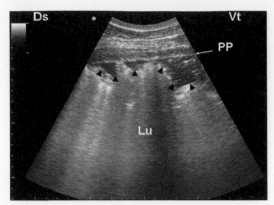

Fig. 19. Ultrasound image of the middle part of the thorax in the sixth intercostal space of a bull with aspiration pneumonia. Several hypoechoic areas of variable size and shape are visible in the superficial part of the lung (*black arrowhead*). Under these consolidated areas of the lung hyperechogenic regions are visible that correspond to inclusions of air. Ds, dorsal; Lu, lung; PP, parietal pleura; Vt, ventral.

bronchoaerograms in this region. They are small bronchi that are filled with air, which makes them appear hyperechoic. They appear as multiple lentil-sized air inlets that measure a few millimeters in diameter (**Fig. 16**) with distal comet-tail artifacts. Another type of structure that can be observed with pulmonary consolidation is a fluid bronchogram (**Figs. 17** and **18**), which appears as an anechoic tubular structure with

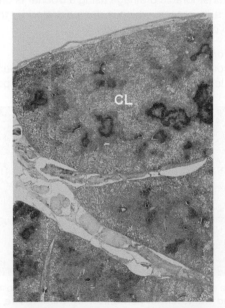

Fig. 20. Histology slide of pulmonary necrosis observed in a case of aspiration pneumonia. This superficial section of necrotic lung corresponds to a fraction of the lesion seen in **Fig. 18**. There is complete absence of normal lung tissue, and no air inclusion is possible. CL, consolidated lung.

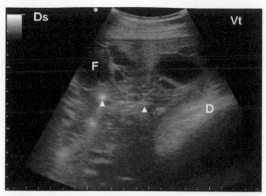

Fig. 21. Ultrasound image of the ventral thorax in the sixth intercostal space of a cow with fibrinous pleuresia and cranioventral peritonitis. The ventral part of the pulmonary lobe is hypoechoic and contains two large anechoic regions (F) and small inclusions of air (*white arrowheads*). This part of the pulmonary lobe is consolidated and seems to be becoming necrotic. D, diaphragm;Ds, dorsal; Vt, ventral.

a hyperechoic wall. Using Doppler ultrasonography, it is distinguishable from a blood vessel because it shows lack of blood flow.

Pulmonary consolidation can be localized, as in the case of aspiration pneumonia (**Figs. 19** and **20**) or it may affect the whole ventral part of a pulmonary lobe (**Figs. 21–23**). The extent of the pneumonia can be evaluated by visualizing either small, localized lesions or lesions that involve the entire part of a pulmonary lobe. It is important to remember, however, that it is not possible to evaluate the deeper parts of the lung if the superficial part is normal because of the presence of air between the probe and the lesion.

It is not uncommon in cattle to observe the presence of pleural effusion associated with pulmonary consolidation that would not be visible or distinguishable on thoracic radiographs (**Fig. 24**). The presence of liquid allows the operator to see the triangular shape of the consolidated extremity of the lung (**Fig. 25**). The diaphragm is also

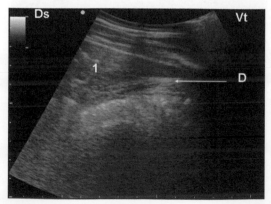

Fig. 22. Ultrasound image of the ventral part of the thorax in the left seventh intercostal space of a cow with aspiration pneumonia. The ventral edge of a consolidated lung lobe (1) appears hypoechoic against the diaphragm (D). Ds, dorsal; Vt, ventral.

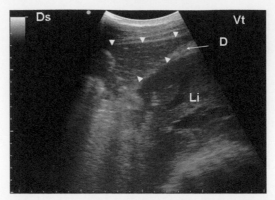

Fig. 23. Ultrasound image of the ventral part of the thorax in the right eighth intercostal space of a cow with aspiration pneumonia. The ventral edge of a consolidated lung lobe (*arrowheads*) appears hypoechoic against the diaphragm (D). Ds, dorsal; Li, liver; Vt, ventral.

sometimes visible. This type of lesion is observed in the case of pleuropneumonia. An ultrasound-guided liquid aspiration can assist in the diagnosis and treatment of the condition.

Atelectasis
Atelectasis of a pulmonary lobe occurs after increased pressure in the pleural cavity caused by pulmonary effusion, a pneumothorax, or the inability to adequately inflate the lung (eg, bronchial obstruction or severe aspiration of amniotic fluid in newborns). In the presence of a pneumothorax, pulmonary atelectasia cannot be diagnosed by ultrasonography because of the presence of air between the two pleura. In the presence of pleural effusion, however, the pulmonary lobe affected by atelectasis is imaged and appears smaller (**Fig. 26**), triangular and well defined, and mildly hyperechoic.[10,12]

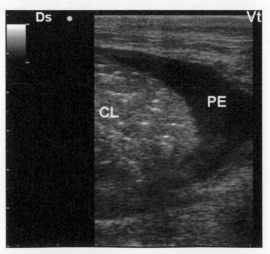

Fig. 24. Ultrasound image of the ventral thorax in the fifth intercostal space of a calf with septicemia. The ventral part of the lung is consolidated (CL) and is floating in an anechogenic pleural effusion (PE). Ds, dorsal; Vt, ventral.

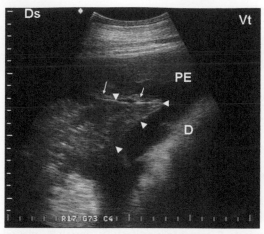

Fig. 25. Ultrasound image of the ventral thorax of a cow with pleuropneumonia. The ventral edge of the pulmonary lobe appears hypoechoic (*white arrowheads*) and is floating in an anechoic pleural effusion (PE). On its parietal surface, a fine layer of more echoic material compatible with fibrin is visible (*white arrows*). Filaments of fibrin are also visible against the diaphragm (D). This part of the lobe is consolidated. Ds, dorsal; Vt, ventral.

The presence of comet-tail artifacts and an interstitial syndrome

As explained elsewhere in this issue, comet tails are artifacts. In human medicine, however, the presence of numerous comet-tail artifacts on a single image can indicate an interstitial syndrome.[17] Diffuse parenchymal lung disease must be considered if multiple comet-tail artifacts are distributed over the entire lung surface and are associated with thickened and irregular pleura.[18] In cattle, Flöck[9] also reported the presence of comet-tail artifacts in the presence of pulmonary emphysema (**Fig. 27**).

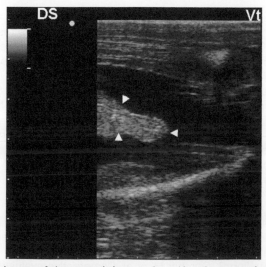

Fig. 26. Ultrasound image of the ventral thorax of a calf with severe pleuropneumonia and atelectasis of a part of the cranial pulmonary lobe. The part of the pulmonary lobe affected (*white arrowheads*) is small and floating in an anechoic pleural effusion. The atelectasia is secondary to the increase in pressure in the pleural space. Ds, dorsal; Vt, ventral.

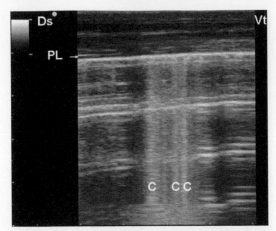

Fig. 27. Comet-tail artifacts. C, comet-tails artifact; Ds, dorsal; PL, pleural line; Vt, ventral.

SUMMARY

Ultrasonographic examination of the pleura and the lung helps detect various lesions. It brings accuracy and complements radiography. Some ultrasound images are characteristic of pathologic processes and can help clinicians with their diagnosis by allowing visualization of the lesion itself or serving as a guide for aspiration. This examination allows evaluation of the extent and severity of pulmonary changes when they are against the pleura. Lesions that are located deeper in the lung tissue are not visible. In current veterinary farm practice, however, in which radiographic examination is impossible, ultrasonography is a diagnostic tool that is available, quickly performed, and noninvasive.

REFERENCES

1. Radostits OM, Gay CC, Hinchcliff KW, et al. Diseases of the respiratory system. In: Radostitis OM, Gay CC, Hinchcliff KW, et al, editors. Veterinary medicine: a textbook of the diseases of cattle, horses, sheep, pigs and goats. 10th edition. Philadelphia: WB Saunders; 2007. p. 471–542.
2. Wilson WD, Lofstedt J. Alterations in respiratory function. In: Smith BP, editor. Large animal internal medicine. 4th edition. St Louis (MO): Mosby; 2008. p. 42–82.
3. Chalmers HJ, Cheetham J, Yeager AE, et al. Ultrasonography of the equine larynx. Vet Radiol Ultrasound 2006;47(5):476–81.
4. Braun U, Föhn J, Pusterla N. Ultrasonographic examination of the ventral neck region in cows. Am J Vet Res 1994;55(1):14–21.
5. Reissig A, Kroegel C. Ultrasound of the lung and pleura. In: Gibson GJ, Geddes DM, Coastabel U, et al, editors. Respiratory medicine. 3rd edition. London: Elsevier Science; 2002. p. 370–7.
6. Braun U, Sicher D, Pusterla N. Ultrasonography of the lungs, pleura, and mediastinum in healthy cows. Am J Vet Res 1996;57(4):432–8.
7. Reinhold P, Rabeling B, Günther H, et al. Comparative evaluation of ultrasonography and lung function testing with the clinical signs and pathology of calves inoculated experimentally with *Pasteurella multocida*. Vet Rec 2002;150(4): 109–14.

8. Rabeling B, Rehage J, Döpfer D, et al. Ultrasonographic findings in calves with respiratory disease. Vet Rec 1998;143(17):468–71.
9. Flöck M. Diagnostic ultrasonography in cattle with thoracic disease. Vet J 2004; 167(3):272–80.
10. Jung C, Bostedt H. Thoracic ultrasonography technique in newborn calves and description of normal and pathological findings. Vet Radiol Ultrasound 2004; 45(4):331–5.
11. Reef VB, Boy MG, Reid CF, et al. Comparison between diagnostic ultrasonography and radiography in the evaluation of horses and cattle with thoracic disease: 56 cases (1984–1985). J Am Vet Med Assoc 1991;198(12):2112–8.
12. Hecht S. Thorax. In: Penninck D, d'Anjou MA, editors. Atlas of small animal ultrasonography. Ames (IA): Blackwell; 2008. p. 119–50.
13. Braun U, Pusterla N, Flückiger M. Ultrasonographic findings in cattle with pleuropneumonia. Vet Rec 1997;141(1):12–7.
14. Mohamed T, Oikawa S. Ultrasonographic caracteristics of abdominal and thoracic abscesses in cattle and buffaloes. J Vet Med A Physiol Pathol Clin Med 2007;54(9):512–7.
15. Braun U, Jehle W, Bart M. Ultrasonographic findings in a beef cow with pulmonary haematoma. Vet Rec 2004;155(3):92–3.
16. Backer JC, Smith JA. Miscellaneous conditions. In: Smith BP, editor. Large animal internal medicine. 4th edition. St Louis (MO): Mosby; 2008. p. 666.
17. Lichtenstein DA, Mezière GA. Relevance of lung ultrasound in the diagnosis of acute respiratory failure: the BLUE protocol. Chest 2008;134(1):117–25.
18. Reißig A, Kroegel C. Transthoracic sonography of diffuse parenchymal lung disease. J Ultrasound Med 2003;22(2):173–80.

Ultrasonography of Bovine Urinary Tract Disorders

Martina Floeck, DVM

KEYWORDS

- Cattle • Sonography • Urinary tract disorders
- Scanning technique

Diseases of the urinary system are less common in cattle than disorders of the gastrointestinal, respiratory, musculoskeletal, and other systems. For this reason and because signs of renal disease may be subtle, the urinary tract often is misdiagnosed as a cause of illness. Most practitioners use the gross appearance of urine, evaluation of abnormal urine constituents based on multiple reagent test strips, and signs found on physical examination as indicators of urinary tract disease. Vague illnesses that originate from the urinary system may require more ancillary data in the form of complete urinalysis, serum electrolytes and chemistry, and complete blood counts for diagnosis.[1]

Many diagnostic imaging techniques can be used for evaluation of the urinary tract of cattle. However, certain radiographic diagnostic procedures, such as intravenous pyelography, contrast cystography, and excretory urography, cannot be performed because of their large size. Ultrasonography, on the other hand, is applicable and valuable diagnostic information can be obtained. Sonography supplements the clinical examination and clinicopathological analysis by providing additional information on urinary tract diseases.[2]

ANATOMY

The right kidney extends from the 13th rib to the third lumbar vertebra. The cranial pole lies in the renal impression of the liver in the 12th intercostal space. Pancreas, colon, and cecum are ventral to the kidney. The left kidney lies caudal and slightly more ventrally to the right kidney and extends from the 2nd to the 5th lumbar vertebra. The dorsal ruminal sac displaces the kidney to the right side with a longitudinal 25° (or more) torsion and dorsal shift of the hilus. The kidneys are surrounded by perirenal fat. The left kidney measures 19 to 25 cm, the right kidney 18 to 24 cm. The lobulated kidney consists of the renal capsule, parenchyma, and sinus. The renal parenchyma

Department for Farm Animals and Veterinary Public Health, Clinic for Ruminants, University of Veterinary Medicine Vienna, Veterinäerplatz 1, 1210 Vienna, Austria
E-mail address: martina.floeck@vu-wien.ac.at

Vet Clin Food Anim 25 (2009) 651–667
doi:10.1016/j.cvfa.2009.07.008
0749-0720/09/$ – see front matter © 2009 Elsevier Inc. All rights reserved.

consists of the renal cortex and medulla with zona interna and zona externa. The apices of the medullary pyramids project singly or multiply as renal papillae into the sinus. There is no renal pelvis in cattle. Urine flows from the renal papillae into the renal calices. All renal calices unite to form the collecting tubules, which join to form the ureter at the hilus.[3]

The urinary bladder is located in the caudal most portion of the abdomen at the pelvic brim and has both an intrapelvic and an abdominal location. The wall of the bladder is muscular and stretches, becoming thinner when the bladder is full.[3]

SCANNING TECHNIQUE
Percutaneous Examination of the Right Kidney

Ultrasonographic examinations are performed on the standing animal. A 5.0 MHz or lower-frequency transducer is usually necessary, and selection of transducer frequency depends on the desirable depth of the field to be examined. The transducer is placed over the right paralumbar fossa and in the last intercostal space (cranial kidney pole, liver window) to examine the kidney and ureter (**Fig. 1**), after shaving and degreasing the skin with alcohol and applying coupling gel. Convex, linear array, and sector transducers can be used.[4]

Transrectal Examination of the Left Kidney and Urinary Bladder

Transrectal sonographic evaluation is performed to visualize the left kidney and the urinary bladder (urethra and ureter). A 5.0 MHz or higher-frequency linear transducer is appropriate for most examinations. All feces should first be removed from the rectum and any air in the rectum should be expelled. Transmission gel is applied to the scanner and it is placed in a plastic rectal glove before being introduced into the rectum. The scanner is placed ventral, lateral, and dorsal on the kidney. Often it is not possible to evaluate the entire left kidney, because the cranial pole cannot be reached, especially in large cattle. For examination of the urinary bladder, the scanner is placed in the area immediately cranial to the symphysis ossis pubis with its beam aimed ventrally. In the pelvic cavity the urethra can be visualized during micturition or after a catheter has been introduced, beginning at the urinary bladder and progressing caudally.[5]

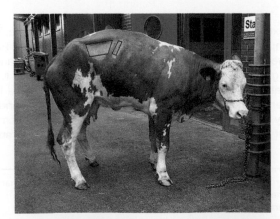

Fig. 1. Percutaneous examination of the right kidney in the right paralumbar fossa and the last intercostal space (*demarcated*). This cow suffered from sacral nerve injury due to riding activity with the clinical signs of bladder atony and tail paralysis (see **Fig. 18**).

Percutaneous Examination of the Left Kidney, Urinary Bladder, and Urethra

Occasionally, in calves and small or thin adult cattle, the left kidney can be visible from the right caudal paralumbar fossa, but it is frequently covered by gas-filled large intestine. With a transcutaneous approach, the cranial pole of the left kidney is visible, in contrast to transrectal examination. However, the image obtained from the left kidney scanned transrectally may be superior to the transcutaneous examination, because the kidney is closer to the focal zone of the transducer and a higher-frequency transducer improves the resolution of the image.

In calves the urinary bladder can also be scanned transcutaneously as described for foals by Traub-Dargatz and Wrigley[2] and Reef.[6] For transcutaneous examination of the bladder, the skin in the caudal ventral abdomen should be prepared by clipping the hair and cleaning extraneous dirt from the area. A suitable couplant gel should then be applied to the skin. A 5.0 MHz convex or linear transducer is appropriate for most examinations. In young calves a higher frequency transducer can be used for better resolution.

The urethra in bull calves is accessible in the ventral midline between scrotum and preputial orifice and can be evaluated with a high-frequency linear transducer (10.0–15.0 MHz) with transverse scans.

The urinary bladder is best examined when it is fluid-filled. It is more readily identified, and the bladder wall is better evaluated in this manner. Additionally, bladder contents are usually best seen when they are suspended in a fluid medium. Ballottement may aid visualization, and it can help to differentiate free-floating material in the lumen from tissue or objects that may be attached to the bladder wall.[2]

INDICATIONS FOR SCANNING

The kidneys should be evaluated sonographically whenever clincal signs or laboratory abnormalities suggest renal disease or dysfunction. Additional indications for ultrasonographic examination of the kidneys include the identification of palpable masses or abnormalities in the region of the kidneys on rectal palpation. Ultrasonography can be useful to differentiate acute from chronic renal disease and to differentiate focal from diffuse renal involvement. It is helpful in identifying sites for biopsy or aspiration of renal tissue, and it can also be used to monitor the progression of renal disease in an individual animal, and prognostic information may be gained.[2]

The most obvious indication for sonographic evaluation of the urinary bladder is the presence of clinical signs of cystitis or production of abnormal urine. Other indications include suspicion of cystic calculi or tumors or masses associated with the bladder wall. Bladder atony may be assessed from the standpoint that failure to void urine usually results in excessive sludging of urine contents. Additionally, the integrity of the bladder wall may need to be evaluated subsequent to an anamnesis of trauma or obstructive urolithiasis.[2]

Imaging of the ureters is indicated when obstruction or enlargement of the ureters are suspected based on rectal palpation.[2]

LIMITATIONS

Some limitations are encountered when scanning the kidneys. Because of the anatomic location of the right kidney, only a lateral approach is possible when scanning transcutaneously. It is difficult to obtain accurate measurements of the dimensions of the kidney, because the entire organ is not visible in a single view. Fat causes the attenuation of the sound and makes imaging tissues difficult in an obese animal. Perirenal fat especially impairs an ultrasonographic examination. In dehydrated animals, dry skin impairs sound transmission. Finally, lower-frequency transducers are required to image the kidneys, and the limitations of the resolving power of these transducers may preclude detection of small changes in architecture and texture. The resolution of a 5.0 MHz convex transducer is usually not sufficient to depict small tissue irregularities of the renal parenchyma, which can be detected at necropsy.[2,7]

ULTRASONOGRAPHIC FINDINGS
Normal Structures

The lobulation of the bovine kidney is obvious ultrasonographically. The renal capsule is not distinctly imaged as a discrete structure. The renal cortex is hypoechoic compared with the surrounding tissues (eg, liver) and is composed of fine homogeneous echoes (with a slightly mottled appearance). The medullary pyramids are less echogenic than the renal cortex (Figs. 2–4). The cortex and the medullary pyramids cannot always be differentiated, depending on the amount of subcutaneous fat and the ultrasound equipment. The medullary pyramids should not be confused with cysts that look similar. The echogenic arcuate arteries are located at the border of the renal cortex and renal medulla, and can be seen with high frequencies only (see Fig. 4). The renal sinus is normally echogenic owing to the presence of fat and fibrous tissue (see Figs. 2 and 3). The renal hilus can be imaged when the transducer is placed in the paralumbar fossa and rotated about its longitudinal axis; however, it is not possible to differentiate between the ureter, renal artery, and renal vein with B-mode. The thickness of the renal cortex and medulla varies between 1.5 and 2.5 cm (left and right kidney). The vertical diameter of the left kidney varies from 4.5 to 7.5 cm and of the right kidney from 4.0 to 7.0 cm. The circumference of the largest medullary pyramid varies from 4.1 to 5.8 cm (left) and 3.6 to 5.9 cm (right). The distance between body surface and right kidney, measured in the paralumbar fossa, varies from 1.2 to 2.9 cm. These measurements have been performed on 11 respectively 12 nonpregnant Swiss Braunvieh cows, between 3 and 4 years old, weighing between 390 and 544 kg.[4,5]

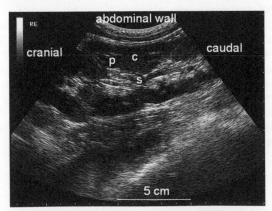

Fig. 2. Longitudinal sonogram of the right kidney of a 7-year-old Simmental cow obtained from the right paralumbar fossa (5.0 MHz). The hyperechoic renal sinus (s) is centrally located and surrounded by the renal parenchyma consisting of the hypoechoic medullary pyramids (p) and the slightly more echogenic renal cortex (c).

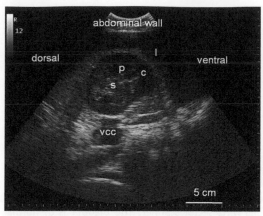

Fig. 3. Transversal sonogram of the right kidney of a 5-year-old Simmental cow (715 kg) obtained from the right dorsal, last intercostal space (3.5 MHz). The kidney lies in the renal impression of the liver; c, renal cortex; l, liver; p, medullary pyramid; s, renal sinus; vcc, caudal vena cava.

The urinary bladder appears as a circumscribed round-to-oval structure in the pelvic area. It usually contains anechoic to hypoechoic urine. The wall of the urinary bladder is echogenic, smooth, and its thickness varies with the amount of bladder distention (**Figs. 5** and **6**). The mucosa and muscular wall of the urinary bladder are separable sonographically only with a high-frequency transducer. In transcutaneous scans, the urinary bladder is usually obscured from view by gas in the interposed large bowel.[5,6]

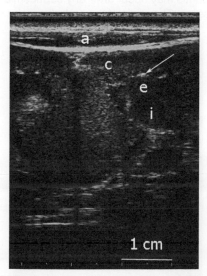

Fig. 4. Transcutaneous longitudinal sonogram of two renal lobes of the right kidney of a 4-month-old male Simmental calf obtained from the right paralumbar fossa (15 MHz): The renal cortex (c) and the medullary pyramid, consisting of zona interna (i) and zona externa (e), are visible. The echogenic arcuate arteries are located at the border of the renal cortex and renal medulla (*arrow*). The abdominal wall (a) is at the top of the sonogram. Cranial is to the left, caudal is to the right.

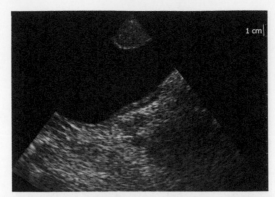

Fig. 5. Sonogram of the urinary bladder of a 1.5-year-old Simmental heifer obtained transrectally with a 3.5 MHz sector scanner: The bladder is of normal size and position, the urine within the urinary bladder is anechoic. Dorsal is at the top, cranial is to the left, caudal is to the right.

In the ventral midline between scrotum and preputial orifice the urethra is a small echogenic round structure within the echogenic penile and preputial tissue. During micturition the anechoic urethral lumen is visible with smooth walls, which collapse after micturition (**Fig. 7**A, B).

Normal ureters generally cannot be imaged ultrasonographically.[2,5,6]

SONOGRAPHIC ABNORMALITIES
Embolic Nephritis

Embolic suppurative nephritis may occur after any septicemia and bacteremia, when bacteria lodge in renal tissues. The origin of the emboli may be valvular endocarditis or

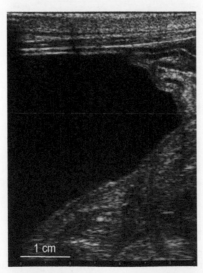

Fig. 6. Transcutaneous sonogram of the urinary bladder of a 17-day-old female Simmental calf obtained with a 10.0 MHz linear scanner: The urine within the urinary bladder is anechoic and the bladder wall is smooth. Ventral is at the top. The right side of the sonogram is the left side of the urinary bladder.

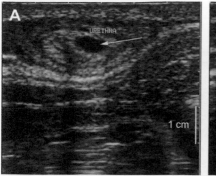 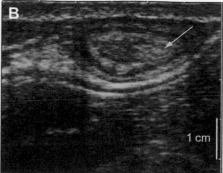

Fig. 7. (A) Transverse sonogram of the normal urethra of a 6-week-old Simmental calf during micturition obtained from the ventral midline between scrotum and preputial orifice (10 MHz). The urethral lumen is distended by anechoic urine (*arrow*). (B) After micturition, the walls of the urethra collapse and the lumen is no longer visible (*arrow*). Ventral is at the top. The right side of the sonogram is the left side of the abdomen.

suppurative lesions in joints, uterus, udder, and navel. Renal infarction can develop secondary to septic embolism.[8] Fever, other signs of septicemia, and specific organ dysfunction (mastitis, joint infections) also may be present. Urine multiple reagent test strips may be positive for blood and protein. Nephritis is seldom the most significant component of disease in these animals but is another sign of septicemia.[1]

With transcutaneous sonography, embolic nephritis is difficult to diagnose owing to the small size of the lesions. Transrectal sonography with a high-frequency transducer may reveal hypoechoic septic infarcts in the renal cortex as a sequel to embolism (**Fig. 8**A, B).

Interstitial Nephritis

In interstitial nephritis, inflammation primarily occurs in the renal stroma, but it can also develop secondarily to glomerular, tubular, or capillary damage. It is a common incidental finding at necropsy but does not present as a clinical urinary tract disease. In pigs, diffuse interstitial nephritis is observed following infection by *Leptospira* spp. In cattle, the kidney is an important reservoir for *Leptospira* spp, but renal disease is not a common clinical problem in carrier animals. Focal interstitial nephritis can also be found in bovine malignant catarrhal fever and bovine virus diarrhea (BVD).[8,9]

Interstitial nephritis may cause increased echogenicity.[6] Concurrent anomalies like septic infarcts, calculi, and changes in kidney size may be visible if the kidneys are examined sonographically (**Fig. 9**A, B).

Pyelonephritis

The inflammation of renal sinus, calices, and interstitial tissue is the most commonly diagnosed disease of the kidney in dairy cattle. It usually develops secondary to ascending urinary tract infection, almost exclusively in females because of their shorter urethra that facilitates passage of bacteria to the bladder.[8,9] In male cattle, pyelonephritis can be a sequel to urolithiasis.[8] Acute primary pyelonephritis causes fever, anorexia, and a precipitous drop in milk production. Some cows with acute pyelonephritis have colic manifested by kicking at the abdomen, restlessness, and treading. Signs of colic usually are associated with renal or ureteral inflammation and pain, but urinary obstruction caused by blood clots blocking urine outflow from

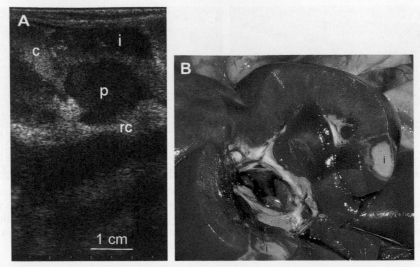

Fig. 8. (*A*) A 14-month-old Simmental heifer (275 kg) presented with a history of anorexia, lethargy, and lameness. A complete blood count of the thin and icteric animal revealed anemia and leukocytosis. Bacteriologic examination of the urine revealed *Streptococcus C* and *E coli*. Transrectal ultrasonography of the left kidney showed oval hypoechoic tissue (i) in the area of the cortex (c), hyperechoic renal sinus and calices (rc), enlargement of the kidney, and dilatation of the ureter (10 MHz). The medullary pyramid (p) is clearly visible. The abdominal wall is at the top of the sonogram. Cranial is to the left, caudal is to the right. A similar, although more severe, change was present in the right kidney. (*B*) Necropsy revealed multiple septic infarcts (i) in both kidneys, septic polyarthritis, and endocarditis of the mitral valve.

a kidney (ureter) or bladder (urethra) also may contribute to colic. Stranguria, polyuria, an arched stance, and gross hematuria, blood clots, fibrin or pyuria also are observed in some patients. Chronic pyelonephritis is associated with weight loss, poor hair coat, anorexia, poor production, diarrhea, polyuria, anemia, and less obvious gross urinary abnormalities. Lordosis and stretching out may be apparent in some cows affected with chronic pyelonephritis because of renal pain. Specific physical signs of pyelonephritis can be minimal unless, upon rectal palpation, the left kidney is large, painful, and has indistinct lobulations – thereby raising the possibility of pyelonephritis.[1]

Gross examination of the urine may be diagnostic in acute cases where fibrin, blood clots, and pus are apparent in voided urine. Urine is alkaline, with sediment containing numerous erythrocytes, leukocytes, and bacteria.[7,10–12] Cattle suffering from pyelonephritis can have a normal blood count[7,12] or a leukocytosis with neutrophilia and mild-to-moderate anemia.[11] Azotemia is not commonly present, even in patients with bilateral pyelonephritis.[7,12] Blood concentrations of blood urea nitrogen and creatinine do not rise appreciably above the normal range until 60%–75% of nephrons are destroyed. Their blood levels can vary with the rate of protein catabolism and are not only dependent on renal function. In cattle, blood urea levels caused by prerenal lesions may be higher than the levels resulting from renal disease, because rumen metabolism may lower plasma urea in chronic disease. Azotemia can be observed at the final stage of the disease.[9] Most cattle with pyelonephritis that also are azotemic have bilateral disease and renal failure. Therefore cattle with bilateral pyelonephritis and azotemia have a guarded prognosis.[1]

Pyelonephritis in cattle has been commonly associated with *Corynebacterium renale* and *Escherichia coli*.[7-12] Conditions that provide physical or chemical damage to mucosa in the lower portion of the urinary tract, such as dystocia, bladder paralysis, or catheterization may predispose the cow to pyelonephritis as a result of ascending infection from the urinary bladder to the ureters and kidneys.[1]

The sonographic finding that is most suggestive of pyelonephritis is the detection of a large amount of echogenic-to-hyperechoic, sometimes fluctuating, debris in the renal sinus and calices. The hyperechoic debris can cast acoustic shadows, associated with the formation of concretions. Gross renal enlargement is commonly present. The renal sinus and renal calices are dilated, and the normal renal architecture is often lost. The dilated renal calices have a cystic appearance.[7,11,12] Uroepithelial thickening, as described in humans with pyelonephritis, can also be seen.[8] Ureteral dilatation with echogenic content can be detected in cattle with pyelonephritis (**Fig. 10**A–C). The urine within the urinary bladder is echogenic and layering of the urine occurs with pyuria because the cellular debris settles to the more ventral aspects of the urinary bladder.[7,11,12]

Nephrosis

Damage to the renal tubules by toxins (heavy metals, plant toxicities such as oxalates, oak, and pigweed), certain drugs (antibiotics), and physiologic events linked to hemoconcentration, endotoxemia, and ischemic changes may cause tubular degeneration, inflammation and, in some instances, interstitial nephritis. Usually, both kidneys are affected equally. Cattle affected with nephrosis usually have nonspecific signs, including depression, anorexia, and dehydration. The cattle usually have more obvious lesions in other body systems, such as septic mastitis, septic metritis, or abomasal disorders. Polyuria may be present in some calves and cattle with nephrosis. Rectal palpation may suggest enlargment of the left kidney. Azotemia is present and RBCs, WBCs, granular casts, and proteinuria usually are confirmed by urinalysis in acute nephrosis. Renal biopsy is the most definitive means of diagnosis

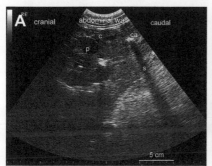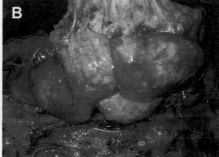

Fig. 9. (*A*) A 2-year-old Limousin feeder steer (588 kg) presented with a history of anorexia, pneumonia, and suspicion for traumatic reticuloperitonitis. Sonography of the right kidney in the paralumbar fossa showed several hyperechoic round-to-oval structures casting strong acoustic shadows in an otherwise normal kidney (3.5 MHz). Blood urea nitrogen and creatinine were within reference ranges. (*B*) Necropsy revealed severe chronic interstitial nephritis, multiple septic infarcts, numerous calculi within the collecting system, and jejunal volvulus. The obvious renal parenchymal changes observed during necropsy could not be depicted with a 3.5 MHz transducer. c, renal cortex; ca, calculus; p, medullary pyramid; s, acoustic shadow.

and can be accomplished through a right flank approach with guidance via rectal palpation or ultrasound.[1]

In acute renal failure, sonographic examination may reveal renal enlargement, with the renal parenchyma appearing less or more echogenic than normal, due to edema or leucocyte infiltration. Occasionally, perirenal edema is detected. Amyloidosis and drug toxicosis may lead to renal enlargement and increased parenchymal echogenicity. Chronic renal disease is characterized by increased parenchymal echogenicity and smaller than normal kidneys with an irregular contour. The increase in parenchymal echogenicity is consistent with chronic inflammation and fibrosis. Renal calculi are frequently imaged in both kidneys in horses with chronic renal disease. The assessment of kidney echogenicity is subjective and hence should be performed only in direct comparison with liver parenchyma.[6,13]

Glomerulonephritis

Glomerulonephritis occurs in association with many primary diseases of animals such as BVD or lead poisoning in cattle. Immunopathological processes play an important role in the pathogenesis. Acute glomerulonephritis is characterized by renal enlargement and distinct hypoechoic medullary pyramids, chronic disease by decreased kidney size. In both, cortical echogenicity is increased (see **Fig. 10**A–C; **11**A, B).[6,8,13]

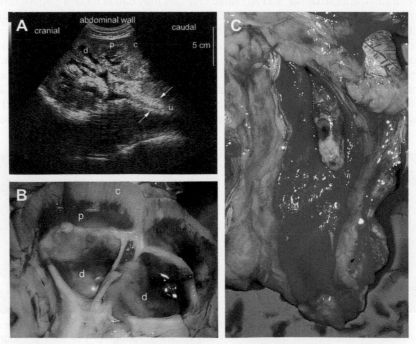

Fig.10. (A) A 6-year-old Braunvieh cow (510 kg) presented with a history of dehydration and bloody urine. Sonography of the right kidney in the paralumbar fossa (5.0 MHz) showed dilated renal calices and ureter (*arrows*), filled with anechoic fluid and echogenic purulent debris. The abdominal wall is at the top of the sonogram. (B) Necropsy revealed severe purulent pyelonephritis, interstitial nephritis, glomerulonephritis, and cystitis. (C) Lumen of the dilated and inflamed ureter, filled with pus. c, renal cortex; d, dilated calices; p, medullary pyramid; u, ureter.

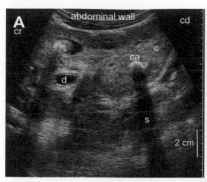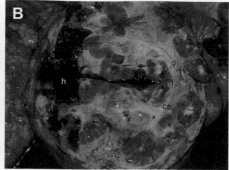

Fig. 11. (*A*) A 6-month-old male Simmental calf presented with a history of distended ventral abdomen and colic. Sonography of the right kidney in the paralumbar fossa (5.0 MHz) showed echogenic renal parenchyma, dilated calices (d) and sinus, filled with echogenic calculi (ca) casting acoustic shadows (s). (*B*) Necropsy revealed urolithiasis with rupture of the urethra and interstitial nephritis and glomerulonephritis. c, renal cortex; cd, caudal; cr, cranial; d, dilated calices ; h, hematoma.

Renal Cysts

Renal cysts are identified readily with ultrasonography and are often incidental findings of no clinical significance in otherwise normal kidneys. They are round to oval anechoic areas with a distinct thin and smooth margin within the renal parenchyma (**Fig. 12**). The cysts are usually solitary and unilateral. Differential diagnoses are abscesses, hematomas, or tumors, which are normally more echogenic and may be thick-walled.[6,9]

Urolithiasis

Urolithiasis is common as a subclinical disorder among ruminants raised in management systems where the rations are composed primarily of grain or where animals graze certain types of pasture. Contributing factors are improper calcium–phosphorus balance, vitamin A deficiency, hypervitaminosis D, reduced water intake, and early castration of male animals. In these situations, 40% to 60% of animals may form calculi in their urinary tract.[9] Urolithiasis becomes an important clinical disease of castrated male ruminants when calculi cause urinary tract obstruction, usually caused by urethral obstruction. Calculi in the renal pelvis or ureters are not usually diagnosed antemortem, although obstruction of a ureter may be detectable on rectal examination, especially if it is accompanied by hydronephrosis. Calculi in the bladder may cause cystitis and are manifested by signs of that disease. Urethral obstruction is characterized clinically by retention of urine, kicking at the belly, tail swishing, frequent unsuccessful attempts to urinate and distention of the bladder. Cattle with incomplete obstruction will pass small amounts of blood-stained urine frequently. A heavy precipitate of crystals is often visible on the preputial hairs. Urethral perforation and rupture of the bladder can be sequelae. Azotemia is usually present in patients with urinary tract obstruction. Mortality is high and treatment is surgical.[9]

The calculi can be found in multiple locations, therefore, a complete sonographic examination of the entire urinary tract is indicated in urolithiasis patients. The kidneys should be examined for evidence of nephrolithiasis or hydronephrosis (see **Fig. 11**A, B; **Fig. 13**), the presence of either justifying a poorer prognosis. The hyperechoic half-moon–shaped or round calculi cast acoustic shadows through the deeper

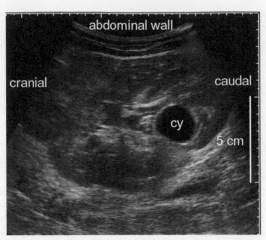

Fig. 12. Transcutaneous sonogram of the right kidney of a 6-year-old Simmental cow obtained from the right paralumbar fossa (5.0 MHz): the anechoic renal cyst (cy) was an incidental finding.

tissues. Some uroliths have no acoustic shadow and must be differentiated from the echogenic renal sinus. In hydronephrotic kidneys, the collecting system is dilated, hypoechoic, and the renal parenchyma is usually very thin (see **Figs. 11**A, B and **13**).[6] Aside from these specific changes, the kidneys can show various sonographic signs of inflammation, secondary to urinary tract obstruction, but can also be normal.

Cystic calculi are easy to image with transrectal ultrasonography.[6] They are commonly multiple and small or represent sandy debris. They are hyperechoic, casting acoustic shadows, and usually have a rough and irregular surface. The urinary bladder wall often appears thickened. In young bull calves that are too small for rectal examination only a transcutaneous approach from the ventral abdominal window is possible. But the urinary bladder is often obscured by gastrointestinal viscera, and gas-filled bowel adjacent to the urinary bladder and reverberation artifacts can mimic concretions. Moreover, ruptured bladders are small and in an intrapelvic location. In these patients a large amount of free peritoneal fluid is sometimes the only sonographic finding suggestive for urolithiasis and urinary bladder rupture.

Urethral calculi are seen in castrated cattle due to the relatively small diameter of the urethra. Urethral obstruction may occur at any site but is most common at the sigmoid flexure in steers.[9] If detected, the sonographic appearance of an urethral calculus is a hyperechoic concretion casting an acoustic shadow wedged in the lumen of the urethra with fluid distention proximal to the urolith (**Fig. 14**).[6]

Uroperitoneum

Uroperitoneum subsequent to urinary bladder rupture is rare in adult cattle, but may occur due to calving injuries or cystitis in cows.[14] More commonly, uroperitoneum is diagnosed in males (beef feeder cattle) with urethral obstruction associated with urethral calculi. Rupture through an incompletely closed urachal remnant can also occur. Osmotic pressure from hypertonic urine promotes movement of extracellular water into the peritoneal cavity. This movement, combined with reduced intake, results in clinical dehydration. Diffusion of urine across the peritoneal membrane results in azotemia with hyponatremia, hypochloremia, hyperkalemia, and hyperphosphatemia. But the blood concentration of urea rises much more slowly in ruminants

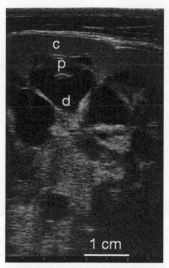

Fig. 13. Transcutaneous sonogram of the right kidney of a 1-month-old Simmental bull calf with urolithiasis obtained from the right paralumbar fossa (15 MHz): The renal calices are dilated (d) and filled with anechoic urine, which compresses the small medullary pyramids (p). The abdominal wall is at the top of the sonogram. Cranial is to the left, caudal is to the right. c, renal cortex.

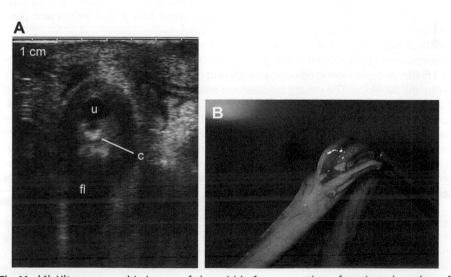

Fig. 14. (*A*) Ultrasonographic image of the midshaft cross-section of penis and urethra of a 1-week-old Simmental bull calf with ventral edema and anuria (10 MHz). The anechoic urethral lumen (u) is visible although no micturition is evident. Notice the small urethral defect filled with echogenic concretions (c). A small amount of anechoic fluid (fl) surrounds the penis. This sonogram was obtained from the ventral midline between scrotum and preputial orifice. The ventral abdominal wall is at the top of the sonogram. (*B*) Necropsy revealed urolithiasis with obstruction and rupture of the distal urethra.

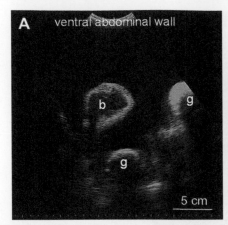
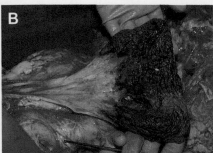

Fig. 15. (*A*) A 4-month-old male Simmental calf (178 kg) presented with a history of distended abdomen, indigestion and sawhorse straddling of the legs. Urea and creatinine levels were 10-fold increased. Transcutaneous ultrasonography of the ventral abdomen (5.0 MHz) showed the urinary bladder (b) with thick and irregular wall and echogenic swirling content, surrounded by gas-filled bowel (g) floating in the anechoic fluid. A defect in the urinary bladder could be detected, where the echogenic urine drained into the anechoic ascites. The kidneys were normal. The right side of the sonogram is the left side of the abdomen. (*B*) Necropsy revealed uroperitoneum, severe hemorrhagic–necrotizing cystitis with rupture of the urinary bladder, urethral obstruction by concretions, and normal kidneys.

compared with other species.[9] Cattle with uroperitoneum often have a pear-shaped abdomen. Ballotement of the abdomen may reveal a fluid wave. The clinical diagnosis can be confirmed by abdominocentesis. The peritoneal fluid is light yellow and clear with urea and creatinine higher than serum values.[9]

With uroperitoneum, the peritoneal cavity is filled with anechoic fluid and the gastrointestinal viscera are imaged floating in and on top of the fluid (**Fig. 15**A, B). The peritoneal fluid may have increased echogenicity and contain strands of fibrin if a secondary peritonitis develops. The urinary bladder can also be imaged floating within the fluid. If the urinary bladder is ruptured, the bladder can appear collapsed, flaccid, and folded upon itself and containing little or no fluid.[6] Cattle produce much fibrin, which closes the defect immediately, and the bladder can be filled well. The defect itself may not be directly imaged during the sonographic examination. The urethra should be evaluated sonographically if urethral obstruction is suspected as the cause of the uroperitoneum (see **Fig. 14**A, B). In males, a subcutaneous edema in the region of the prepuce is considered diagnostic for ruptured urethra (**Fig. 16**A, B).[6,9]

The most difficult defect to diagnose sonographically is the ureteral defect because the ureters are not normally visible throughout their length. Sonographic evaluation of the kidneys should be performed because retroperitoneal fluid (urine) may be imaged surrounding the kidney in patients with a ruptured ureter (**Fig. 17**).[6]

Cystitis

Inflammation of the bladder is usually caused by bacterial infection and is characterized clinically by frequent, painful urination, and the presence of blood, inflammatory cells, and bacteria in the urine.[9]

In cattle with cystitis, the bladder contains multiple echogenic areas swirling in the bladder, or there is a region of medium-to-high echogenicity in the cranioventral

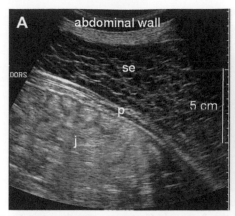
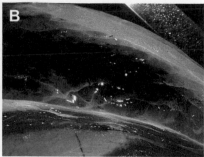

Fig. 16. (*A*) Sonogram of the ventral abdomen of the calf of **Fig. 14** (5.0 MHz) with severe subcutaneous edema. The right side of the sonogram is ventral and the left side dorsal. (*B*) Necropsy revealed subcutaneous accumulation of urine following urethral rupture. j, jejunum; p, peritoneum; se, subcutaneous edema.

portion of the bladder, which is consistent with blood or exudate.[7] Diffuse thickening of the bladder wall is a common sonographic abnormality detected in affected animals (see **Fig. 15**A, B).[6]

Urinary Bladder Neoplasms

Tumors of the urinary bladder are commonly associated with bracken poisoning. Clinical signs include hematuria, anemia, weight loss, stranguria, and the secondary

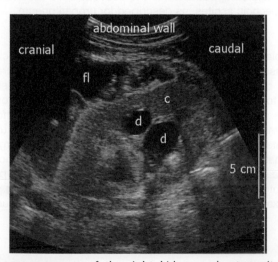

Fig. 17. Transcutaneous sonogram of the right kidney and retroperitoneal space of a 3-year-old Simmental cow obtained from the right paralumbar fossa (5.0 MHz): The kidney is surrounded by hypoechoic fluid (fl) with echogenic loculations, associated with ureteral rupture. The renal parenchyma is inhomogeneous, cortex (c) and medulla cannot be differentiated, the dilated calices (d) are filled with anechoic fluid. The abdominal wall is at the top of the sonogram. Necropsy revealed purulent embolic interstitial nephritis and pyelonephritis, ureteral obstruction, and blood and urine in the retroperitoneal space.

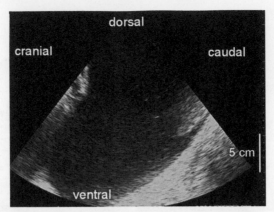

Fig. 18. Sonogram of the urinary bladder of the 3-year-old Simmental cow shown in **Fig. 1** obtained transrectally with a 3.5 MHz sector scanner. The urine within the urinary bladder is hypoechoic with multiple swirling echoes. The dilated bladder measures 29 cm in longitudinal diameter. The cow showed lameness, arching of the back and urinary retention. At necropsy, the bladder paralysis following sacral fracture was confirmed.

development of cystitis.[9] Sonographically, an increased bladder wall thickness and irregular sessile masses extending into the bladder lumen can be detected.[15]

Congenital Defects of the Urinary Tract

Congenital defects of the urinary tract include patent urachus, rupture of the bladder, urethral atresia, ureteral defect, polycystic kidneys, hypospadias, renal hypoplasia, and dysplasia and ectopic ureter.[2,9] Sonographically, some of these conditions can result in a multiloculated appearance of the subcutaneous accumulation of urine or anechoic-to-hypoechoic ascites, as described for uroperitoneum.

Bladder Atony

Paralysis of the bladder is uncommon in large animals. It usually occurs as a result of neurologic diseases affecting the lumbosacral spinal cord.[9] Sacral nerve injuries causing bladder dysfunction are caused by dystocia with intrapelvic injury or by crushing injuries to the sacrum and tail head at the vertebral level from riding activity. Dribbling of urine and voiding of small amounts of urine despite efforts at complete urination are the major signs of bladder dysfunction. Urine is normal unless secondary cystitis (and crystalluria) occurs. Rectal palpation confirms an enlarged bladder, and the affected animal cannot empty the bladder when stimulated.[1] Sonographic appearance usually reveals a markedly distended urinary bladder with hyperechoic sludge accumulating ventrally in the bladder or multiple swirling echoes (**Fig. 18**). The kidneys should also be examined as the prognosis is poor in cases with recurrent cystitis and pyelonephritis.[6]

SUMMARY

Many patients with urinary tract disorders are presented with a history pointing to another disease. In these patients, urine constituents commonly are abnormal, but this is often missed. Blood urea nitrogen and creatinine can be within reference ranges, although severe parenchymal anomalies are present. Moreover, serum biochemical profiles are often not performed in cattle due to cost reasons. Ultrasonography has the potential to aid in the diagnosis of several urinary tract abnormalities.

However, an accurate diagnosis of urinary tract disease can only be ensured by careful and thorough ultrasonographic examination of the entire urinary tract since only one kidney may be affected. The limitations are diffuse or small parenchymal changes that are not visible because of poor resolution of low-frequency transducers, and the time-consuming examination of the complete urinary tract.

ACKNOWLEDGMENTS

The author thanks the personnel of the Institute of Pathology and Forensic Veterinary Medicine of the University of Veterinary Medicine, Vienna, for performing the necropsies.

REFERENCES

1. Divers TJ. Urinary tract diseases. In: Divers TJ, Peek SF, editors. Rebhuńs diseases of dairy cattle. 2nd edition. Philadelphia: W.B. Saunders; 2007. p. 447–66.
2. Traub-Dargatz JL, Wrigley RH. Ultrasonographic evaluation of the urinary tract. In: Rantanen NW, McKinnon AO, editors. Equine diagnostic ultrasonography. 1st edition. Philadelphia: Williams & Wilkins; 1998. p. 613–8.
3. Vollmerhaus B. Urinary system. In: Frewein J, Gasse H, Leiser R, editors. Textbook of the anatomy of domestic animals, Band 2. 9th edition. Berlin, Hamburg: Paul Parey; 2004. p. 308–40 [in German].
4. Braun U. Ultrasonographic examination of the right kidney in cows. Am J Vet Res 1991;5211:1933–9.
5. Braun U. Ultrasonographic examination of the left kidney, the urinary bladder, and the urethra in cows. Zentralbl Veterinarmed A 1993;4012(1):1–9.
6. Reef VB. Adult abdominal ultrasonography. In: Reef VB, editor. Equine diagnostic ultrasound. Philadelphia: W.B. Saunders; 1998. p. 273–363.
7. Floeck M. Sonographic application in the diagnosis of pyelonephritis in cattle. Vet Radiol Ultrasound 2007;48(1):74–7.
8. Weiss E. Urinary system. In: Dahme E, Weiss E, editors. Textbook of the pathologic anatomy of domestic animals. Stuttgart: Enke Verlag; 2007. p. 173–201 [in German].
9. Radostits OM, Gay CC, Hinchcliff KW, et al. Diseases of the urinary system. In: Radostits OM, Gay CC, Hinchcliff KW, editors. Veterinary medicine. A textbook of the diseases of cattle, horses, sheep, pigs, and goats. 10th edition. Edinburgh: Saunders Elsevier; 2007. p. 543–73.
10. Rebhun WC, Dill SG, Perdrizet JA. Pyelonephritis in cows: 15 cases (1982–1986). J Am Vet Med Assoc 1989;194(7):953–5.
11. Hayashi H, Biller DS, Rings DM, et al. Ultranonographic diagnosis of pyelonephritis in a cow. J Am Vet Med Assoc 1994;205(5):736–8.
12. Gufler H. Kidney abscesses, pyelonephritis, and purulent cystitis in a 5-month-old calf—diagnosed by sonography. Wiener Tierärztliche Monatsschrift 1999; 86:247–51 [in German].
13. Schmidt G. Renal failure. In: Schmidt G, editor. Checklist sonography. 3rd edition. Stuttgart: Thieme; 2005. p. 138–52 [in German].
14. Braun U, Wetli U, Bryce B, et al. Clinical, ultrasonographic and endoscopic findings in a cow with bladder rupture caused by suppurative necrotising cystitis. Vet Rec 2007;161(20):700–2.
15. Hoque M, Somvanshi R, Singh GR, et al. Ultrasonographic evaluation of urinary bladder in normal, fern fed and enzootic bovine haematuria-affected cattle. J Vet Med A 2002;49(8):403–7.

Ultrasonography of the Bovine Udder and Teat

Sonja Franz, DVM[a],*, Martina Floek, DVM[a],
Margarete Hofmann-Parisot, DVM[b]

KEYWORDS

- Ultrasonography • Teat • Udder • Cattle • Teat stenosis
- Diagnosis

Udder health plays an important role in modern dairy farming and is the basis for an economical and hygienic milk production process.[1,2] In the dairy industry, prophylactic procedures are just as important as therapeutic ones. Milk flow disorders are a central problem in the field of udder health. They give rise to different kinds of mastitis, which consequently leads to a loss in milk production, detrimental changes to the milk components and raw milk quality, increased costs for the treatment of the animal, early culling of dairy cows, and, hence, a negative economic impact. Therefore, a rapid and accurate diagnosis and prognosis is mandatory in patients with udder diseases, and requires the use of state-of-the-art examination techniques and therapeutic treatments.

STRUCTURE OF UDDER AND TEATS

The adult bovine mammary is a skin gland and is therefore external to the body cavity. The gland comprises four quarters, each with an individual secretory gland drained by a teat. Strong and dense suspensory ligaments carry the heavy weight of the udder (udder suspensory system). The median suspensory ligament partially separates the left and right halves of the udder. Front and rear quarters are separated by a thin membrane. There is no internal crossover of the milk duct system within the quarters.

Glandular Parenchyma

The milk is synthesized in the secretory cells, alveoli, which are arranged as a single layer on a basal membrane in a spherical structure. The alveoli are surrounded by myoepithelial cells and participate in the oxytocin-induced milk ejection. Several alveoli

[a] Department for Farm Animals and Veterinary Public Health, Clinic for Ruminants, University of Veterinary Medicine Vienna, Veterinärplatz 1, 1210 Vienna, Austria
[b] Department for Biomedical Sciences, Institute for Physics and Biostatistics, University of Veterinary Medicine Vienna, Veterinärplatz 1, 1210 Vienna, Austria
* Corresponding author.
E-mail address: sonja.franz@vetmeduni.ac.at (S. Franz).

Vet Clin Food Anim 25 (2009) 669–685
doi:10.1016/j.cvfa.2009.07.007
0749-0720/09/$ – see front matter © 2009 Elsevier Inc. All rights reserved.

together form a lobule. Ducts are the tubes by which milk drains from the alveoli down to the gland cistern. There are intra- and interlobular ducts.

Teat

The teat consists of the teat canal and the teat cistern. The teat canal is located between the teat cistern and the outside ending of the teat. It is lined with a skin-like epidermis (stratified squamous epithelium) that forms the keratin material that has antibacterial properties and, therefore, is the main barrier against intramammary infection. At the level of the teat canal, the circular muscle is well developed, forming the teat sphincter, whose function is to retain milk in the intervals between suckling or milking. The mucous membrane of the teat canal has longitudinal folds, and there also are folds at the junction of the teat canal and teat cistern (rosette of Fürstenberg). The rosette of Fürstenberg represents the proximal delineation of the teat canal. The teat cistern is the cavity within the teat and is lined with numerous longitudinal and circular folds in the mucosa. The teat wall consists of the outer skin (epidermis), the middle muscle–connective tissue and the inner mucous membrane. The middle layer carries the blood and lymph vessels and nerves; however, the sensory nerve endings are in the epidermis.

Proximally to the teat cistern there is the gland cistern of the corresponding quarter. There are large venous vessels forming the erectile venous plexus at the teat base (boundary between teat cistern and gland cistern), called the venous ring of Fürstenberg.

EXAMINATION TECHNIQUES

The udder is a very sensitive organ and therefore very susceptible to disease. An early diagnosis of any kind of udder disease is of medical and economic importance.[3] Diseases of the udder should be recognized first in the single animal by performing a physical examination, including inspection and palpation. Several additional examination techniques should help to give a correct diagnosis:

    Examination of milk secretion by hand and/or machine milking
    California Mastitis Test, microbiological examination of milk
    Probing the teat canal, injecting methylene blue dye
    Diagnostic imaging techniques: radiography, sonography, endoscopy

Examination techniques that allow visualization of inner parts of the teat are preferable to techniques such as palpation of the teat, examination of the teat with a probe, or even diagnostic thelotomy. In the 1970s and 1980s radiography of the teat was performed as diagnostic tool in patients with milk flow disorders.[4–8] In recent years, radiography has been totally replaced by sonography and endoscopy. The advantage of sonography is that it is noninvasive and it is possible to visualize all structures of the bovine udder (teat and glandular parenchyma) without the use of ionizing radiation.[9,10] The big advantage of theloscopy (endoscopic examination of the teat) is that pathologic findings are visualized truthfully. However, the endoscopic technique only permits examination of the teat cistern and the teat canal. The anatomic structures located more proximally cannot be visualized. Theloscopy is mainly used for surgical intervention in cases of teat stenosis.[9]

ULTRASONOGRAPHY OF THE BOVINE MAMMARY GLAND

Reviewing the literature, several reports about ultrasonographic examination of the bovine mammary gland can be found.

In 1967, ultrasonography of the bovine teat in A-mode, with 1 MHz frequency, was first performed.[11] Later on, B-mode (real-time mode) was tested.[12] Upon recognition of the economic importance of hygienic milk from healthy cows, further studies followed, namely in the field of milk machine technology and the diagnosis of milk flow disturbances.[13–24] Nearly all investigations were done directly on the animal, although some were performed on the extirpated organ. Vertical and horizontal sonographic scanning was performed with 3.5 MHz or 5.0 MHz using a sector and a linear array transducer, the latter proving to be more useful. The achieved image quality was evaluated in various ways. Some investigators have described the teat canal (using a 3.5 MHz linear array transducer) as a hypoechoic, unclearly demarcated zone.[15] By using a 5.0 MHz linear array transducer the sonographic image of the teat canal was interpreted as one or two hyperechoic lines.[17,21] In part, the image quality was considered satisfactory by coupling of the probe directly to the teat skin.[14] Other investigators remarked that ultrasonography was only satisfactory when the teat was held in a water bath during ultrasonography.[15,17] Filling of the teat (after oxytocin application), either with normal saline solution or with milk, was also an important criterium for achieving optimal image quality.

The teat canal is a very delicate structure with a length of approximately 8 to 12 mm and a lumen approximately 0.4 mm at the distal opening.[15,17,21]

For some time there was no explanation as to which tissue structures are responsible for the different echogenicity in the image section of the teat canal. Some researchers supported the opinion that the hypoechoic part is caused by vessels in the teat wall.[15] When the isolated teats of cows were examined,[25] histologic studies of the tissues whose removal led to the disappearance of this characteristic ultrasonographic appearance showed that it was associated with the stratified keratinized squamous epithelium with distinct papillae. The content of keratin in the stratum corneum was apparently responsible for the bright zone; the stratum lucidum was not visible, and the surrounding dark, less echoic area was associated with the stratum granulosum. Color Doppler echography in live animals confirmed this designation.[25] This method proved that the two parallel thick hypoechoic bands (dark, gray-black image sections in vertical scan) could not be identified as vessels, because there was no registration of blood flow, despite the sensivity of this method even for very slow blood flow. In the remaining sonographic areas of the teat wall, vessels and blood flow were visible in both vertical and horizontal scans.

In contrary to the sonographic examination of the teat that is now performed routinely, the sonographic examination of the glandular parenchyma rarely is described. Few studies deal with descriptions of physiologic and pathologic sonographic findings of the glandular parenchyma.[10,12,14,24,26,27]

INDICATIONS FOR ULTRASONOGRAPHY OF THE BOVINE MAMMARY GLAND

Ultrasonography of the udder parenchyma is a diagnostic aid in mastitis, enlargement of the udder (**Fig. 1**) without clinical signs of mastitis (eg, hematoma, neoplasia), and, occasionally, detection of penetrating foreign bodies. Ultrasonography does not replace bacteriologic criteria or somatic cell counts but gives additional information on the status of the udder and, consequently, aids in determining a prognosis. It is more objective than palpation of the gland. Furthermore, parallels can be found between the sonographic image of the affected udder parenchyma and certain species of bacteria, particularly *Arcanobacterium pyogenes* and gram-negative bacteria.[27]

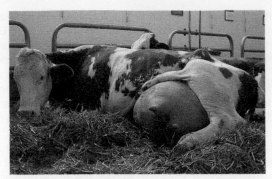

Fig. 1. A cow with severe enlargement of the udder.

Ultrasonography of the teat is generally performed in the single animal for diagnosis of pathologic changes in the area of the teat canal, the teat, and the gland cistern.[9,10,12,15,17,18,20,21,26,28,29] Milk flow disorders (**Fig. 2**) are the main indications in the field setting for ultrasonographic examination of the teat. In these patients, the first demand is a rapid restoration of good milkability and a healthy udder. In the literature, teat injuries and milking technique, such as improper manipulation of the teat, are common reasons for the disturbance of milk flow.[30–32] Inflammation with swelling and sensitivity develop and lead to partial or total stenosis. Teat stenosis can be localized in the proximal part (boundary between gland and teat cistern), in the middle part (teat cistern), and distal part (teat canal).

Relationships between susceptibility to mastitis in cows and age, number of lactations, stage of lactation, and physical characteristics of teats and teat canal development have been reported and correlations exist between characteristics of the udder and parameters of udder health, productivity, ease of milking, and milk quality.[33–41] In several studies, sonographic examination of the bovine teat proved to be a useful method to measure teat and teat canal structures. This diagnostic imaging technique was used to look for breed differences such as number of lactations, lengthening of the teat canal along with the teat as a result of the mechanical exposure to milking, and for the influence of the teat parameters on the development of mastitis.[24,42–46]

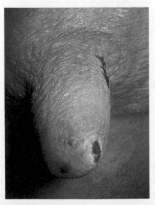

Fig. 2. Milk flow disorders due to traumatic covered teat injuries are the main indications for ultrasonography of the bovine teat.

SCANNING TECHNIQUE

By using suitable equipment (2D ultrasonography) it is possible to differentiate morphologic structures such as the glandular parenchyma, the gland cistern, the teat cistern, and the teat canal.

Ultrasonographic examinations of the glandular parenchyma are performed with a 5.0 MHz or lower-frequency transducer. The transducer is placed lateral and caudal directly onto the udder skin to examine the parenchyma, after shaving and degreasing the skin with alcohol and applying coupling gel. Convex, linear array, and sector transducers can be used.[12,27]

To visualize the border between the gland cistern and the teat cistern, the probe must be applied directly to the organ. To examine the teat, the teat is dipped in a water-filled plastic cup (Fig. 3). In order to get good quality sonographic images, it is necessary to use a linear ultrasound probe with a frequency of at least 7.5 MHz. Contact gel has to be applied between the probe and the skin or plastic cup to guarantee optimal contact. The water-filled plastic cup enables the examiner to keep a hand free to move the teat into position and/or to handle the machine, while the other hand is used to hold the cup and to move the probe simultaneously in a vertical plane. Another reason for using a water-filled plastic cup is to prevent any deformation of the tip of the teat and to visualize the teat canal in its entire length. The filling of the teat in lactating cows with aqua ad injectabila or normal saline solution does not seem to be necessary.[25]

NORMAL SONOGRAM
Glandular Parenchyma

The normal bovine mammary gland is uniformly echogenic with a granular structure (Fig. 4). This characteristic image is a result of the even distribution of connective tissue with a higher echoic density and gland parenchyma with less echoic density. The anechoic antra can either correspond to blood vessels or lactiferous ducts. The milk in the gland cistern is anechoic or may contain echogenic particles. The entries of the large lactiferous ducts into the gland cistern are clearly visible. The degree of echogenicity of the lactiferous gland is also dependent upon fill volume.[12,27]

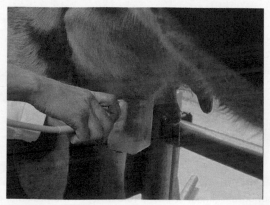

Fig. 3. Ultrasonography of the bovine teat using a water-filled plastic cup in order to examine the distal parts of the teat.

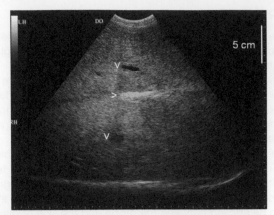

Fig. 4. Sonogram obtained with a 5.0 MHz convex transducer of a physiologic gland parenchyma with homogeneous echogenicity and isolated anechoic vessels (v). An echogenic septum (*arrowhead*) separates the rear quarters. The udder skin is on the top of the sonogram, the dorsal portion of the udder is to the left, ventral to the right.

Teat

The boundary between the gland cistern and the teat cistern is marked by the presence of large, round-shaped anechoic structures in the teat wall that represent large vessels of the venous ring of Fürstenberg (**Fig. 5**). The gland cistern itself is anechoic and demarcated by a hyperechoic line (mucosal membrane).

The teat wall appears as a triple-layered construction, with a thin, bright, echoic line internally, followed by a thicker, homogeneous, hypoechoic layer with characteristic anechoic cavities within (vessels), and a thin, bright, echoic line externally. These layers are related, respectively, to the mucous membrane, to the muscle–connective tissue, and the skin (**Fig. 6**). When filled with milk, the lumen of the teat cistern is anechoic. The hyperechoic mucosal membrane of the teat cistern is demarcated regularly from the lumen.

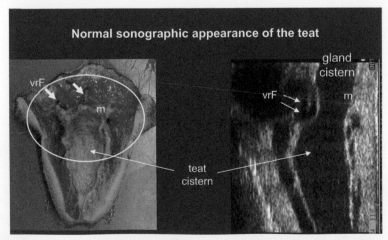

Fig. 5. Physiologic sonogram (linear scanner, 10.0 MHz) of the proximal part of the bovine teat (horizontal scan) presenting the boundary between the gland and the teat cistern. m, mucosal membrane; vrF, venous ring of Fürstenberg.

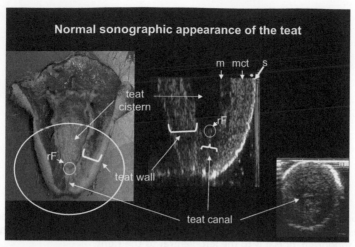

Fig. 6. Physiologic sonogram (linear scanner, 10.0 MHz, horizontal and vertical scan) of the distal part of the bovine teat. m, mucosal membrane; mct, muscle–connective tissue; rF, rosette of Fürstenberg; s, skin.

The junction between the teat canal and teat cistern (rosette of Fürstenberg) is homogeneous and hyperechoic and displays as two parallel white echoic lines (see **Fig. 6**).

The teat canal appears as a thin, white line, bordered on each side by parallel, thick, hypoechoic bands (see **Fig. 6**). A comparable image is obtained in the vertical and horizontal planes.

SONOGRAPHIC ABNORMALITIES

This section presents the most frequent pathologic sonographic findings of the glandular parenchyma and the teat diagnosed by 2D ultrasonography.

Glandular Parenchyma

Mastitis

The sonographic image of the udder in cases of mastitis depends on the degree of structural changes that occur in the tissue. The parenchyma may be inhomogeneous with a decreased or increased echogenicity, but can also have a normal sonographic appearance (eg, in infections with coagulase-negative staphylococci).[26,27] Inhomogeneity with hyperechoic spots or with bands casting dirty shadows is an indicator for gas formation in the parenchyma, and can be connected with gram-negative bacteria (**Fig. 7**). In such cases, a regular parenchyma structure is rarely found in the affected quarter and the changes extend mostly all across the entire quarter. Another finding can be hypoechoic round spots that measure, on average, 1 cm and have a small hyperechoic center, as a sequel to infection with A pyogenes (**Fig. 8**). A pyogenes, Klebsiella spp and E coli can be responsible for distinctive sonographic changes in the parenchyma, but can also be connected with a normal sonographic appearance.[27]

The milk shows increased echogenicity with an increased cellular content as a result of mastitis. The interchanging pattern of echogenic connecting tissue and anechoic edema fluid yields an image of the subcutis that resembles the skin of an onion.[26,27]

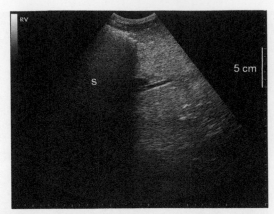

Fig. 7. Sonogram (5.0 MHz) of an inhomogeneous parenchyma with a strap-shaped hypere-choic zone casting a dirty shadow in a case of infection with *E coli*. The udder skin is on the top of the sonogram, dorsal is to the left, ventral to the right.

Hematoma

For hematomas of the udder, the sonographic image shows large anechoic or hypo-echoic spaces with thin, echoic free-floating septae or large clots (**Fig. 9**). The gland parenchyma is compressed by the pressure of the fluid. The differential between hematoma and edema of the udder is found in a larger extension of the spaces filled with fluid. Udder hematoma is often caused by a trauma.[27]

Foreign body

It can be difficult to palpate a foreign body in a lactating udder. Sonography can reveal hyperechoic linear structures casting acoustic shadows, even deep inside the paren-chyma (**Fig. 10**).

Teat

Teat canal and rosette of Fürstenberg

Normally, the teat canal appears as a central echoic line that is bordered on each side by two parallel hypoechoic bands. In cases of severe inflammation due to acute

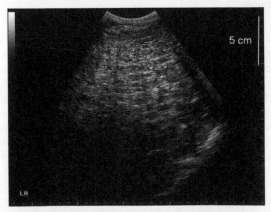

Fig. 8. Characteristic echo pattern of parenchyma in a case of an infection with *A pyogenes*: multiple hypoechoic round spots that measure a few mm in diameter (5.0 MHz). The udder skin is on the top of the sonogram, dorsal is to the left, ventral to the right.

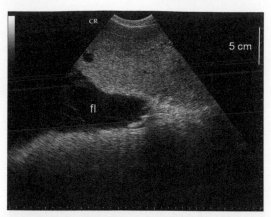

Fig. 9. Sonogram (5.0 MHz) of an udder hematoma between the front quarters. The hypo-echoic loculated fluid (fl) represents blood. The udder skin is on the top of the sonogram, cranial is to the left, caudal to the right.

trauma, however, the area appears as an inhomogeneous hypoechoic region. In some cases, this is combined with the existence of sonographically visible echoic mucosal lesions in the area of the rosette of Fürstenberg (**Fig. 11**).

Teat cistern
Common pathologic findings in the teat cistern diagnosed by means of ultrasonography are severe inflammation, mucosal lesions, tissue proliferation, foreign bodies, milkstones, and congenital changes.

In cases of inflammation, the mucosal membrane of the teat cistern is thickened and humpy. Often, the middle layer is inhomogeneous and the vessels have an increased diameter (**Fig. 12**).

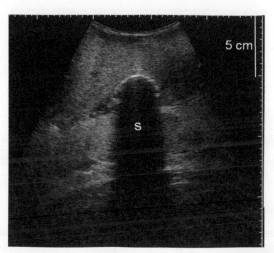

Fig. 10. Sonogram (5.0 MHz) of a traumatic perforation of the udder parenchyma by a foreign body. The hyperechoic half-moon–shaped transverse section of the broomstick is casting a strong acoustic shadow (S). The udder skin is on the top of the sonogram, dorsal is to the left, ventral to the right.

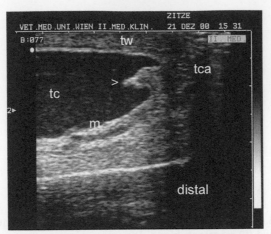

Fig. 11. A cow with covered teat injury showing disturbance of milk flow: the normal sonogram of the teat canal (tca) is not visible; in the area of the rosette of Fürstenberg, an echoic mucosal lesion can be diagnosed (>); in addition, the mucosal membrane (m) of the distal part of the teat cistern is thickened and lumpy, a sign of inflammation. The milk in the teat cistern (tc) shows an increased echogenicity; tw, teat wall.

Frequently, signs of inflammation caused by covered teat injuries can be observed in combination with mucosal lesions in the area of the teat cistern (see **Fig. 12**). Ultrasonography helps to localize and determine the amount of pathologic alteration and to diagnose an upper teat stenosis.

Milk stones can be completely free or attached to the mucosal membrane. By means of sonography it is possible to identify the milk stone and look for localization and size (**Fig. 13**). Due to the density of the lactolith, the milk stone is of echoic pattern.

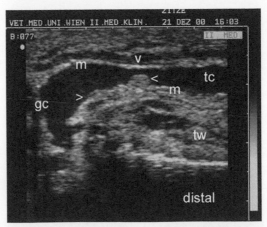

Fig. 12. An upper teat stenosis (linear scanner, 10.0 MHz) caused by a covered teat injury was diagnosed by means of ultrasonography. In the proximal part [boundary between gland cistern (gc) and teat cistern (tc)], several echoic mucosal lesions (>, <) are visible. The mucosal membrane (m) is thickened and lumpy, as is the middle layer of the teat wall (tw). Here the muscle–connective tissue shows an inhomogeneous structure. Anechoic vessels (v) can be recognized.

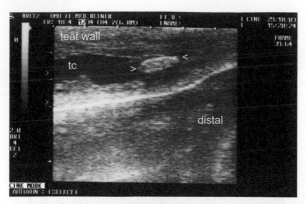

Fig. 13. This cow showed a disturbance of milk flow due to the existence of a free milk stone (>) in the anechoic teat cistern (tc). Ultrasonographically (linear scanner, 7.5 MHz), the milk stone is of echoic structure. Depending on the size of the milk stone, it can be removed under ultrasound guidance using a foreign body forceps inserted via teat canal.

It is the same as diagnosing proliferation tissue localized in the teat, such as polyps and papilloma (**Fig. 14**). If present, in some cases it can be difficult to detect a pedunculus.[9]

Congenital changes that may cause disturbance of milk flow can be intraluminal membranes (**Fig. 15**) or agenesis of the teat cistern. Most intraluminal membranes run transversally in the teat cistern and are recognized initially after the first calving. They can be responsible for partial or complete obstruction.[9]

In primiparous heifers, the congenital degeneration of the gland cistern and ducts associated with congenital teat obstruction (**Fig. 16**) that causes blind quarters is a common pathologic finding. These cows give only small amount milk, if at all, from a normal-sized quarter.

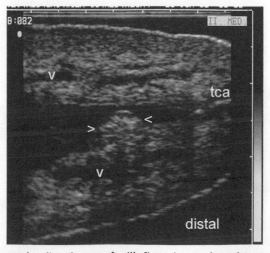

Fig. 14. This cow showed a disturbance of milk flow due to the existence of a papilloma of echoic structure in the anechoic teat cistern fixed to the teat wall (linear scanner, 7.5 MHz). The teat canal (tca) and the teat wall with vessels (v) in the middle layer are visible.

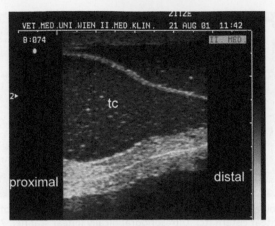

Fig. 15. Diagnosis of an congenital septum in the teat cistern (tc) of a cow using a linear 10.0 MHz scanner. The milk in the teat cistern shows an increased echogenicity.

Teat wall
Ultrasonography is a very helpful tool for diagnosis of teat wall alterations such as hematoma (**Fig. 17**) or abscess, which also can lead to disturbance of milk flow depending on the location. A hematoma is identifiable as a hypoechoic and inhomogeneous area, whereas an abscess often displays an echoic structure.

Conjoined teats
A conjoined teat is a supernumerary teat adjoined to the main teat. The conjoined teat has its own gland and teat cistern. The teat canal can be functional or not.[47–49] Conjoined teats show an increase incidence of mastitis due to incomplete emptying and insufficient development and function of the teat canal and teat sphincter. Therefore, diagnosis of a conjoined teat and differentiation from a teat fistula is of great importance. Ultrasonography may assist in differentiating a suspected conjoined teat.

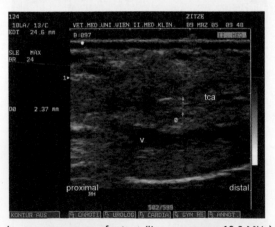

Fig. 16. This figure shows a sonogram of a teat (linear scanner, 10.0 MHz) with a congenital teat obstruction: at the distal part of the teat, the teat canal (tca) is still visible. Proximal to the teat canal, no anechoic lumen, normally representing the teat cistern, can be viewed. The anechoic structures in this figure represent vessels (v) in the teat wall.

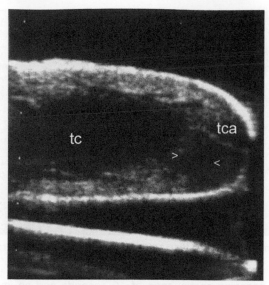

Fig. 17. Patient with covered teat injury showing disturbance of milk flow caused by a hematoma in the distal part of the teat wall that was diagnosed using ultrasonography (linear scanner, 7.5 MHz). The distal part of the teat shows an inhomogeneous hypoechoic structure and marks the localization of the hematoma (>). The anechoic teat cistern (tc) and the teat canal (tca) with the central white echoic line are also visible.

CLINICAL RELEVANCE OF TWO-DIMENSIONAL ULTRASONOGRAPHY OF THE BOVINE UDDER

Ultrasonography of the bovine mammary gland is a noninvasive diagnostic imaging technique and can be performed without any difficulties. The main indications for ultrasonography of the bovine mammary gland are milk flow disorders caused by various reasons, mainly traumatic covered teat injuries.[9,10] Using suitable equipment, it is possible to visualize the teat canal, the rosette of Fürstenberg, the teat cistern, the gland cistern, and the glandular parenchyma. With this noninvasive technique, it is possible to diagnose upper, middle, and lower teat stenosis. In many cases, physical examination of the teat alone cannot help determine exact diagnosis nor prognosis. Owing to important medical and economic factors, the use of ultrasonography is imperative because different pathologies require different therapeutic procedures and prognoses.

Ultrasonography of the teat allows for the localization and demarcation of the extent of teat stenosis and other abnormalities. Ultrasonography is also useful for monitoring the healing process after surgical removal of proliferative tissue. Additionally, it aids in the diagnosis of mastitis and thus promotes efficient therapy.

THREE-DIMENSION ULTRASONOGRAPHY OF THE BOVINE TEAT

In an experimental study, 3D ultrasonography of bovine mammary gland, including the glandular parenchyma, gland cistern, teat cistern, and teat canal, was evaluated.[50] Ultrasonography was performed using a conventional 2D, 50-mm linear array transducer with a frequency range of 8.5 to 10 MHz. The transducer was used without a position sensor (spatial locator). All regions of interest were examined by way of freehand scanning. The transducer was moved with an estimated speed of 5 mm per

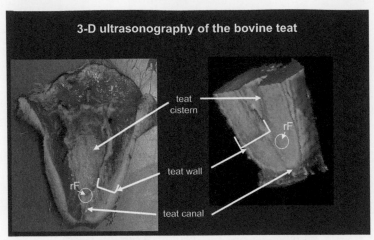

Fig. 18. 3D sonogram of the bovine teat: teat canal, rosette of Fürstenberg (rF), teat cistern.

second. Within a scanning continuance of 10 seconds and an image rate of 12.5 images per second, a series of parallel slices of approximately 0.4 mm thick were obtained.

The acquired 2D data (ie, output of the scanner in analog format) were downloaded to an offline system and a frame grabber was used to capture the images. An appropriate software program for 3D image reconstruction was used to digitize each image and produce a 3D block of digitized information. The selected anatomic area was displayed as a 3D volume cube. The software made it possible for the ultrasonographer to manipulate the image by rotating and slicing the volume cube in all planes and directions.

The technique used (freehand scanning without position sensor) does not provide constant data density, however; some areas may easily be under- or overscanned, and slice spacing may vary. The volume data acquired cannot be used for accurate measurement of structures of interest. The method is known as "cosmetic 3D ultrasonography." The technique provides a good-quality 3D section from the glandular parenchyma and gland cistern to the teat cistern, the rosette of Fürstenberg, and the teat canal (**Fig. 18**).

Three-dimensional ultrasonography can produce complete tomographic images of organs and provide valuable images of anatomic structures. In human medicine, the enhanced visualization of the examined organ can help reduce the variability in diagnoses. The cost of 3D ultrasonography varies depending on the technology used. Many scanners routinely used in veterinary practice have the resolution required to produce satisfactory images, and the cost of refitting a standard ultrasonographic unit with 3D software is affordable. The cost of a volume transducer with a positioning system and mechanical sweep strategy, however, may be prohibitive. Nevertheless, 3D ultrasonography is a new imaging technique with promising applications in a variety of fields of veterinary medicine and research.

REFERENCES

1. Wendt K, Bostedt H, Mielke H, et al. Udder and teat diseases. Stuttgart: Gustav Fischer Verlag Jena; 1994. p. 229–31.

2. Kossaibati MA. The costs of clinical mastitis in UK dairy herds. Cattle Practice 2000;8:323–7.
3. Winter P. Ziele der Mastitisdiagnostik [Aims of diagnosing mastitis]. In: Winter P, editor. Praktischer Leitfaden Mastitis [Practical guide mastitis]. Stuttgart: Parey; 2009. p. 30–6.
4. Kubicek J. The radiographical view of the bovine teat. Attribution to physical findings in the teat of dairy cows. Tierarztl Umsch 1972;27(3):119–24.
5. Witzig P, Hugelshofer J. Clarification of teat stenoses using radiography double contrast staining. Schweiz Arch Tierheilkd 1984;126(3):155–63.
6. Witzig P, Rusch P, Berchtold M. Diagnosis and treatment of the teat stenoses in dairy cattle with special reference to radiography and thelotomy. Vet Med Rev 1984;2:123–32.
7. Stocker H, Bättig U, Duss M, et al. [Clarification of teat stenoses in cattle by ultrasound]. Tierarztl Prax 1989;17(3):251–6 [in German].
8. Alacam D, Dinc A, Güler M, et al. Incidence and radiographic examination of different pathological findings in the teat of dairy cows. Dtsch Tierarztl Wochenschr 1990;97(12):523–5.
9. Hospes R, Seeh C. Sonographie. In: Hospes R , Seeh C, editors. Sonographie und Endoskopie an der Zitze des Rindes [Sonography and endoscopy of the bovine teat]. Stuttgart: Schattauer; 1999. p. 29–48.
10. Stocker H, Rüsch P. Euter und Zitzen. In: Braun U, editor. Textbook of ultrasonography in cattle. 1st edition. Berlin: Parey; 1997. p. 163–75.
11. Caruolo EV, Mochrie RD. Ultrasonograms of lactating mammary glands. J Dairy Sci 1967;50(2):225–30.
12. Cartee RE, Ibrahim AK, Mc Leary D. B-mode ultrasonography of the bovine udder and teat. J Am Vet Med Assoc 1986;188(11):1284–7.
13. Worstorff H, Steib JD, Prediger A, et al. Assessment of ultrasonography for examination of teat changes in cows during milking. Milch Wissenschaft 1986; 41:12–5.
14. Jenninger S. Ultrasonography of the bovine udder–physiological and pathological findings. Thesis 1989; München.
15. Stocker H, Battig U, Duss M, et al. Clarification. Tierärztl Prax 1989;17(3):251–6.
16. Takeda T. Diagnostic ultrasound of the bovine udder. Jpn J Vet Res 1989;37:133.
17. Will S, Würgau ST, Fraunholz J, et al. Ultrasonographic findings of the bovine teat. Dtsch Tierarztl Wochenschr 1990;97(10):403–6.
18. Dreyfuss DJ, Madison JB, Reef VB. Surgical treatment of a mural teat abscess in a cow. J Am Vet Med Assoc 1990;197(12):1629–30.
19. Duvelsdorf A, Duck M, Scheidemann B. Method and device for the mechanical attachment of one teat cup at a time. Deutsche Patentschrift; 1991. DE 3938 077 A1.
20. Saratis P. Zur Diagnostik von Zitzenstenosen des Rindes mit Hilfe der Ultraschalltomographie (Literaturübersicht). Dtsch Tierarztl Wochenschr 1991;98(12): 441–76.
21. Saratis P, Grunert E. Ultrasonography in the cow for determination of dimension and localization of pathological teat changes. Dtsch Tierarztl Wochenschr 1993;100(4):159–63.
22. Bruckmaier RM, Rothenanger E, Blum JW. Measurement of mammary gland cistern size and determination of the cisternal milk fraction in dairy cows. Milch Wiss 1994;49:543–6.

23. Seeh C, Hospes R, Bostedt H. Use of diagnostic imaging techniques (sonography/endoscopy) for diagnosis of a conjoined teat–case report. Tierärztl Prax 1996;24:438–42.
24. Banting A. Ultrasonographic examination of the mammary gland in cows with induced S. aureus mastitis: a criteria for prognosis and evaluation of therapy. Cattle Pract 1998;6:121–4.
25. Franz S, Hofmann-Parisot M, Baumgartner W, et al. Ultrasonography of the teat canal in cows and sheep. Vet Rec 2001;149(4):109–12.
26. Trostle SS, ÓBrien RT. Ultrasonography of the bovine mammary gland. Compendium on Continuing Education for the Practicing Veterinarian 1998;20:64–71.
27. Floeck M, Winter P. Diagnostic ultrasonography in cattle with diseases of the mammary gland. Vet J 2006;171(2):314–21.
28. Dinc DA, Sendang S, Aydin I. Diagnosis of teat stenosis in dairy cattle by real time ultrasonography. Vet Rec 2000;147(10):270–2.
29. Flöck M, Klein D, Hofmann-Parisot M. Ultrasonographic findings of pathological teat changes in cattle. Wiener Tierärztliche Monatsschrift [Veterinary Medicine Austria] 2004;91(7):184–95.
30. Seeh C, Melle T, Medl M, et al. [Systematic classification of milk flow obstruction in cattle using endoscopic findings with special consideration of hidden teat injuries]. Tierarztl Prax Ausg G Grosstiere Nutztiere 1998;26(4):174–86 [in German].
31. Bleul UT, Schwantag SC, Bachofner CH, et al. Milk flow and udder health in cows after treatment of covered teat injuries via theloresectoscopy: 52 cases (2000–2002). J Am Vet Med Assoc 2005;226(7):1119–23.
32. Geishauser T, Querengässer K, Querengässer J. Teat endoscopy (theloscopy) for diagnosis and therapy of milk flow disorders in dairy cows. Vet Clin North Am Food Anim Pract 2005;21(1):205–25.
33. McDonald JS. Radiographic method for anatomic study of the teat canal: characteristics related to resistance to new intramammary infection during lactation and the early dry period. Cornell Vet 1975;65(4):492–9.
34. Binde M, Bakke H. Relationships between teat characteristics and udder health. Nord Vet Med 1984;36(3–4):111–6.
35. Seykora AJ, McDaniel BT. Udder and teat morphology related to mastitis resistance: a review. J Dairy Sci 1985;68(8):2087–93.
36. Michel G, Rausch B. Change in teat dimensions of cattle udder during several periods of lactation. Monatshefte Veterinärmedizin 1998;43:337–9.
37. Grindal RJ, Walton AW, Hillerton JE. Influence of milk flow rate and streak canal length on new intramammary infection in dairy cows. J Dairy Res 1991;58(4):383–8.
38. Seyfried G. The sonographic measurement of teat structures and the significance for udder health of 'Braun-and-Fleckvieh' cows. Thesis, 1992; University of Veterinary Medicine Vienna, Austria.
39. Scherzer J. Ultrasound examination of the bovine teat—influence of teat canal length and other factors on the udder health. Thesis, 1992; University of Veterinary Medicine Vienna, Austria.
40. Hamann J, Østeras O. Special aspects. Teat tissue reactions to machine milking and new infection risk. Bulletin of the International Dairy Federation 1994;297:51–60.
41. Lacy-Hulbert SJ, Hillerton JE. Physical characteristics of the bovine teat canal and their influence on susceptibility to streptococcal infection. J Dairy Res 1995;62(3):395–404.
42. Neijenhuis F, Klungel GH, Hogeveen H. Recovery of teats after milking as determined by ultrasonographic scanning. J Dairy Sci 2001;84(12):2599–606.

43. Ayadi M, Caja G, Such X, et al. Use of ultrasonography to estimate cistern size and milk storage at different milking intervals in the udder of dairy cows. J Dairy Res 2003;70(1):1–7.
44. Klein D, Flöck M, Khol JL, et al. Ultrasonographic measurement of the bovine teat: breed differences, and the significance of the measurements for udder health. J Dairy Res 2005;72(3):296–302.
45. Khol JL, Franz S, Klein D, et al. Influence of milking technique and lactation on the bovine teat by means of ultrasonographic examination. Berl Münch Tierarztl Wochenschr 2006;119(1–2):68–73.
46. Rovai M, Kollmann MT, Bruckmaier RM. Incontinentia lactis: physiology and anatomy conducive to milk leakage in dairy cows. J Dairy Sci 2007;90(2):682–90.
47. Steiner A. Teat surgery. In: Fubini SL, Ducharme NG, editors. Farm Animal Surgery. 1st edition. Philadelphia: Saunders Elsevier; 2004. p. 408–19.
48. Couture Y, Mulon PY. Procedures and surgeries of the teat. Vet Clin Food Anim Pract 2005;21(1):173–204.
49. George LW, Divers TJ, Ducharme N, et al. Diseases of the Teats and Udder. In: Divers TJ, Peek SF, editors. Rebhun's diseases of dairy cattle. 2nd edition. Philadelphia: Saunders Elsevier; 2008. p. 327–94.
50. Franz S, Hofmann-Parisot M, Baumgartner W. Evaluation of three-dimensional ultrasonography of the bovine mammary gland. Am J Vet Res 2004;65(8): 1159–63.

Ultrasonography as a Diagnostic Aid in Bovine Musculoskeletal Disorders

Johann Kofler, DVM

KEYWORDS

- Ultrasonography • Musculoskeletal disorders • Arthritis
- Tenosynovitis • Bursitis

In the last 15 years, ultrasonography of the bovine musculoskeletal system has become an established diagnostic method used routinely in many veterinary teaching hospitals worldwide.[1–31] Ultrasonography is ideal for the evaluation of musculoskeletal disorders, such as arthritis, tenosynovitis, bursitis, and muscle disorders, because they are often associated with extensive soft tissue swelling and inflammatory exudation, usually attributable to infection.[2,4–8,13–15,18,19,21,23,24,27,31,32] For the diagnosis of conditions limited to soft tissues, ultrasonography is superior to radiography.[33,34]

Diagnosis of bovine musculoskeletal disorders starts with a thorough clinical and orthopedic examination before ultrasonography to identify the "region of interest" for the sonographer. Other clinical diagnostic techniques include exploration of wounds with a probe, centesis of synovial or other fluid-filled cavities and macroscopic, microscopic, and bacteriologic examination of the aspirated fluid.[33,35–38]

Making a diagnosis in cases with diffuse soft tissue swelling and in cases with disorders of the proximal limb is often challenging. It is frequently impossible to identify with certainty the affected anatomic structures in patients with severe diffuse swelling, concurrent disease of two or more adjacent synovial structures (joints, tendon sheaths, bursae), or concurrent myositis. Identification of the anatomic structures affected in the proximal limb can also be problematic for the clinician.

For many veterinarians in bovine practice, radiographic equipment is not available. Radiography is ideal for evaluation of bones and joints, but does not allow detection of early stages of septic joint disease. For technical and anatomic reasons, radiography of the proximal limb and trunk is seldom feasible, especially in adult cattle.[39] Centesis is only successful if the material to be aspirated is sufficiently liquid; however, cattle

Clinical Department of Horses and Small Animals, Clinic of Horses, Large Animal Surgery and Orthopedics, University of Veterinary Medicine Vienna, Veterinärplatz 1, A-1210 Vienna, Austria
E-mail address: johann.kofler@vetmeduni.ac.at

Vet Clin Food Anim 25 (2009) 687–731
doi:10.1016/j.cvfa.2009.07.011
0749-0720/09/$ – see front matter © 2009 Elsevier Inc. All rights reserved.

frequently have semisolid inflammatory exudates because of marked fibrin production.[5,7,8,35,38]

In contrast to radiography, ultrasonography has been used for many years in bovine practice for the diagnosis of pregnancy and gynecologic disorders. Ultrasound machines with 5.0 and 7.5 MHz linear transducers used for bovine reproduction can also be used for evaluation of orthopedic diseases.

The goal of this article is to encourage veterinarians to use ultrasonography for the evaluation of bovine orthopedic disorders. Not only does ultrasonography improve the likelihood of a definitive diagnosis, added use of the machine helps recoup expenses.

An in-depth understanding of the anatomy of the musculoskeletal system is critical for correct interpretation of the sonographic images. The examiner must be familiar with the three-dimensional structure of the anatomic region. This can be practiced by comparing longitudinal and transverse sonograms with corresponding frozen longitudinal and transverse sections, with intraoperative findings or by studying carcass specimens during postmortem examination.

PREPARATION OF THE PATIENT

Ultrasonographic examination of the proximal regions of the musculoskeletal system is best achieved in the standing patient. For evaluation of the digit, particularly the metacarpophalangeal, metatarsophalangeal, and interphalangeal joints, the animal can be confined in a chute with the affected limb raised and secured. However, placing the patient in lateral recumbency on a claw trimming or surgical table is preferred for examination of these distal regions. In most cattle, sedation is not required. For fractious animals, xylazine (0.05–0.1 mg/kg) or detomidine (10 μg/kg), intravenously, is recommended.[40] Calves can be examined standing or restrained in lateral recumbency.

To optimize coupling, the region of interest, especially on the limbs, is carefully clipped, washed, and cleaned with alcohol, and a liberal amount of transmission gel is applied to the skin and transducer. Penetration of the ultrasound waves can be substantially impaired by surfaces with crusts, calluses, and scars.

METHOD OF ULTRASONOGRAPHIC EXAMINATION

A 7.5 MHz linear transducer is recommended for examination of superficial structures of the musculoskeletal system that are up to approximately 6 cm from the skin surface. This frequency can also be used to examine all the joints of calves that are only a few weeks old. For evaluation of deeper structures or large swellings, a 5.0 or 3.5 MHz convex or sector transducer is advised because of the greater depth of penetration.[1–21,27,29,30,32,40,41] These latter frequencies are required for assessment of thick muscle bellies in the trunk, the hip, thigh, and shoulder region in adult cattle and severe swelling anywhere on the limb.[29,30,42]

Ultrasonographic evaluation of healthy joints in the distal limb can be problematic because of a paucity of soft tissue and the uneven limb surface, which tends to prevent good contact between the transducer and skin.[11,40] Imaging can be improved by using a silicone stand-off pad in these areas. However, this aid is usually not required for evaluation of prominent localized swelling and is never needed for the examination of healthy or diseased regions proximal to the carpus or tarsus. Linear transducers provide images that are geometrically accurate, whereas convex and sector transducers yield better images of deep layers and allow a better overview of proximal joints, large muscle bellies and large swellings.[29,30,41,42]

The examiner starts by obtaining a general overview of the affected region for orientation purposes. This is achieved by locating and imaging certain anatomic landmarks, such as bone surfaces, joint spaces, tendons, ligaments, or large blood vessels that are easy to identify because of their location, shape, or surface characteristics. Once the anatomic landmarks in the area of interest have been identified, one can search for pathologic changes.[8]

The transducer must always be placed perpendicular or parallel to the fiber direction when examining tendons and ligaments in transverse or longitudinal planes.[8–11,41] The region of interest (eg, the carpus) is examined longitudinally, transversely, and sometimes obliquely from all sides and from proximal to distal, cranial to caudal, dorsal to ventral, and medial to lateral. The entire length of ligaments, tendons, and tendon sheaths is examined, and all pouches of a joint (eg, dorsal, palmar) are inspected.

Just as the clinical examination follows a standardized systematic protocol, so should the ultrasonographic examination. This ensures that all anatomic structures in the region of interest are thoroughly inspected.[28,34]

The following criteria should be evaluated: the exact anatomic location of the lesion, the echogenicity; echo pattern; size; type of border of the lesion or cavity and of the soft tissue swelling; and the presence or absence of flow phenomena and of artifacts such as acoustic enhancement or acoustic shadowing.[8] Flow phenomena can be elicited by balloting or compressing a fluid-filled cavity manually or with the transducer.[8,34] The presence of flow phenomena indicates liquid content, which may be serous, serofibrinous, purulent, or hemorrhagic.[2,5–8,18,19] Absence of flow phenomena indicates a semisolid to solid content, such as fibrinous clotted exudate or clotted blood.[5–8,18,19,32] Flow phenomena can be elicited in joint recesses by passive flexion or extension of the joint.[9,10,34] Joints should be examined in the normal and flexed position to allow inspection of as much articular surface as possible and to detect possible subchondral lesions.[5,7,8] The size of distended synovial cavities, abscesses, and hematomas as well as the distance between the skin surface and lesion can be accurately measured using the electronic cursors (see below discussion on ultrasound-guided centesis); comparison with the contralateral normal extremity is recommended in difficult cases or cases of doubt. These measurements provide important information for subsequent centesis or surgery.[8]

Many large vessels, such as the medial and lateral saphenous artery and vein, and the median artery and vein, and smaller distal vessels can be examined ultrasonographically in cattle.[2,13,17,43] Transrectal ultrasonography can be used to assess the abdominal aorta and its branches.[42] Each vessel is evaluated along its course, noting pulsation of arteries, compressibility of veins and the presence of intraluminal thrombi, which are associated with loss of compressibility and increased intraluminal echogenicity.[3,13,17] Modern ultrasound machines also have built-in color Doppler capabilities for the evaluation of blood flow.[13,28]

Ultrasonographic Examination of Important Regions of the Musculoskeletal System

In principle, the region of interest and the anatomic structures within should always be viewed longitudinally and transversely in their entirety. However, for practical purposes, there are certain sonographic planes that facilitate orientation, making identification and evaluation of the region of interest easier for the sonographer.

Distal and proximal interphalangeal joints

The standard examination plane of choice is longitudinal, in which the transducer is placed over the dorsal pouches so that the bone contours of the first (P1), second (P2), and third (P3) phalanges, and each joint space in between, can be seen (**Figs. 1** and **2**).[4,11,40] The longitudinal plane produced by placing the transducer on the heel bulb or in the pastern region does not always provide good images for anatomic reasons (concave contour, skin folds).

Easily identifiable anatomic landmarks include the extensor process of P3; the joint spaces of proximal and distal interphalangeal joints; and the bone surfaces of P1 and P2.

Metacarpophalangeal or metatarsophalangeal joint

The longitudinal plane produced by placing the transducer over the dorsal recess (**Figs. 3** and **4A**), and the transverse plane with the transducer placed in the palmar or plantar aspect proximal to the sesamoid bones are the standard planes of choice. The latter enables simultaneous visualization of the digital flexor tendon sheath, the suspensory ligament branches (SLB), and the joint recess in the same plane (**Figs. 4B, 5–7**).[11,22] The collateral ligaments are best seen in the longitudinal plane with the transducer held parallel to the direction of the fibers, which run slightly obliquely (dorsoproximal to palmar distal or plantar distal).

Easily identifiable anatomic landmarks include the bone surfaces of P1 and the metacarpus or metatarsus; joint space; the condyles of the distal metacarpus or metatarsus with the sagittal ridge; and the cartilaginous growth plates in calves.

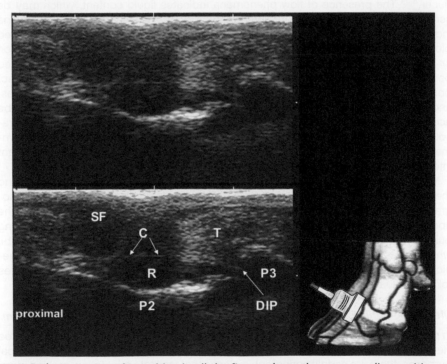

Fig. 1. Each anatomic probe position in all the figures shows the corresponding position of the probe in the standing animal. Longitudinal sonogram (7.5 MHz linear transducer) of the dorsal aspect of the left digital region showing the normal appearance of the distal interphalangeal joint (=DIP) in a 4-year-old Simmental cow. C, joint capsule; DIP, joint space between phalanx 2 (P2) and phalanx 3; P3, extensor process of phalanx 3; R, dorsal pouch of the DIP-joint showing the normal small amount of synovial fluid; SF, subcutaneous and fatty tissue; T, extensor tendon.

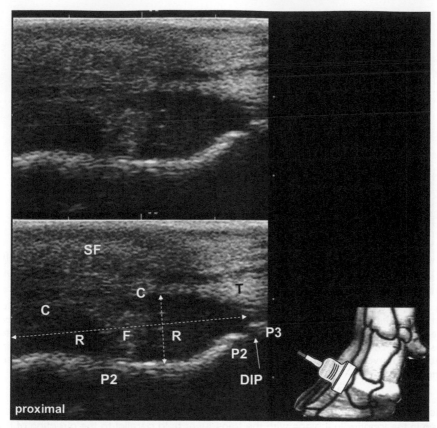

Fig. 2. Longitudinal sonogram (7.5 MHz linear transducer) of the dorsal aspect of the DIP-joint of the right forelimb showing a serofibrinous arthritis in a 3-year-old Simmental cow; capsule and dorsal border (C) of the distended dorsal joint pouch (R), which contains a predominantly anechoic effusion with a hypoechoic fibrin clot (F). The maximum dorso-palmar length of the pouch is 9 mm, the maximum proximo-distal length is 30.1 mm. Extensor tendon (T); joint space (DIP) between the extensor process of phalanx 3 (P3), and the articular surface of phalanx 2 (P2).

Tendons and ligaments of the metacarpus or metatarsus and digital flexor tendon sheath

The transverse plane is recommended for examination of these structures; the transducer is placed in a palmar or plantar position starting at the accessory carpal bone or tuber calcanei and then moved distally to view the superficial digital flexor tendon (SDFT), deep digital flexor tendon (DDFT), the branch of the suspensory ligament to the SDFT (BSL-S), the BSL-S, and the suspensory ligament (SL) with five branches and the entire digital flexor tendon sheaths of the medial and lateral digits to the pastern and heels (see **Figs. 4B, 5, 7, 8A, B and 9A, B**).[1,6,11,22]

Easily identifiable anatomic landmarks include the SDFT, DDFT, and the bone surfaces.

Carpal region

The transducer is placed over the dorsal aspect of the carpus at the distal radius in the longitudinal plane to view the individual joint recesses, which include the antebrachio-carpal (ABC), intercarpal (IC), and the carpometacarpal (CMC) joints (**Figs. 10, 11A–C,**

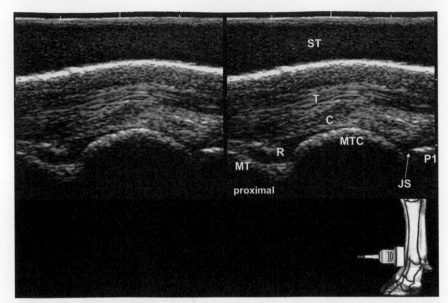

Fig. 3. Longitudinal sonogram (7.5 MHz linear transducer) showing the normal appearance of the dorsal aspect of the right metatarsophalangeal joint in a 4-year-old Simmental cow. C, echoic joint capsule (which lies directly on the articular surface); JS, joint space; MT, metatarsus; MTC, condyle of the metatarsus; P1, phalanx 1; R, dorsal pouch of the fetlock joint (showing the very small normal amount of synovial fluid); ST, stand-off pad; T, extensor tendon.

and **12A, B**). The lateral and medial collateral ligaments of the carpus are also best seen in the longitudinal plane with the transducer held parallel to the direction of the fibers. The plane of choice for evaluation of all tendons and tendon sheaths situated on the dorsal, dorsolateral, lateral, and palmar aspects of the carpus is the transverse plane,[10,15,18,25,27] (**Figs. 13B, C–15**) but they should be imaged in the longitudinal plane too (**Figs. 10–12A and 16**).

Easily identifiable anatomic landmarks include bone surfaces; joint spaces of the ABC, IC, and CMC joints; flexor and extensor tendons; and cartilaginous growth plates in calves.

Elbow region

The joint recess and collateral ligaments of the elbow are best viewed in the longitudinal plane with the transducer held on the lateral side immediately cranial or caudal to the lateral collateral ligament (**Fig. 17**) or precisely over the lateral or medial collateral ligaments.[5,7] In calves, the cranial aspect should also be scanned (**Fig. 18**).

Easily identifiable anatomic landmarks include bone surfaces, joint space, collateral ligaments, and cartilaginous epiphyseal and apophyseal growth plates in calves.

Shoulder region

The joint recess is best imaged in the longitudinal plane with the transducer placed over the craniolateral aspect in the region of the greater tubercle of the humerus (**Figs. 19–21**) or caudal to the insertion of the infraspinatus muscle.[23,29] The insertion of the infraspinatus muscle and its bursa are imaged best in both planes.

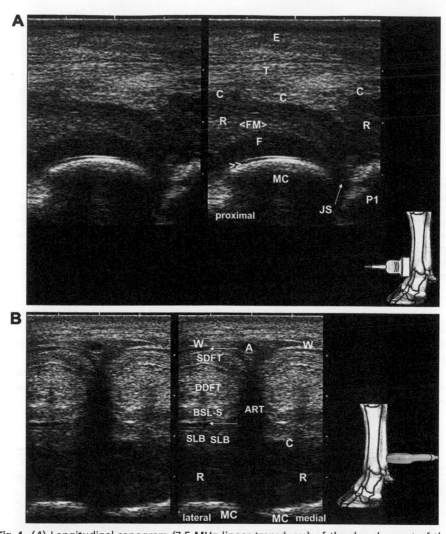

Fig. 4. (*A*) Longitudinal sonogram (7.5 MHz linear transducer) of the dorsal aspect of the metacarpophalangeal joint of the right, lateral digit with a septic, fibrinopurulent arthritis in a 3-year-old Simmental cow. Severely distended dorsal recess (R) of the fetlock joint containing anechoic fluid (F) and a large hypoechoic clotted fibrin mass (FM) dorsally in the pouch. Thin anechoic seam of the articular cartilage (*arrowheads*). C, joint capsule; E, subcutaneous inflammatory edema; JS, joint space; MC, convex condyle of the metacarpus; P1, phalanx 1 with irregular dorsal contour due to osteolysis; T, extensor tendon. (*B*) Transverse sonogram (7.5 MHz linear transducer) of the palmar aspect of the right metacarpal region of the cow in part *A* showing the normal appearance of the lateral and medial digital flexor tendon sheaths (DFTS) and the severely distended palmar pouch of the fetlock joint caused by fibrinopurulent arthritis. Small lumina of the normal DFTS compartments (*white arrows*). A, common digital palmar artery III; ART, edge shadowing artifact; BSL-S, branch of the suspensory ligament to the SDFT; C, palmar joint capsule of the fetlock joint; DDFT, deep digital flexor tendon; MC, plantar surface of the metacarpus; R, severely distended palmar recess of the fetlock joint containing mainly anechoic fluid; SDFT, superficial digital flexor tendon; SLB, suspensory ligament branches; W, wall of DFTS.

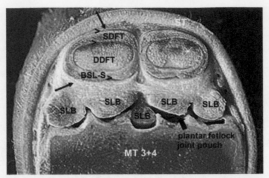

Fig. 5. Transverse anatomic section of a frozen specimen 2 cm proximal to the proximal sesamoid bones showing the lateral and medial digital flexor tendons and the DFTS compartments in an adult cow. Small, normal lumen (*arrowheads*) of the DFTS compartment; DFTS wall (*long black arrows*); metatarsus 3 and 4 (MT3+4);. BSL-S, branch of the suspensory ligament to the SDFT; DDFT, deep digital flexor tendon; SDFT, superficial digital flexor tendon; SLB, five suspensory ligament branches (which are less echoic than the flexor tendons).

The transverse plane is used to evaluate the tendon of the brachial biceps muscle and its bursa in the cranial shoulder region. The musculature of the scapula, which includes the supraspinatus and infraspinatus muscles, and the surface of the scapula are imaged in both planes.[44]

Easily identifiable anatomic landmarks include the greater tubercle, joint space, bicipital tendon, bone surface, and spine of the scapula; and cartilaginous epiphyseal and apophyseal growth plates in calves.

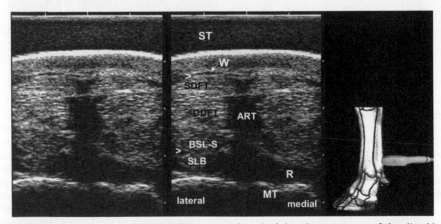

Fig. 6. Transverse sonogram (7.5 MHz linear transducer) of the plantar aspect of the distal left metatarsus showing the normal appearance of the lateral and medial DFTS, the digital flexor tendons and the plantar pouch of the fetlock joint in a 4-year-old Simmental cow. Small lumen of the DFTS compartments (*arrowheads*). ART, edge shadowing artifact; BSL-S, branch of the suspensory ligament to the superficial flexor tendon; DDFT, deep digital flexor tendon; MT, plantar surface of the metatarsus; R, normal plantar pouch of the fetlock joint; SDFT, superficial digital flexor tendon; SLB, abaxial branch of the suspensory ligament (which is less echoic than the flexor tendons); ST, stand-off pad; W, DFTS wall.

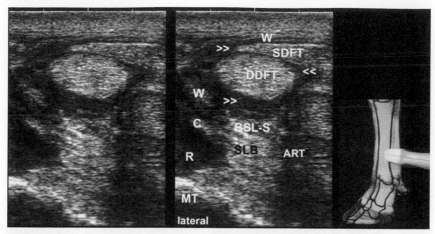

Fig. 7. Transverse sonogram (7.5 MHz linear transducer) of the plantar aspect of the distal right metatarsal region of a 19-month-old Charolais bull showing the lateral DFTS and the plantar pouch of the fetlock joint with serofibrinous arthritis and a concurrent septic serofibrinous tenosynovitis of the lateral DFTS. Distended compartments of DFTS with anechoic fluid (*arrowheads*). ART, edge shadowing artifact; BSL-S, branch of the suspensory ligament to the SDFT; DDFT, deep digital flexor tendon; MT, plantar surface of metatarsus; R, distended plantar recess of the fetlock joint with predominantly anechoic effusion; SDFT, superficial digital flexor tendon; SLB, abaxial branch of the suspensory ligament; W, DFTS wall.

Tarsal region

For imaging the four joint recesses of the tarsocrural joint, the transverse plane is used with the transducer placed on the dorsomedial and dorsolateral aspects and over the caudal pouches laterocaudally and mediocaudally, where the caudal contour of the tibia meets the cranial contour of the calcaneus (**Figs. 22, 23, 24**A, **25**B, C and

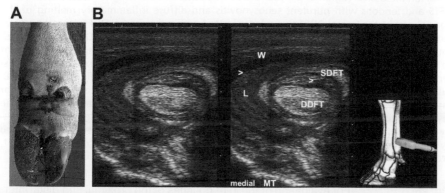

Fig. 8. (*A*) Septic fibrinous tenosynovitis of the medial DFTS of the left hindlimb in a 10-month-old Holstein-Friesian heifer; the causative puncture wound and the distension of the DFTS from the bulbs of the heels to the mid-metatarsus are apparent. (*B*) Transverse sonogram (7.5 MHz linear transducer) of the plantar aspect of the distal left metatarsal region of the heifer in **Fig. 8**A showing the medial DFTS with a septic, fibrinous tenosynovitis. Distended compartments of DFTS (*arrowhead*). L, severely distended lumen of DFTS with predominantly hypoechoic effusion; MT, plantar surface of the metatarsus; W, DFTS wall.

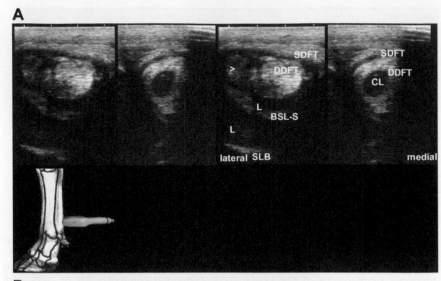

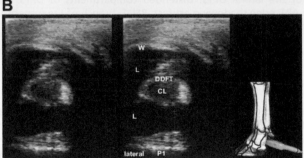

Fig. 9. (*A*) Transverse sonograms (7.5 MHz linear transducer) of the plantar aspect of the distal left metatarsal region of a 4-year-old Brown-Swiss cow showing the lateral and medial DFTS and tendons with purulent tenosynovitis and diffuse inflammatory melting of the abaxial part of the lateral DDFT and a "core lesion" within the medial DDFT caused by purulent inflammation of the tendinous tissue. Large lesion on the lateral DDFT (*arrowhead*) caused by purulent inflammation and necrosis. BSL-S, branch of the suspensory ligament to the SDFT; CL, core lesion within the medial DDFT; DDFT, deep digital flexor tendon; L, distended lumen of DFTS with heterogeneous fluid; SDFT, superficial digital flexor tendon; SLB, suspensory ligament. (*B*) Transverse sonogram (7.5 MHz linear transducer) of the plantar aspect of the lateral pastern region of the left hindlimb of patient of part *A* showing the severely distended distal compartment of the lateral DFTS with purulent tenosynovitis. Deep digital flexor tendon (DDFT) showing a centrally located "core lesion" (CL) caused by the purulent infection. L, distended lumen of DFTS with mainly anechoich effusion; P1, proximal phalanx.

Fig. 26).[5,7,8,16,19,21] For evaluation of the joint pouches of the proximal and distal intertarsal and tarsometatarsal joints and the collateral tarsal ligaments, the longitudinal plane with the transducer placed on the medial, dorsal or lateral sides (**Figs. 25D, E** and **Fig. 27**) has been described.[16,19] Tendons (extensor, flexor, and Achilles) and tendon sheaths (see **Figs. 22** and **25C, D**),[5,7,8,16,19,24] inflammation of the bursa subtendinea and bursa subcutanea calcanei and the bursa tarsalis lateralis should always be examined in both planes (see **Figs. 25C, D, 27** and **28A, B**).[16,19,27,45]

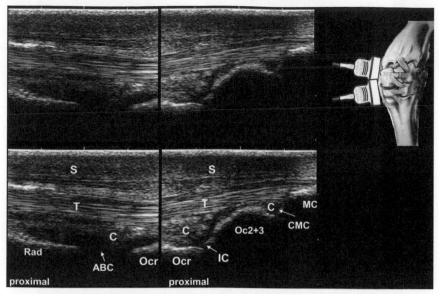

Fig. 10. Longitudinal sonogram (7.5 MHz linear transducer) of the dorsal aspect of the normal left carpus in a 4-year-old Simmental cow. Joint spaces of antebrachiocarpal (ABC), intercarpal (IC), and carpometacarpal (CMC) joints. C, joint capsules that are lying close to the articular surface; MC, surface of the metacarpus; Oc2+3, carpal bones 2+3; S, subcutis; Ocr, radial carpal bone; Rad, surface of the radius; T, extensor carpi radialis tendon with parallel fiber bundles.

Easily identifiable anatomic landmarks include bone surfaces; medial and lateral trochlear ridges of the talus; intertrochlear groove; joint spaces; extensor and flexor tendons; and cartilaginous epiphyseal and apophyseal growth plates in calves.

Stifle region
The longitudinal plane is the plane of choice for evaluation of the individual joint recesses, collateral ligaments, and the menisci. For imaging the femoropatellar joint, the transducer is placed cranial to the patella and moved from proximal to distal toward the tibial tuberosity (**Figs. 29** and **30**A). The distal sac of the lateral femorotibial joint in the sulcus extensorius on the lateral tibial tuberosity, with the tendons of origin of the extensor digitalis longus and fibularis tertius muscles, is best viewed in the transverse plane (**Fig. 30**B).[5,7,8,9,20] For evaluation of the medial and lateral femorotibial joints, the menisci and collateral ligaments, the transducer is placed on the medial-lateral aspect cranial or over the collateral ligaments in the longitudinal plane; this position allows visualization of the joint pouches; proximal and distal bone contours; the joint space in between; and the menisci as echoic triangular structures (**Figs. 31** and **32**A, B). The medial meniscus is easy to image, but the lateral meniscus is somewhat more difficult to visualize because it is situated farther from the skin surface.

Easily identifiable anatomic landmarks include bone surfaces of the patella, femur, and tibia; medial and lateral trochlear ridges of the femur; intertrochlear groove; tibial tuberosity; joint spaces; and cartilaginous epiphyseal and apophyseal growth plates in calves.

Coxofemoral joint and pelvis
The oblique longitudinal plane along the femoral neck axis is best suited for evaluation of the coxofemoral joint. The transducer is placed on the trochanter major and moved

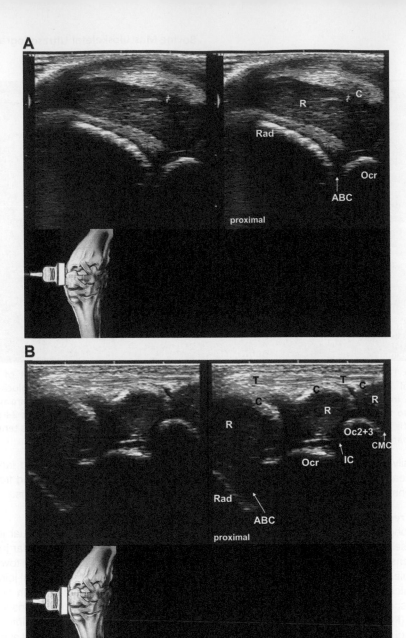

Fig. 11. (*A*) Longitudinal sonogram (7.5 MHz linear transducer) of the dorsal aspect of the left carpus of an 8-week-old Simmental calf with septic, fibrinous arthritis of the antebrachiocarpal (ABC) joint; distended joint recess (R) with heterogeneous hypoechoic effusion without acoustic enhancement and without flow-phenomena. ABC, joint space of ABC-joint; C, joint capsule; Ocr, radial carpal bone; Rad, surface of radius. (*B*) Longitudinal sonogram (7.5 MHz linear transducer) of the dorsal aspect of the left carpus of the calf in **Fig. 11**A with all 3 carpal joints. Joint spaces of ABC, IC, and CMC joints. C, joint capsule; R, distended joint recesses; Oc2+3, carpal bones 2+3; Ocr, radial carpal bone; Rad, surface of radius; T, extensor carpi radialis tendon. (*C*) Longitudinal sonogram (7.5 MHz linear transducer) of the dorsal aspect of the left carpus of the calf in **Fig. 11**A showing the flexed ABC-joint with septic fibrinous arthritis. ABC, joint space; BO, subchondral bone osteolysis with a bone fragment; C, joint capsule; Ocr, radial carpal bone; R, distended recess of ABC-joint; Rad, surface of radius; T, extensor carpi radialis tendon.

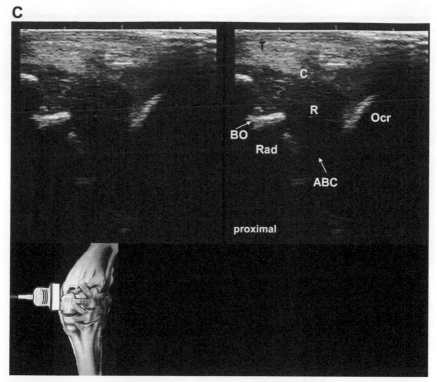

Fig. 11. (*continued*)

craniomedially toward the point where a line drawn between the two tuber coxae intersects the longitudinal axis of the vertebral column. This allows assessment of the trochanter major; femoral neck and head; coxofemoral joint space; joint capsule; and the surface of the acetabulum (**Figs. 33–35**). In adult cattle, a 3.5 MHz convex or sector transducer is required to image the coxofemoral joint because it is usually 12 to 18 cm from the skin surface.[30,42]

Transrectal ultrasonography using a multifrequency rectal transducer (4–8 MHz) allows evaluation of the entire bony pelvic girdle; the ventral aspect of the caudal lumbar vertebrae and sacrum; the iliosacral joints; and the abdominal aorta and its proximal branches.[42]

Easily identifiable anatomic landmarks include trochanter major; surfaces of femoral neck and head; cartilaginous epiphyseal and apophyseal growth plates in calves; outer and inner surfaces of the pelvic bones; and vertebrae and abdominal aorta.

ULTRASONOGRAPHIC APPEARANCE OF NORMAL STRUCTURES OF THE MUSCULOSKELETAL SYSTEM
Joints and Bones

Anatomy
Joints are formed by the union of two or more bones, which are covered with hyaline cartilage forming the joint space, a fibrous joint capsule that is closely associated with the joint surfaces, a joint cavity that usually has one or multiple recesses, and the joint ligaments.[46] The interphalangeal, elbow, and shoulder joints have dorsal and palmar or plantar or cranial and caudal recesses. The palmar or plantar recesses of the

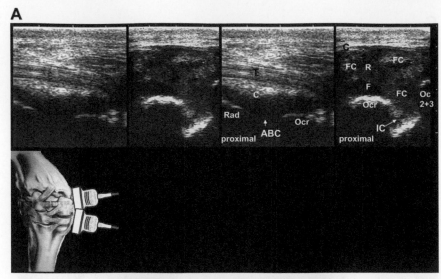

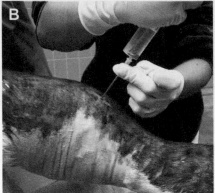

Fig. 12. (*A*) Longitudinal sonograms (7.5 MHz linear transducer) of the dorsal aspect of the right carpus of a 9-month-old bull calf with a normal ABC-joint and a serofibrinous arthritis of the IC-joint. Distended joint recess (R) of the IC-joint with predominantly hypoechoic, clotted fibrin masses (FC) and a small amount of anechoic fluid (F). Joint spaces of ABC and IC joint. C, joint capsule; Oc2+3, carpal bones 2+3; Ocr, radial carpal bone; Rad, surface of radius; T, extensor carpi radialis tendon. (*B*) Arthrocentesis and aspiration of a small amount of inflammatory exudate from the intercarpal joint seen in **Fig. 12A**. The needle was placed in this seldom-used lateral position for centesis after ultrasonographic inspection and detection of fluid accumulation within the joint pouch in this area.

interphalangeal joints are immediately dorsal to the digital flexor tendon sheath. Large composite joints, such as the carpal, tarsal, and stifle joints have recesses for each individual joint; these may communicate with each other or be completely separate, and their size varies greatly depending on the degree of mobility of the joint.[46]

Normal ultrasonographic appearance
The anatomic landmarks for ultrasonographic examination of joints have been listed. In young cattle, the cartilaginous growth plates of long bones and the apophyseal growth plates of the olecranon, the greater tubercle of the humerus, calcaneus, tibial tuberosity, and trochanter major are easily identified and appear as short anechoic

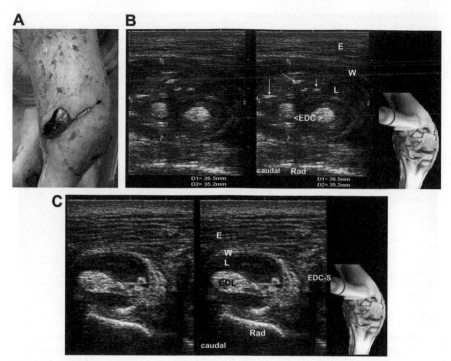

Fig. 13. (A) The right carpus of a 5-year-old Simmental cow with septic, fibrinopurulent teno-synovitis of the tendon sheaths of the lateral and common digital extensor tendons caused by a penetrating laceration wound 10 days before sonography. (B) Transverse sonogram (7.5 MHz linear transducer) of the laterodorsal aspect of the right carpal region of the cow in **Fig. 13**A with fibrinopurulent inflammation of the tendon sheath of the common digital extensor tendon. Severely distended tendon sheath lumen (L) with heterogeneous hypo-echoic effusion and small echoic particles (*arrows*). The diameters of the distended tendon sheath were 26.5 mm and 35.2 mm; common digital extensor tendon (<EDC>) composed of two branches within the tendon sheath. E, subcutaneous edema; Rad, surface of radius; W, wall of the tendon sheath. (C) Transverse sonogram (7.5 MHz linear transducer) of the lateral aspect of the right carpal region of the cow in **Fig. 13**A with fibrinopurulent tenosynovitis of the lateral digital extensor tendon sheath. E, inflammatory subcutaneous edema; EDC-S, tendon sheath of the adjoining common digital extensor tendon; EDL, lateral digital extensor tendon; L, severely distended lumen with heterogeneous hypoechoic effusion; Rad, surface of radius; W, wall of the tendon sheath.

interruptions of the hyperechoic bone surface in the longitudinal plane (see **Figs. 33** and **34**).[5,7,8,9,10,20,25,29,42]

In an ideal situation, the bones forming the joint, joint space, cartilage, ligaments (collateral, patellar), periarticular tendons, and large blood vessels can be visualized in healthy cattle. Passive flexion and extension of the joint allows evaluation of joint mobility and visual assessment of a maximum amount of the articular surface (see **Fig. 11**C).[4,5,7,8,11,18,19,20,47,48,49] In some joints, the hyaline cartilage appears as a delicate anechoic seam on the hyperechoic bone surface when the ultrasound beam is aimed perpendicularly. Visualization of the articular cartilage depends on its thickness, the age of the patient, and the resolution capacity of the ultrasound machine. In adult cattle, the noncalcified layer of hyaline cartilage is 1 to 2 mm thick or less (see **Figs. 4**A, **19, 21,** and **29**).[9,42,46,50] In one- to six-week-old calves, the joint cartilage may be 6 to 10 mm

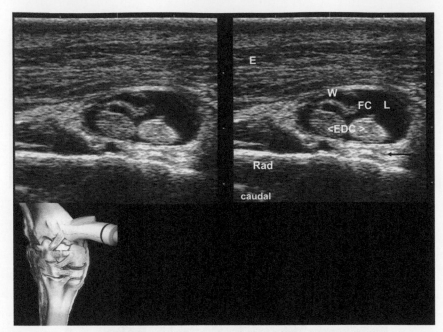

Fig.14. Transverse sonogram (7.5 MHz linear transducer) of the laterodorsal lateral aspect of the right carpal region of a 5-year-old Simmental cow with septic serous inflammation of the common digital extensor tendon sheath caused by a hematogenous infection (polysynovitis; traumatic reticuloperitonitis). Severely distended lumen (L) with anechoic fluid. Acoustic enhancement (*arrow*) and flow-phenomena with a floating fibrin clot (*FC*) were visible. E, inflammatory subcutaneous edema; EDC, common digital extensor tendon with its two branches; Rad: surface of radius; W, tendon sheath wall.

thick and appears homogeneously hypoechoic with small pinpoint anechoic and mildly echoic areas (see **Fig. 34**).[16,29,42] The same applies to the thick cartilage layer on the apophyses (trochanter major, tibial tuberosity; see **Fig. 33**).[9,16,29,42] The increased cartilage thickness in very young calves may be easily mistaken for pathologic synovial fluid. However, cartilage does not yield under pressure and produces no flow phenomena. In doubtful cases, the contralateral limb should be examined for comparison.

In the longitudinal plane, the joint spaces of all joints appear as a short interruptions in the hyperechoic bone surfaces or are funnel-shaped because of the slightly inward curved contours of the joint-forming bones (see **Figs. 1–4**A, **10–12**A, **16–21**, **25**E, **26**, **27, 31, 32**B, and **33–35**, **Table 1**).[9,10,11,16,18,19,25,29,42] With concave or convex bone or joint surfaces, or by directing the ultrasound beam tangentially, artifacts that look like subchondral lesions (see **Figs. 22, 23**, and **24**A) may be produced because the waves are not reflected sufficiently.[47]

The joint capsule appears as a thin echoic structure that lies close to the articular surface in healthy joints, and is rather difficult to differentiate from the adjoining soft tissue owing to the similar echogenicity (see **Figs. 1–3, 10, 19, 22, 29, 33**, and **34**).[5,8,9,10,11,16,25,29,42] Because the normal amount of synovial fluid is small, ultrasonographic visualization of healthy joint pouches is limited in general (see **Figs. 1, 3, 10, 17, 19, 22, 29, 33**, and **34**, see **Table 1** and **2**).[5,11,16,47,51] The recesses of the normal interphalangeal and fetlock joints usually cannot be imaged. However, sometimes a small part of the dorsal or palmar, or plantar pouches of these digital joints can be

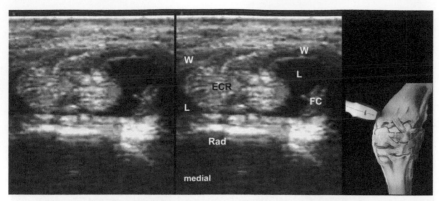

Fig. 15. Transverse sonogram (7.5 MHz linear transducer) of the dorsal aspect of the left distal antebrachial region showing the tendon and tendon sheath of the extensor carpi radialis muscle with a chronic, serous, aseptic tenosynovitis in a 3-year-old Simmental cow. ECR, extensor carpi radialis tendon; FC, hypoechoic fibrin clot within the tendon sheath cavity; L, severely distended lumen with anechoic fluid; Rad, surface of radius; W, tendon sheath wall.

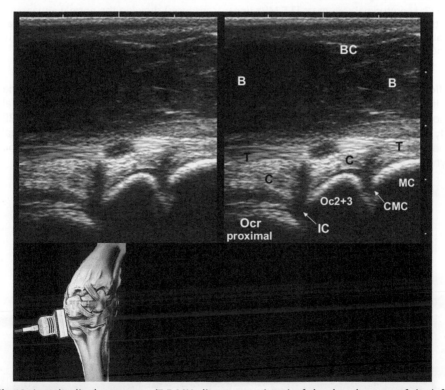

Fig. 16. Longitudinal sonogram (7.5 MHz linear transducer) of the dorsal aspect of the left carpal region showing normal intercarpal and carpometacarpal joints and a purulent carpal hygroma (bursitis) in a 4-week-old Simmental calf. Severely distended bursal cavity (B) with mainly anechoic effusion proximally and heterogeneous hypoechoic exudate distally. Joint space of IC and CMC joints, and Oc2+3 carpal bones. BC, capsule of the bursa; C, joint capsule in direct contact with the articular surface; MC, surface of the proximal metacarpus; Ocr, radial carpal bone; T, extensor carpi radialis tendon.

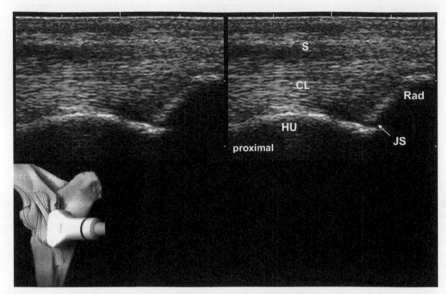

Fig. 17. Longitudinal sonogram (7.5 MHz linear transducer) showing the normal appearance of the lateral aspect of the left elbow joint in a 4-year-old Simmental cow. CL, lateral collateral ligament with the parallel fiber bundles; HU, humeral surface; JS, joint space of the elbow joint; Rad, surface of radius with the insertion site of the lateral CL; S, subcutis.

differentiated in both planes; it appears as a narrow, up to 2 mm wide anechoic zone, indicating synovial fluid (see **Figs. 1, 3,** and **6**).[11] The recesses of the hip, stifle, tarsal, shoulder, elbow, and carpal joints can not be differentiated (see **Figs. 10, 17, 19, 29, 31, 33,** and **34**), although part of a pouch may sometimes be imaged as a small anechoic area. This is because no amount or only a small normal amount of anechoic synovial fluid can be seen at the level of the joint space.[9,10,11,16,20,25,29,42]

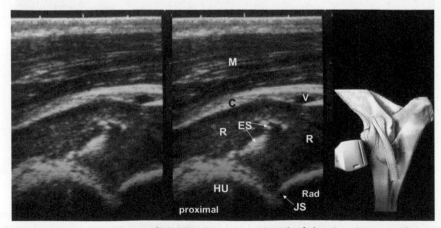

Fig. 18. Longitudinal sonogram (7.5 MHz linear transducer) of the dorsal aspect of the left elbow joint of a 4-week-old Simmental calf with a septic fibrinopurulent arthritis. Severely distended dorsal pouch (R) with heterogeneous hypoechoic effusion and small echoic spots (ES). C, joint capsule; HU, convex surface of the humeral condyle; JS, joint space of the elbow joint; M, biceps brachii muscle; Rad, surface of radius; V, blood vessel.

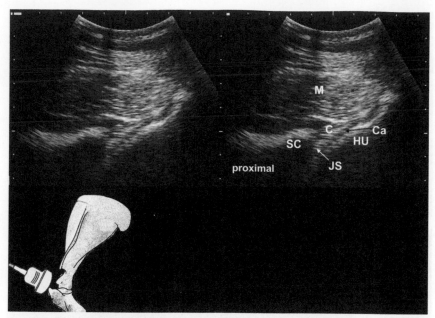

Fig. 19. Longitudinal sonogram (4 MHz convex transducer) showing the normal appearance of the craniolateral aspect of the right scapulohumeral joint of a 4-year-old Simmental cow. C, the joint capsule lies directly on the articular surface; Ca, small anechoic band of the articular cartilage; HU, humeral surface; JS, joint space of the scapulohumeral joint; M, supraspinatus muscle; SC, surface of scapula.

Tendon Sheaths, Bursae, Tendons, and Ligaments

Anatomy

Tendon sheaths contain synovia and are tube-like structures that guide extensor and flexor tendons as they change direction or over hard surfaces, for example in the digital, carpal, and tarsal regions.[46] The walls of tendon sheaths are structurally the same as joint capsules.

Tendons and ligaments consist of bundles of fibers arranged parallel to one another. The digital flexor tendon sheath of the superficial and deep flexor tendons extends from the lower third of the metacarpal or metatarsal bone to slightly proximal to the distal sesamoid bone, and does not communicate with the tendon sheath of the adjacent digit.[52] The unique anatomic arrangement of the tendons within this sheath gives rise to spatial divisions consisting of an inner and outer proximal compartment (see **Fig. 5**) and a distal compartment distal to the dewclaws. The inner proximal compartment envelops the DDFT proximal to the dewclaws, and is bordered by the superficial flexor tendon and the BSL-S (manica flexoria). The outer proximal compartment surrounds the manica flexoria and has a palmar or plantar and a dorsal cavity.[46,52] Along the metacarpal or metatarsal bone the SL divides into five branches (see **Fig. 5**), four of which insert on the proximal sesamoid bones. It is composed almost entirely of muscle fibers in young cattle but becomes ligamentous with age.[46] The extensor tendons originate from muscles located dorsal or lateral on the radius, humerus, femur, and tibia; and travel within tendon sheaths over the carpus or tarsus. The common and lateral extensor tendons insert dorsally on P3.

Bursae are fluid-filled encapsulated sacs within loose connective tissue and act as cushions between bone and tightly associated tendons and ligaments, or between

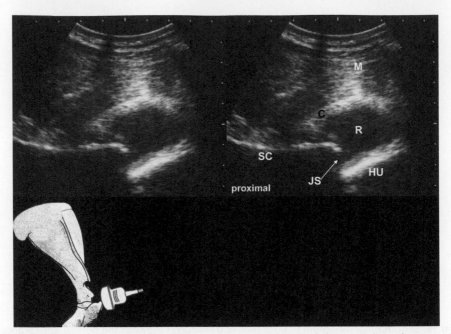

Fig. 20. Longitudinal sonogram (3.5 MHz convex transducer) of the craniolateral aspect of the right scapulohumeral joint of a 2.5-year-old Simmental cow with fibrinopurulent arthritis. The joint capsule (C) is severely distended because of marked heterogeneous hypo-echoic effusion in the joint recess (R). HU, humeral surface; JS, joint space of the scapulo-humeral joint; M, supraspinatus muscle; SC, hyperechoic surface of the scapula and HU.

bone and skin.[46] A bursa is interposed between the tendon of the biceps femoris muscle and the lateral femoral condyle. The bursa calcanea subcutanea is located between the skin and SDFT and the bursa calcanea subtendinea lies between the SDFT and the tuber calcanei. The bicipital bursa (bursa intertubercularis) at the cranial aspect of the shoulder cushions the tendon of the biceps brachii muscle, and a bursa is interposed between the tendon of the infraspinatus muscle and the lateral part of the greater tubercle of the humerus. Reactive (trauma-induced) bursae in the subcutis may be caused by excessive pressure on the dorsal aspect of the carpus (carpal hygroma) or lateral aspect of the tarsus (bursitis tarsalis lateralis).[46]

Normal ultrasonographic appearance

Tendons and ligaments appear as homogeneous echoic structures of varying sizes. They are round to ovoid or ring-shaped (manica flexoria) in cross section, and longitu-dinally, they have a strong linear and parallel fiber arrangement (see **Figs. 3, 4**B, **6, 7, 8**B, **10, 13**B–**17, 22, 25**C, D, **28**A, **29,** and **30**A, B, see **Table 1**).[1,6,9,10,11,22,25,47,53,54,55] The transducer must be held parallel or perpendicular to the direction of fibers for optimal longitudinal or transverse images. This is critical to avoid artifacts[41,53] in pla-ces where tendons have a curved rather than a straight course (see **Fig. 25**D). In contrast to the flexor tendons, the SL is slightly less echoic because of its connective tissue and muscle tissue content (see **Figs. 4**B and **6**).[6,22] The extensor tendons have the same echogenicity as the flexor tendons, but are considerably smaller in cross section (see **Figs. 3, 10,** and **16**).[3,10,25,40] The collateral ligaments of the fetlock, carpal,

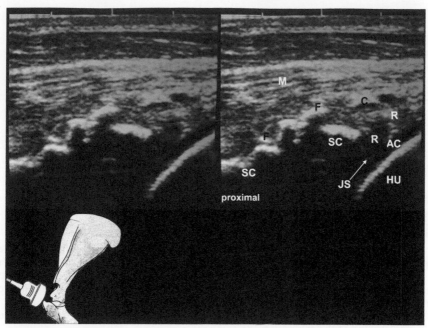

Fig. 21. Longitudinal sonogram (7.5 MHz linear transducer) of the craniolateral aspect of the left scapulohumeral joint of a 10-week-old Simmental calf with serofibrinous arthritis, osteitis, and osteomyelitis of the distal scapula. Distended joint recess (R), anechoic articular cartilage (AC) covering the humeral head (HU). Irregular rough surface of the scapula (SC) with small bone fragments (F) indicating osteolysis and periosteal proliferation. C, joint capsule; JS, joint space; M, supraspinatus muscle.

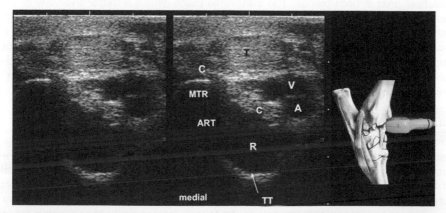

Fig. 22. Transverse sonogram (7.5 MHz linear transducer) of the dorsal aspect of the left tarsocrural joint showing the normal appearance of the dorsomedial joint pouch in a 4-year-old Simmental cow. A, dorsal pedal artery; ART, artifact (this part of the bone contour of the talus cannot be imaged because of its parallel position to the ultrasound waves); C, joint capsule; MTR, medial ridge of the talus; R, recess with normal amount of anechoic synovial fluid; T, tendon of insertion of fibularis tertius muscle; TT, concave contour of the trochlea tali; V, dorsal pedal vein.

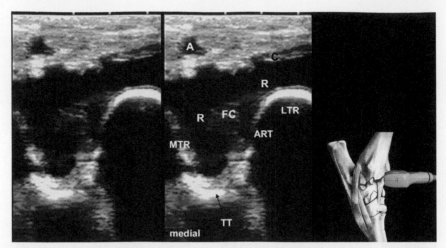

Fig. 23. Transverse sonogram (7.5 MHz linear transducer) of the dorsal aspect of the left tarsocrural joint showing the dorsal joint pouch with septic serofibrinous arthritis (polyarthritis) in a 3-month-old Simmental calf. Severely distended joint recess (R) with anechoic effusion and acoustic enhancement indicated by the broad hyperechoic band of reflection from the lateral ridge of the talus and the trochlea tali (TT). ART is the same artifact as in **Fig. 22**. A, dorsal pedal artery; C, joint capsule; FC, fibrin clot; LTR, lateral ridge of the talus; MTR, medial ridge of the talus.

elbow, tarsal, and stifle joints are echoic and the parallel fiber arrangement is apparent in the longitudinal plane (**Figs. 17, 27, 31,** and **32**B).[9,10,16,20,25]

Tendon sheaths
Normally, the lumina and borders of the individual compartments of the digital flexor tendon sheath cannot be visualized (see **Figs. 4**B and **6**) with the exception of the dorsal part of the outer proximal compartment, which appears as a narrow ($\leq$ 2 mm) anechoic area in both planes. The transverse plane allows a better overview of the tendon sheath. Furthermore, the directly adjoining tendon sheath of the other digit can be visualized simultaneously for comparison, provided the linear transducer is long enough. Ultrasonographic studies of the normal tendon sheaths over the carpus and tarsus have shown that their lumina and walls are extremely difficult or impossible to visualize (see **Figs. 10** and **22**) because of the small amount of synovia.[2,5,10,16,25] This also applies to the previously mentioned bursae.[9,16,29]

Muscles

Anatomy
Large muscle groups are associated with the passive musculoskeletal system in the proximal limb and trunk. Skeletal muscles are well-delineated organs, which consist of the tendons of origin, muscle belly, and tendons of insertion. The muscle fibers run longitudinally and parallel to each other within the muscle belly and, in many, muscles are accompanied by muscle septa. Muscle fasciae are tight connective tissue layers of varying thickness that surround individual muscles or divide into various leaves that run between the muscles as muscle septa.[46]

Normal ultrasonographic appearance
When viewed longitudinally, muscles are less hypoechoic with characteristic echoic to hyperechoic branching caused by the muscle septa. In the transverse plane, the septa

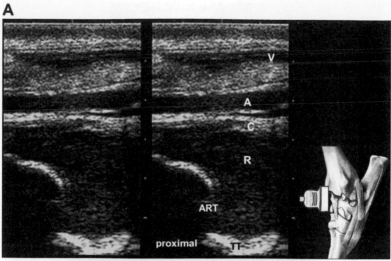

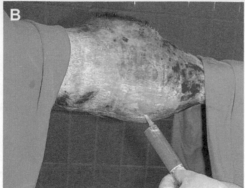

Fig. 24. (*A*) Longitudinal sonogram (7.5 MHz linear transducer) of the dorsal aspect of the left tarsocrural joint showing the dorsal joint pouch with septic, serous arthritis in a 3-year-old Simmental cow. Distended dorsal joint recess (R) with acoustic enhancement indicated by the broad hyperechoic band of reflection from the trochlea tali (TT). ART is the same artifact as in **Fig. 22**. A, dorsal pedal artery; C, joint capsule; V, dorsal pedal vein. (*B*) Dorsal view of the left tarsus (same cow as in **Fig. 24**A) showing arthrocentesis and aspiration of abnormal synovial fluid from the dorsomedial pouch of the tarsocrural joint with septic, serous arthritis. The aspirated sample is a yellow, turbid liquid containing small fibrinous floccules.

appear as small, irregular pinpoints with echoic to hyperechoic reflections (see **Figs. 18–21** and **33–35, Table 1**). Muscle fasciae appear as hyperechoic lines of varying width. The transition from muscle to tendinous insertion is characterized by an increase in echogenicity. Several septa and fasciae converge from various directions to form the echoic and parallel tendon fiber arrangement.[10,25,29,47,55,56,57,58,59]

ULTRASONOGRAPHIC FINDINGS IN MUSCULOSKELETAL DISORDERS

Fluid is the ideal transmission medium for ultrasound waves and is responsible for differences in acoustic impedance, which is a prerequisite for the differentiation of

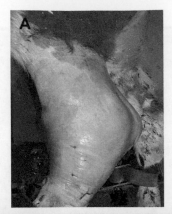

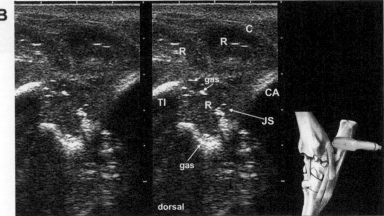

Fig. 25. (*A*) Dorsolateral view of the left tarsus of a 12-week-old Simmental calf with puru-lent arthritis of the tarsocrural, intertarsal and the tarsometatarsal joints caused by a pene-trating wound on the dorsomedial aspect. The dorsal and caudal joint pouches are easy to recognize because of severe effusion. (*B*) Transverse sonogram (7.5 MHz linear transducer) of the laterocaudal aspect of the left tarsocrural joint of the calf in **Fig. 25**A showing puru-lent exudate in the laterocaudal joint pouch. Severely distended joint recess (R) in the triangle between the hyperechoic tibial surface (TI) cranially and the hyperechoic calcaneal surface (CA) caudally. The joint recess is filled with a heterogeneous, mainly hypoechoic effusion and some large and small gas bubbles. C, joint capsule; JS, joint space. (*C*) Trans-verse sonogram (7.5 MHz linear transducer) of the mediocaudal aspect of the left tarsus of the calf in **Fig. 25**A showing the mediocaudal joint pouch of the tarsocrural joint and the directly adjoining tarsal flexor tendon sheath with purulent arthritis and tenosynovitis. Distended joint recess (R), DDFT, and flexor hallucis longus tendon. Large gas accumulation. A, saphenous artery; C, joint capsule; L, distended lumen of the tendon sheath; W, wall of tendon sheath. (*D*) Longitudinal sonogram (7.5 MHz linear transducer) of the same region as in **Fig. 25** C. DDFT and flexor hallucis longus tendon with the parallel fiber bundles. Large gas accumulation within the joint pouch with artifacts distal to the gas that impedes imaging of the synovial effusion. L, distended lumen of tendon sheath; R, distended joint recess; W, wall of tendon sheath. (*E*) Longitudinal sonogram (7.5 MHz linear transducer) of the lateral aspect of the left tarsus of the calf in **Fig. 25**A showing the joint pouch of the tarsometatarsal joint distended with purulent effusion. Distended joint pouch (R) with heterogeneous effu-sion. C, joint capsule; MT, metatarsal surface; Otc, centroquartal tarsal bone; TMT, joint space of the tarsometatarsal joint.

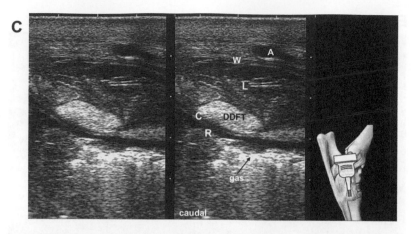

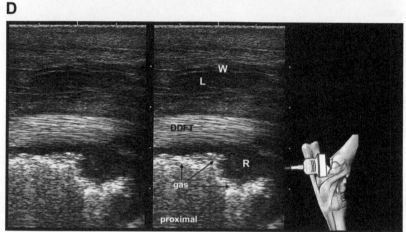

Fig. 25. (*continued*)

tissues. Fluid also improves the propagation of sound waves.[41] Inflammatory (septic) processes are especially suited to ultrasonography because of the accumulation of fluid in the tissues during the exudative phase.[60] In cattle, septic disorders of the musculoskeletal system are common. Traumatic soft tissue swellings and delayed wound healing are other indications for ultrasonography.[2,3,5,6,7,18,19,49,51,61] Radiography often provides little useful information in the early stages of septic processes because only soft tissues are affected.[5,33,34,39] The ultrasonographic findings are very similar for all inflamed synovial cavities; thus, they will be discussed as one.

Arthritis, Tenosynovitis, and Bursitis

Septic disorders of synovial cavities may be caused by direct infection from a puncture wound, from an adjacent septic process, or from hematogenous spread of infection (see **Figs. 8**A, **12**B, **13**A, **24**B, and **25**A).[35,62] Traumatic arthritis usually affects large joints and is often associated with tearing or rupture of the joint capsule, collateral ligaments, or cruciate ligaments; and luxation or subluxation.[30,33,36,51,62] The most commonly affected tendon sheath in cattle is the digital flexor tendon sheath of the hind limbs.[1,6,52,63,64,65]

E

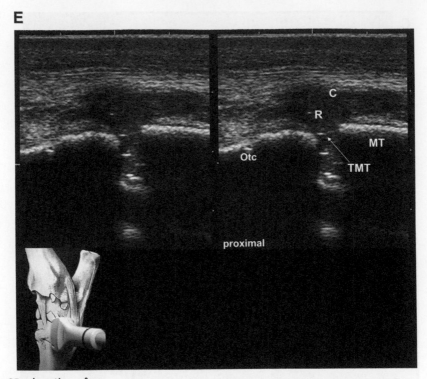

Fig. 25. (*continued*)

The increased volume of synovial fluid (effusion) can be reliably detected using ultrasonography.[1,2,4,5,6,7,8,11,16,18,19,20,21,23,24,27,47,48,49,51,66] The diseased synovial cavity (joint recess, tendon sheath, bursa) appears as a mildly to severely dilated cavity at the expected location with a thin echoic capsule or wall, which is distinctly displaced from the articular surface by 6 to 42 mm (see **Figs. 2, 4**A, B, **11**A, B, C, **12**A, **18, 20, 21, 23, 24**A, **25** B, C, E, **26, 30**A, B, **32**A, B, and **35**, see **Table 2**). The echogenicity of the effusion ranges from anechoic to echoic depending on its nature (serous, serofibrinous, fibrinous, purulent; **Table 3**). Anechoic or hypoechoic content allows good differentiation of the synovial cavity from surrounding tissues (see **Figs. 4**A, B, **11**A, B, C, **20, 24**A, **26, 30**A, B, and **32**A, B), which are generally echoic, whereas echoic content does not (see **Figs. 21, 25**B). Liquid content can be identified based on flow phenomena, which are characterized by small and large hypoechoic to echoic particles, or clots that are set in motion and are seen floating in the anechoic fluid (see **Figs. 4**A, **12**A, **18, 23, 25**B, C, **30**B, and **35**).[1,2,4,5,6,7,8,18,19,21,27,47,66] In longstanding cases of septic inflammation, large amounts of fibrinogen are present in the synovial fluid, and the precipitated gelatinous masses of fibrin impair or prevent aspiration of fluid. In sonograms, these semisolid masses appear hypoechoic to echoic, depending on the duration of the disease (see **Figs. 11**A–C, and **26**). Although it may be possible to compress these masses, they show no flow phenomena.[1,2,4,5,6,7,8,18,19,27] The ability to differentiate the content of fluid-filled cavities from the surrounding echoic soft tissues depends on the density and cellular content, and echogenicity of the inflammatory exudate (see **Figs. 2, 4**A, B, **11**A, B, C, **12**A, **18, 20, 21, 23, 24**A, **25** B, C, E, **26, 30**A, B, **32**A, B, and **35**).[5,6,7,18,19]

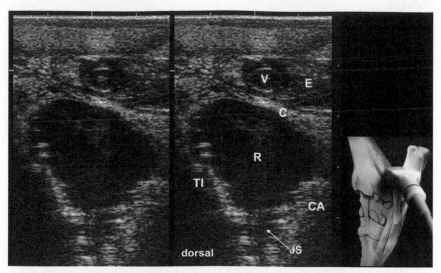

Fig. 26. Transverse sonogram (7.5 MHz linear transducer) of the laterocaudal aspect of the left tarsocrural joint of a 5-year-old Simmental cow with septic fibrinous arthritis of the laterocaudal joint pouch and vein thrombosis. Distended joint recess (R) with mainly hypoechoic effusion without acoustic enhancement and without flow-phenomena indicating a fibrinous exudate. C, joint capsule; CA, calcaneal surface; E, subcutaneous inflammatory edema; JS, joint space; TI, tibial surface; V, dilated venous lumen filled with a hypoechoic thrombus.

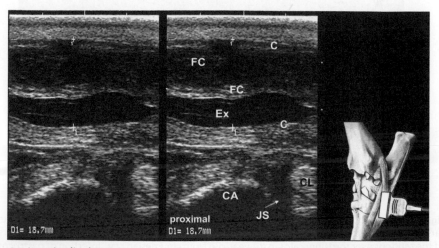

Fig. 27. Longitudinal sonogram (7.5 MHz linear transducer) of the lateral aspect of the tarsus showing septic serofibrinous bursitis (bursitis tarsalis lateralis) in a 6-year-old Holstein-Friesian cow. The bursa is filled with fibrin clots (FC) and anechoic serous exudate (Ex). The lateromedial width of the distended bursa (D1) was 18.7 mm. C, capsule of bursa; CA, bone surface of the distal calcaneus; CL, lateral collateral ligament; JS, joint space between the calcaneus and the centroquartal tarsal bone.

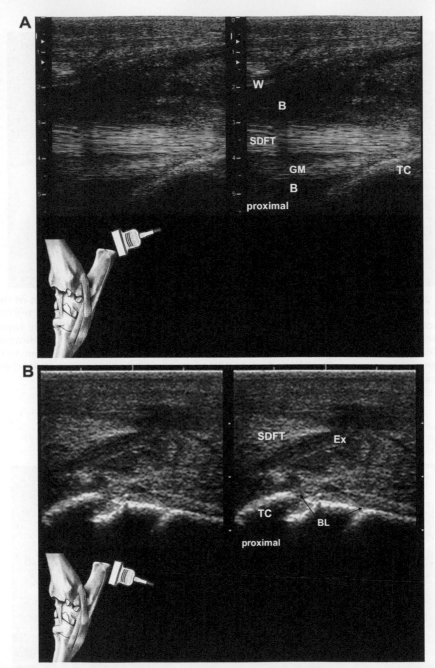

Fig. 28. (*A*) Longitudinal sonogram (7.5 MHz linear transducer) of the caudal aspect of the left tarsus showing septic fibrinous inflammation of the bursa subtendinea calcanei and the course of the tendons over the tuber calcis in a 4-year-old Holstein-Friesian cow. Insertion of gastrocnemius tendon (GM) at the tuber calcis (TC). B, distended bursal cavity with hypoechoic effusion; SDFT, superficial digital flexor tendon; W, wall of the bursa. (*B*) Longitudinal sonogram (7.5 MHz linear transducer) of the caudal aspect of the left tarsus showing septic fibrinous inflammation the bursa subtendinea calcanei and the course of the SDFT over the tuber calcis in the cow of **Fig. 28**A. BL, lysis of the fibrocartilage and surface of the tuber calcis; Ex, fibrinous exudate and destruction of the tendon fibers; SDFT, superficial digital flexor tendon; TC, tuber calcis.

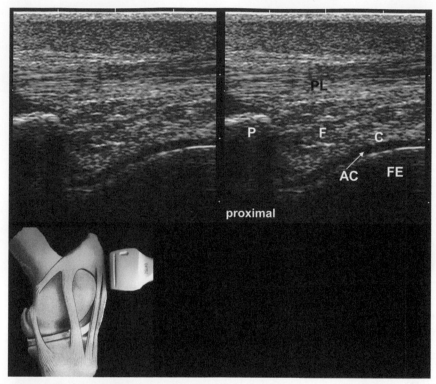

Fig. 29. Longitudinal sonogram (7.5 MHz transducer) showing the normal appearance of the dorsal aspect of the right femoropatellar joint of a 4-year-old Simmental cow. AC, anechoic band of the articular cartilage of the medial trochlear ridge; C, joint capsule of the femoropatellar joint lying directly on the articular cartilage; F, fatty tissue; FE, convex subchondral bone surface of the medial trochlear ridge of the femur; P, hyperechoic surface of the basis of the patella; PL, medial patellar ligament with the parallel fiber arrangement.

Table 3 shows that ultrasonography cannot definitively characterize the type of exudate. Based on history, physical examination and the cause of the disorder, the experienced clinician has a relatively good idea about the consistency and nature of the synovial fluid before centesis is performed. A definitive answer is provided by the aspirated sample (see **Fig. 24**B).

Fresh blood in the joint cavity caused by trauma appears homogenously anechoic, similar to hematomas that are only a few hours old.[32] However, cattle are not usually presented for examination at this stage. Later in the disease process, the ultrasonographic appearance becomes similar to that of coagulated blood, characterized by heterogeneous hypoechoic masses with well-demarcated anechoic areas.[5,32] Sometimes an accurate sonographic diagnosis of traumatic arthritis can be made when lesions in the joint capsule, the collateral and cruciate ligaments, or the menisci (see **Fig. 32**B) can be identified[47,51] and a hemorrhagic sample can be collected by arthocentesis.[38,63]

In septic disorders of synovial cavities, there may be inflammatory edema in the surrounding connective tissue, characterized by irregular areas of anechoic fluid accumulation separated by thin, weakly echoic septa (honeycomb appearance; **Figs. 4**A, **13**B, C, **14**, and **26**). In cattle with swollen joints, the differential diagnosis includes

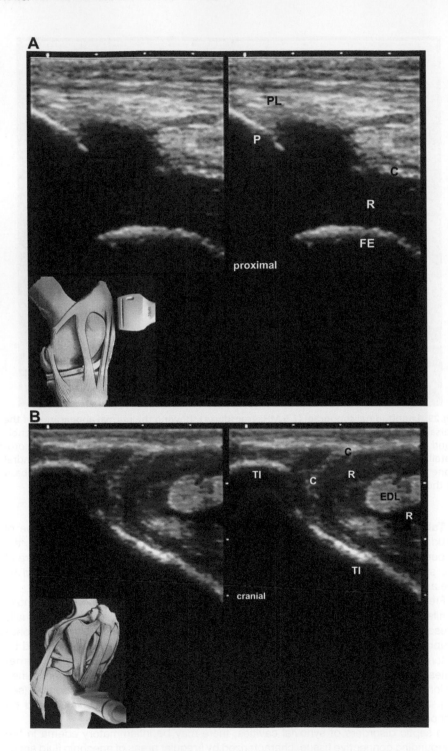

concurrent tenosynovitis and periarticular abscess, hematoma, or phlegmon. The exact location of the swelling and the incriminated structures can be determined quickly and reliably by ultrasonography.[1,2,5,6,15,18,19,21,24,27,30,31,32,34,44,45] Pathologic communications between adjacent synovial cavities, such as tendon sheaths and joints, especially in the digit, carpus, or tarsus of cattle, can also be detected (see **Figs. 7, 9**A, B, and **25**C, D).[1,2,4,5,6,18,19]

Septic disorders of tendon sheaths other than the digital flexor tendon sheath are uncommon in cattle but occasionally occur in the sheaths of the tendons of the extensor carpi radialis muscle and the common and lateral digital extensor muscles, the carpal flexor muscles and the tendons of the flexor hallucis longus and tibialis caudalis muscles in the tarsus (see **Figs. 13**B, C, **14**, and **25**C, D).[2,19,24,63,65] Aseptic tenosynovitis of the tendon of the extensor carpi radialis muscle (see **Fig. 15**) has also been described.[2,18,64]

Orthopedic and internal diseases that lead to prolonged recumbency and other factors, such as insufficient bedding, poor flooring, and muscle atrophy, all predispose cattle to decubital ulcers in areas such as the carpus, tarsus, and stifle. These can be chronic and aseptic or they may lead to septic bursitis.[27,63,67] The most commonly observed are the bursitis praecarpalis (carpal hygroma) (see **Fig. 16**), bursitis tarsalis lateralis (see **Fig. 27**), bursitis subcutanea and subtendinea calcanei (see **Fig. 28**A, B). The bursa intertubercularis and the bursa of the tendon of the infraspinatus and the biceps femoris muscle are less commonly affected. The involved bursae can be identified using anatomic landmarks such as tendons that run below or above them, or characteristic bone surfaces.[2,14,18,19,27,63,67]

Abscess and Hematoma

Causes of abscesses, hematomas, and seromas include decubital ulcers, iatrogenic factors, and sharp or blunt trauma.[63] The clinical examination of space-occupying lesions situated over large muscle groups or near joints often allows only a tentative diagnosis.

Depending on their morphologic makeup (cell debris, microvesicles, cell conglomerates), abscesses generally have a heterogeneous appearance on sonograms.[14,18,19,32,59,61,66] An ultrasonographic study of abscesses in various locations in 14 cattle revealed two main types.[32] Type-1 abscesses were characterized by a large dorsal gas accumulation, which appeared as a broad hyperechoic reflective band (similar to what is shown in **Fig. 25**C, D). Associated with the gas pocket were acoustic shadows with reverberation and ring-down artifacts. The liquid exudate was seen distal or ventral to the gas accumulation and had a heterogeneous hypoechoic to echoic appearance. These abscesses generally were not well demarcated

---

Fig. 30. (A) Longitudinal sonogram (7.5 MHz linear transducer) of the dorsal aspect of the right femoropatellar joint showing serofibrinous inflammation (polyarthritis) of the femoropatellar joint pouch in a 6-week-old Simmental calf. The joint capsule (C) of the femoropatellar joint is markedly elevated by a large heterogeneous effusion in the femoropatellar joint recess (R). FE, convex hyperechoic surface of the medial trochlear ridge of the femur. P, surface of the basis of the patella; PL, medial patellar ligament. (B) Transverse sonogram (7.5 MHz linear transducer) of the craniolateral stifle region of the calf in **Fig. 30**A showing the distal sac of the lateral femorotibial joint pouch with a serofibrinous arthritis. Distal sac of the lateral femorotibial joint recess (R) located in the sulcus extensorius of the tibia. Long digital extensor tendon (EDL) surrounded by heterogeneous effusion (anechoic, hypoechoic). C, joint capsule; TI, surface of the tibia.

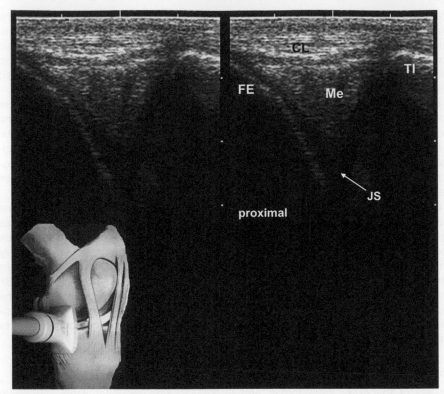

Fig. 31. Longitudinal sonogram (7.5 MHz linear transducer) showing the normal appearance of the medial aspect of the right femorotibial joint in a 4-year-old Simmental cow. Medial collateral ligament (CL) of the medial femorotibial joint, which is attached to the triangular shaped, homogeneous, hypoechoic medial meniscus (Me). FE, surface of the femur; JS, joint space of the medial femorotibial joint; TI, surface of the tibia.

from surrounding structures, but flow phenomena could be elicited. Type-2 abscesses were characterized by a predominantly anechoic content that was well demarcated from the surrounding tissues and contained unevenly distributed, small, floating hypoechoic reflections and many minute echoic to hyperechoic reflections, and flow phenomena were seen (**Figs. 36** and **37**).[32,66]

Hematomas occur when blood escapes from injured blood vessels into the surrounding tissue, and fibrin deposits form at the site of the defect, giving rise to adhesions.[63] Fresh hematomas have an almost anechoic appearance (**Fig. 38**), and flow phenomena and acoustic enhancement can be seen. With progressive coagulation and organization of the hematoma, heterogeneous areas are seen with alternating anechoic (fluid) and hypoechoic and echoic (organized) zones (**Fig. 39**).[32,61,68] In cattle with normal hemostasis, the hematoma starts to become heterogeneous within a few hours because of coagulation; infiltration of fibroblasts causes the mass to become more echoic. Parameters that are important for coagulation and thus the resulting sonographic image are the packed cell volume, the fibrinogen concentration of blood, resorption processes, and fibrinolysis.[32,68] It is possible to diagnose abscesses and hematomas clinically, but when they are located near joints, tendon sheaths, bones, and vessels, it is not clinically possible to confidently rule out involvement of these structures. Based on history and clinical findings, ultrasonography facilitates differentiation of abscesses,

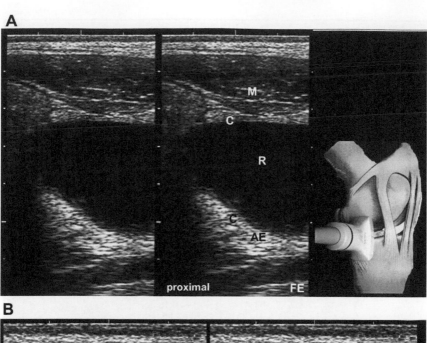

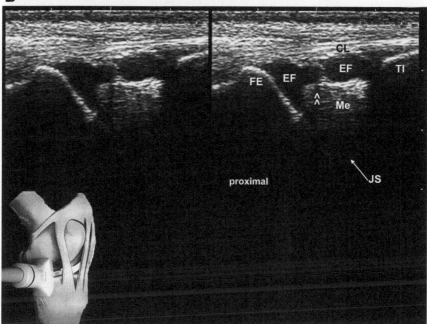

Fig. 32. (*A*) Longitudinal sonogram (7.5 MHz linear transducer) of the medial aspect of the stifle of a 13-month-old Simmental heifer with severe effusion in the medial femorotibial joint pouch caused by trauma. Severely distended recess (R) with serous effusion and acoustic enhancement (AE) caused by anechoic fluid. C, joint capsule of the medial femorotibial joint; FE, surface of the femur; M, gracilis muscle. (*B*) Longitudinal sonogram (7.5 MHz linear transducer) of the medial aspect of the stifle of the heifer in **Fig. 32**A showing detachment of the medial meniscus from the medial collateral ligament and joint effusion. Triangular shaped medial meniscus (Me) with a fine horizontal lesion (*arrowheads*). CL, medial collateral ligament of the femorotibial joint; EF, anechoic effusion between the meniscus and the medial CL; FE, hyperechoic surface of the femur; JS, joint space; TI, hyperechoic surface of the tibia.

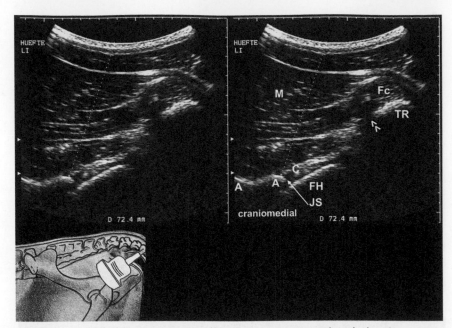

Fig. 33. Longitudinal-oblique sonogram (3.5 MHz convex transducer) showing a normal appearance of the left hip joint region in a 7-month-old Simmental calf; the transducer was placed parallel to the long axis of the femoral neck by moving it on an imaginary line from the trochanter major craniodorsally toward the point where a line drawn between the two tuber coxae intersects the longitudinal axis of the vertebral column. Fibrocartilage layer (Fc) with heterogeneous hypoechoic appearance covering the trochanter major, apophyseal growth plate (*arrowheads*). Joint space (JS) between the acetabular rim and the femoral head (FH); the distance from the skin surface to the joint is 72.4 mm. A, rim and bone surface of the acetabulum; C, coxofemoral joint capsule covering the articular surface; M, gluteal muscles; TR, hyperechoic surface of the trochanter major.

hematomas, and tumors. Centesis or biopsy of the swelling confirms the diagnosis.[28] Hematomas do not have a dorsal gas cap, which is frequently seen in abscesses. In contrast to abscesses and acute hematomas, tumors are usually solid masses.[69]

Tendinitis and Desmitis

Indications for ultrasonography
Indications for ultrasonography include swellings along the course of tendons or ligaments (collateral and patellar ligaments) with a history of trauma, wounds with possible damage to tendons or ligaments, and suspected tenosynovitis.

Ultrasonography is used to evaluate tendons in horses and can be used to assess the structure, echogenicity, and fiber direction of tendons and ligaments in cattle. In horses, tendinitis and desmitis are often characterized by focal circumscribed lesions with anechoic to hypoechoic areas (core lesions) in the tendon or ligament.[53,54,55] Most are attributable to excessive stress leading to rupture of individual fiber bundles.

Although ultrasonographic diagnosis of aseptic tendinitis or desmitis with partial fiber rupture has not been yet documented in cattle, the sonographic appearance can be expected to be similar to that in horses.[53,54,55]

The sonographic appearance of diseased flexor tendons has been well documented in cattle, including infection of the digital flexor tendon sheaths with purulent necrosis

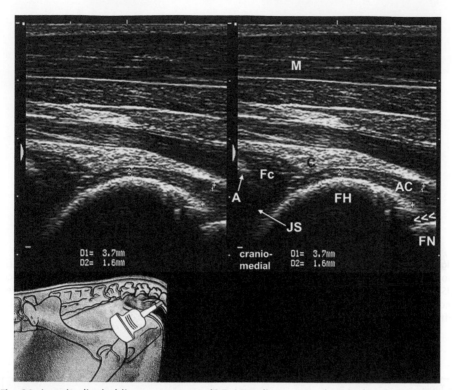

Fig. 34. Longitudinal-oblique sonogram (7.5 MHz linear transducer) showing a normal appearance of the left hip joint region in a 7-day-old Simmental calf. Joint space (JS) between the acetabulum and femoral head; the hyaline articular cartilage (AC) covering the femoral head and neck has a hypoechoic appearance in this young calf; the thickness of the articular cartilage is 3.7 mm and 1.6 mm, epiphyseal growth plate (*arrowheads*) between the femoral head and neck (FN). A, acetabular surface; C, coxofemoral joint capsule; Fc, fibrocartilaginous labium with heterogeneous hypoechoic appearance covering the acetabular rim; FH, convex surface of femoral head; M, gluteal muscles.

of the tendon, and tendons with circular defects caused by a penetrating foreign body. These defects were characterized by a circumscribed, diffuse decrease or complete loss of echogenicity; loss of the parallel fiber arrangement; or the presence of anechoic focal lesions extending over a considerable length, caused by purulent infection or necrosis (see **Figs. 9**A, B, and **28**B).[1,6]

Muscle Lesions

Indications for ultrasonography include swellings involving muscles (eg, rupture of the gastrocnemius muscle), decubital ulcers on the skin over muscle bellies, intertrigo on the medial crural skin, decubital ulcer on the lateral thigh, septic tendinitis, and tenosynovitis at the transition from muscle to the tendon of origin (eg, on the extensor carpi radialis muscle).

Muscle lesions in cattle may result from acute trauma, an iatrogenic origin, or from chronic ischemia and hypoxia caused by continuous pressure on muscles in cows with decubital skin ulcers caused by increased recumbency on hard ground or, sometimes, by severe udder edema. Depending on the causative event, muscle trauma may

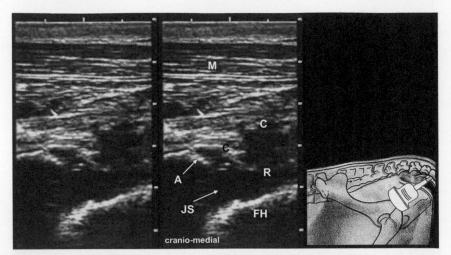

Fig. 35. Longitudinal-oblique sonogram (7.5 MHz linear transducer) showing septic serofibrinous arthritis of the left coxofemoral joint in a 4.5-month-old Brown-Swiss calf. Joint space (JS) between the acetabulum and femoral head (FH). A, surface of acetabulum; C, coxofemoral joint capsule; M, gluteal muscles; R, distended joint recess with heterogeneous effusion.

Table 1
Ultrasonographic appearance of important structures of the musculoskeletal system

Skin	Thin Echoic Line
Connective tissue	Echogenicity varies from hypoechoic to echoic, depending on the density of the tissue
Fat tissue	Echogenicity varies from nearly anechoic to hypoechoic
Muscle	Less hypoechoic with characteristic echoic to hyperechoic striations caused by the muscle septa in longitudinal planes; and small irregular, pinpoint, echoic to hyperechoic reflections of the septa in transverse planes
Tendon, ligament	Homogeneous echoic structure of varying size with a distinct, linear, and parallel arrangement of the fiber bundles
Bone surface	Smooth hyperechoic reflective band with total acoustic shadowing distally
Articular cartilage	Thin anechoic seam over the subchondral hyperechoic bone of the joint
Joint space	Narrow interruption of the hyperechoic bone surfaces with funnel-shaped, inward-curved contours of the joint-forming bones
Joint recess (pouch)	Normally, the joint cavity cannot be imaged; sometimes only very small anechoic zones at the level of the joint space can be identified
Joint capsule	Thin echoic structure lying close to the articular surface in healthy joints
Meniscus	Homogeneous hypoechoic to echoic triangular-shaped structure
Vessels	Anechoic tubular or band-shaped structures enveloped by thin echoic lines (wall; seen especially in arteries); arteries show pulsations, veins can be compressed completely

Table 2
Ultrasonographic measurements of the maximum width of distended joint pouches of 133 joints suffering with septic or traumatic arthritis

Joint	Age of cattle	Number of joints	Maximum Width of Dorsal/Cranial Pouches in Millimeters	Maximum Width of Palmar/Plantar/Caudal pouches in Millimeters
Coxofemoral[a]	4 mo	1	10	—
Shoulder[a]	1 wk–3 y	6	20	—
Elbow	1 wk	1	—	11
Antebrachiocarpal	1 wk–10 y	28	17–32	16–32
Intercarpal	3 wk–6 mo	4	13	—
Carpometacarpal	3 wk–6 mo	3	9.5	—
Femoropatellar	2 mo–7 y	4	28–36	—
Tarsocrural	1 wk–11 y	61	21–42	21–34
Distal intertarsal	7 mo–7 y	4	13	—
Tarsometatarsal	10 mo–8 y	4	9.5	—
Fetlock	1 wk–6 y	7	6–17	12–22
Proximal interphalangeal	14 mo–4 y	3	7–12	6–9
Distal interphalangeal	6 mo–6 y	7	6–17	8–14

[a] Johann Kofler and Birgit Altenbrunner-Martinek, unpublished data, 2009.
Data from Refs.[4,5,7,18,19]

Table 3
Comparison of ultrasonographic findings with macroscopic findings of aspirated synovial fluid and intraoperative or necropsy findings in 155 joints with septic or traumatic arthritis in 118 cattle

Echogenicity of Joint Effusion	Flow-Phenomena	Acoustic Enhancement	Differentiation From Adjoining Tissue	Type of Aspirated Fluid, Type of Exudative Inflammation
Homogeneous anechoic	Present	Present	Clear	Serous, serofibrinous
Homogeneous anechoic	Not present	Not present	Clear	Fresh coagulated gelatinous fibrin masses
Heterogeneous anechoic to hypoechoic	Not present	Not present	Unclear or difficult	Chronic fibrinous inflammation, fibrin clots undergoing organization
Heterogeneous hypoechoic with dispersed anechoic areas and small hyperechoic reflexes of various size	Present	Not present	Fairly clear	Serofibrinous effusion with small fibrin clots or liquid purulent exudate
Heterogeneous hypoechoic areas with some anechoic zones	Not present	Only distal to anechoic zones	Anechoic zones clearly differentiable	Serum-like, reddish, clotted blood and fibrin masses, hemarthrosis

Data from.[5,18,19]

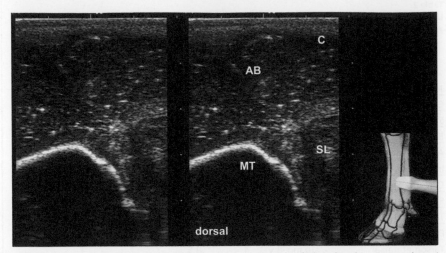

Fig. 36. Transverse sonogram (7.5 MHz linear transducer) of the distal metatarsal region showing an abscess on the lateroplantar edge of the left metatarsus in a 5-year-old Simmental cow. AB, abscess cavity; C, abscess capsule; MT, hyperechoic, convex surface of the metatarsus with no periosteal reaction.

result in the formation of hematomas, muscle tears, compartment syndrome, muscle necrosis, or abscess.[54,56,59,63,70] Depending on the type of causative disorder various sonographic patterns have been identified. These include anechoic fluid accumulation in fresh muscle hematomas (see **Fig. 36**), small or large, irregularly shaped lesions with scattered low-level echoes (in muscle tears), ill-defined echoic areas with loss of normal muscle striations, and overall increase in muscle echogenicity (in muscle compartment syndrome, postanesthetic myopathy, or muscle necrosis), and highly reflective zones with acoustic shadowing and loss of normal muscle architecture (in muscular abscesses).[54,55,56,57,58,59,70] Chronic muscle injuries develop fibrosis and scarring characterized by heterogeneous areas of increased echoes that do not increase in size with contraction.[54,55,59]

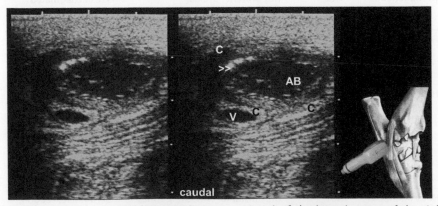

Fig. 37. Transverse sonogram (7.5 MHz linear transducer) of the lateral aspect of the right tarsus showing an abscess located very close to a vein in a 6-year-old Simmental cow. Hyperechoic reflexes indicating gas or dense debris (*arrowheads*). AB, abscess cavity; C, abscess capsule; V, caudal branch of the lateral saphenous vein.

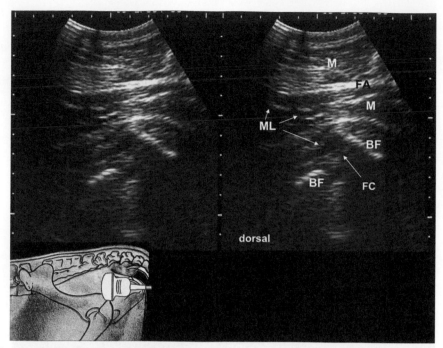

Fig. 38. Transverse sonogram (3.5 MHz convex transducer) of the left hip joint region showing a fracture of the ischial spine dorsal to the coxofemoral joint in a 5-year-old Simmental cow; the transducer was placed in a dorso-ventral position. BF, fractured bone fragments of the rim of the ischial spine with distal shadowing; FA, muscle fascia; FC, fracture cleft; M, normal gluteal muscles; ML, muscle lesion with a fresh hematoma with anechoic areas.

Fractures, Periostitis, Osteitis, and Osteomyelitis

Indications for ultrasonography include regions that are difficult to access by way of radiography, such as the scapula, ribs, and pelvis. These can be examined by way of ultrasonography; the latter may be examined transcutaneously or transrectally.[42]

Obviously, radiography is the method of choice for the evaluation of bone lesions. Ultrasound waves are reflected by the bone surface and are completely absorbed so that the normal bone contour appears as a smooth hyperechoic reflective band.[41,47,48,49] Fractures are characterized by an interruption or a step in the smooth contour of the bone. Small bone fragments in the soft tissues produce hyperechoic reflections with a distal acoustic shadow (**Figs. 38** and **39**).[41,45,47,55,71,72] Concurrent fracture-associated hematomas appear as anechoic to hypoechoic areas of varying size around the fracture site.[47,71,72]

Osteolysis and osteomyelitis are associated with alterations in the surrounding soft tissue; bone sequestra or periosteal reactions occur later. Early signs of osteitis and osteomyelitis, before they are detected by radiography, include thickening and displacement of the periosteum from the bone by anechoic inflammatory exudate and swelling of the surrounding soft tissue.[55,59,73] Small anechoic areas are seen between the surface of the bone, which is still smooth and hyperechoic, and the surrounding hypoechoic to echoic soft tissues.[7,8,55,73] Bone lysis and periosteal reaction appear later as irregular roughening of the bone surface (see **Figs. 4, 11C, 21,** and **28B**).[2,8]

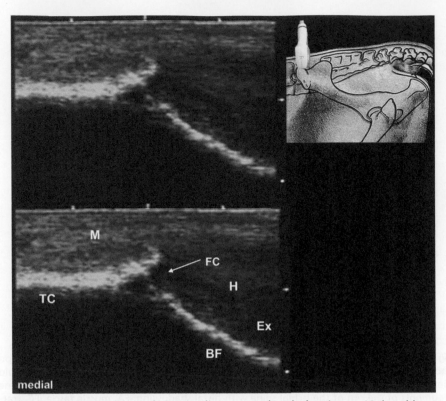

Fig. 39. Transverse sonogram (7.5 MHz linear transducer) showing a 14-day-old, open fracture of the tuber coxae in a 6-year-old Holstein-Friesian cow; the transducer was held in a lateromedial position. BF, fractured and displaced bone fragment of the tuber coxae. Ex, liquid exudate; FC, fracture cleft; H, coagulated hematoma; M, gluteus medius muscle.

ULTRASOUND-GUIDED CENTESIS

Centesis of diseased synovial cavities and other fluid accumulations (abscess, hematoma) is an established and straightforward diagnostic technique.[33,36,38,62,74] Only liquid content can be aspirated by way of centesis with a large gauge needle.[2,5,32,33,38]

Indications for Ultrasound-Guided Centesis

Large diffuse swellings in the region of a synovial cavity, which hamper or preclude the identification by palpation of the optimal site for centesis. This is particularly applicable to swellings in which two or more adjacent synovial cavities are involved and synovial cavities in the proximal limb where centesis is rarely performed (eg, shoulder and hip joints, bicipital bursa). If the equipment is available, ultrasonographic inspection of the structure of interest should always be performed before centesis.

Ultrasonography allows exact localization of a dilated cavity and the consistency of the content can be determined based on the presence or absence of flow phenomena and acoustic enhancement.[8] The position and size of the distended cavity and the location of liquid effusion within (see **Fig. 12**A, B) and its distance and direction from a set point on the skin surface can be determined accurately using the electronic cursors. After determining the direction and depth for centesis by way of ultrasonography,[8,14] the needle can be inserted with or without (freehand) ultrasonographic guidance.[28,73–75] The same technique can also be used for biopsy collection from suspicious tissue[76] or for centesis of veins of the limb or neck suspected of having septic thrombosis.[14]

CONCLUSIONS FOR USE IN CLINICAL PRACTICE

Ultrasonography is an imaging modality that can be used anywhere and allows rapid noninvasive differentiation of soft tissue structures of the bovine musculoskeletal system. It is an extremely useful adjunct to the clinical examination. In practice, there are numerous indications for ultrasonography of the musculoskeletal system in cattle. It should always be used for evaluation of soft tissue swellings that cannot be diagnosed based on clinical examination. Ultrasonography provides accurate information about the location and size of lesions or fluid-filled cavities, the surrounding tissues, and the nature of the content (fluid or semisolid). Targeted centesis of synovial cavities or other cavities can be done freehand or under the guidance of ultrasound after a preliminary ultrasonographic inspection.

Normal synovial cavities in cattle are difficult or impossible to visualize by way of ultrasonography because of the very small amount of synovial fluid. Thus, effusion that is easily visualized usually indicates an inflammatory process (see **Table 2**). In contrast to radiography, ultrasonography can detect early stages of joint inflammation, based on an increased amount of effusion and distension of the synovial pouch. An early diagnosis, accurate anatomic differentiation of the soft tissue structures involved, characterization of the lesions, and a thorough preoperative inspection of affected regions are of enormous benefit for planning surgery and treatment and for determining the prognosis.

Other applications include the diagnosis of muscle and tendon lesions or rupture, monitoring of abnormal postoperative wound healing; detection of foreign bodies in the limbs or trunk that cannot be diagnosed by radiography; and identification of fractures of proximal bones (such as the pelvis, scapula or ribs) that cannot be accessed by radiography. However, the clinician should be aware of the limitations of ultrasonography such as the depth of penetration of the ultrasound waves and the anatomic intricacies of the bovine musculoskeletal system.

Ultrasound machines with 5.0 to 7.5 MHz linear transducers, which are commonly used in large animal reproduction, are well suited for rapid and straightforward differentiation of soft tissue swelling in the musculoskeletal system of cattle.

REFERENCES

1. Kofler J. Sonography as a new diagnostic tool for septic tenosynovitis of the digital flexor tendon sheath in cattle—therapy and long term follow-up. Dtsch Tierarztl Wschr 1994;101(6):215–22.
2. Kofler J. Application of ultrasonic examination in the diagnosis of bovine locomotory system disorders. Schweizer Archiv fur Tierheilkunde 1995a;137(8):369–80.
3. Kofler J. Description and determination of the diameter of arteries and veins in the hindlimb of cattle using B-mode ultrasonography. J Vet Med 1995b;42(4):253–66.
4. Kofler J. Septic arthritis of the proximal interphalangeal (pastern) joint in cattle— clinical, radiographic, ultrasonographic findings and treatment. Berliner und Munchener Tierarztliche Wochenschrift 1995c;108(8):281–9.

5. Kofler J. Arthrosonography: the use of diagnostic ultrasound in septic and traumatic arthritis in cattle—a retrospective study of 25 patients. Br Vet J 1996a; 152(6):683–98.
6. Kofler J. Sonographic imaging of pathology of digital flexor tendon sheath in cattle. Vet Rec 1996b;139(2):36–41.
7. Kofler J. Ultrasonography in haematogeneous septic arthritis, polyarthritis and osteomyelitis in calves. Wien Tierarztl Mschr 1997a;84(5):129–39.
8. Kofler J. Ultraschalluntersuchung am Bewegungsapparat. In: Braun U, editor. Atlas und Lehrbuch der Ultraschalldiagnostik beim Rind. Berlin: Parey Buchverlag; 1997b. p. 253–68 [in German].
9. Kofler J. Ultrasonographic examination of the stifle region in cattle—normal appearance. Vet J 1999;158(1):21–32.
10. Kofler J. Ultrasonographic examination of the carpal region in cattle—normal appearance. Vet J 2000;159(1):85–96.
11. Kofler J, Edinger H. Diagnostic ultrasound imaging of the soft tissues in distal bovine limb. Vet Radiol Ultrasound 1995;36(3):246–52.
12. Kofler J, Kuebber P, Henninger W. Ultrasonographic imaging and thickness measurement of the sole horn and the underlying soft tissue layer in bovine claws. Vet J 1999;157(3):322–31.
13. Kofler J, Martinek B, Kuebber-Heiss A, et al. Generalised distal limb vessel thrombosis in two cows with digital and inner organ infections. Vet J 2004;167(1): 107–10.
14. Kofler J, Breinreich B, Altenbrunner-Martinek B. Phlegmon of the distal limb—an exact diagnosis? Revista Romana Medicina Veterinaria 2007;17(2 Suppl):34–5 [in German].
15. Munroe GA, Cauvin ER. The use of arthroscopy in the treatment of septic arthritis in two highland calves. Br Vet J 1994;150(5):439–49.
16. Flury S. Ultrasonographische Darstellung des Tarsus beim Rind [Ultrasonographic imaging of the tarsus in cattle]. 1996; Thesis: Veterinary Medicine, Bern, Switzerland.
17. Kofler J, Kuebber-Heiss A. Long-term ultrasonographic and venographic study of the development of tarsal vein thrombosis in a cow. Vet Rec 1997;140(26):676–8.
18. Kofler J, Martinek B. Ultrasonographic imaging of disorders of the carpal region in 42 cattle—arthritis, tenosynovitis, precarpal hygroma, periarticular abscess. Tierarztl Prax Ausg G Grosstiere Nutztiere 2004;32(2):61–72.
19. Kofler J, Altenbrunner-Martinek B. Ultrasonographic findings of disorders of the tarsal region in 97 cattle—arthritis, bursitis, tenosynovitis, periarticular abscess and vein thrombosis. Berl Munch Tierarztl Wschr 2008;121(3-4):145–58.
20. Schock B, Nuss K, Koestlin R. Ultrasonographic examination of the stifle in the calf. In: Proceedings of the 10th International Symposium on Lameness in Ruminants. Lucerne, Switzerland; 1998. p. 311–3.
21. Roth M, Nuss K. Der klinische Fall: septische Arthritis beider Tarsokruralgelenke metastatischen Ursprungs bei einem Kalb. Tierarztl Prax 1999;21(5):(287), 379–81 [in German].
22. Tryon KA, Clark CR. Ultrasonographic examination of the distal limb of cattle. Vet Clin North Am Food Anim Pract 1999;15(2):275–300.
23. Nuss K. Septic arthritis of the shoulder and hip joint in cattle: diagnosis and therapy. Schweiz Arch Tierheilkd 2003;145(19):455–63.
24. Nuss K, Maierl J. Tenosynovitis of the deep flexor tendon sheath (M. flexor digitalis lateralis et M. tibialis caudalis) at the bovine tarsus (16 cases). Tierarztl Prax (G) 2000;28(6):299–306.

25. Saule C, Nuss K, Köstlin RG, et al. Ultrasonographic anatomy of the bovine carpal joint. Tierarztl Prax 2005;33(G):364–72.
26. Van Amstel SR, Palin FL, Rohrbach BW, et al. Ultrasound measurement of sole horn thickness in trimmed claws of dairy cows. J Am Vet Med Assoc 2003; 223(4):492–4.
27. Seyrek-Intas D, Celimli N, Gorgul OS, et al. Comparison of clinical, ultrasonographic, and postoperative macroscopic findings in cows with bursitis. Vet Radiol Ultrasound 2005;46(2):143–5.
28. King AM. Development, advances and applications of diagnostic ultrasound in animals. Vet J 2006;171(3):408–20.
29. Altenbrunner-Martinek B, Grubelnik M, Kofler J. Ultrasonographic examination of important aspects of the bovine shoulder—physiological findings. Vet J 2007; 173(2):317–24.
30. Starke A, Herzog K, Sohrt J, et al. Diagnostic procedures and surgical treatment of craniodorsal coxofemoral luxation in calves. Vet Surg 2007;36(2):99–106.
31. Starke A, Heppelmann M, Meyer H, et al. Diagnosis and therapy of septic arthritis in cattle. Cattle Pract 2008;16(1):36–43.
32. Kofler J, Buchner A. Ultrasonic differential diagnostic examination of abscesses, haematomas and seromas in cattle. Wien Tierarztl Mschr 1995;82(5):159–68.
33. Weaver AD. Joint conditions. In: Greenough PR, Weaver AD, editors. Lameness in cattle. 3rd edition. Philadelphia: WB Saunders; 1997. p. 162–70.
34. Kofler J, Hittmair K. Diagnostic ultrasonography in animals—continuation of the clinical examination? Vet J 2006;171(3):393–5.
35. Bailey JV. Bovine arthritides: classification, diagnosis, prognosis, treatment. Vet Clin North Am Food Anim Pract 1985;1(1):39–51.
36. Dirksen G. Bewegungsapparat. In: Dirksen G, Gründer H-D, Stöber M, editors. Die klinische Untersuchung des Rindes. 3rd edition. Berlin: Parey; 1990. p. 549–91 [in German].
37. Stanek C. Examination of the locomotor system. In: Greenough PR, Weaver AD, editors. Lameness in cattle. 3rd edition. Philadelphia: WB Saunders; 1997. p. 14–23.
38. Rohde C, Anderson DE, Desrochers A, et al. Synovial fluid analysis in cattle: a review of 130 cases. Vet Surg 2000;29(4):341–6.
39. Farrow CS. The radiologic investigation of bovine lameness associated with infection. Vet Clin North Am Food Anim Pract 1999;15(1):411–23.
40. Heppelmann M, Rehage J, Kofler J, et al. Ultrasonographic diagnosis of the septic arthritis of the distal interphalangeal joint in cattle. Vet J 2009;179(1): 407–16.
41. Gladisch R. Einführung in die sonographische Diagnostik. Sonderheft. Tierarztl Prax 1993;41:3–9 [in German].
42. Grubelnik M, Kofler J, Martinek B, et al. Ultrasonographic examination of the hip joint and the pelvic region in cattle. Berliner und Munchener Tierarztliche Wochenschrift 2002;115(5–6):209–20.
43. Kofler J, Buchner A, Sendlhofer A. Application of real-time ultrasonography for the detection of tarsal vein thrombosis in cattle. Vet Rec 1996;138(2):34–8.
44. Martinek B, Zoltan B, Floeck M, et al. Chondrosarcoma in a Simmental cow—clinical, ultrasonographic, radiographic and pathological findings. Vet J 2006; 172(1):181–4.
45. Martinek B, Huber J, Kofler J, et al. Bilateral avulsion fracture (apophyseolysis) of the calcaneal tuber in a heifer. Berl Munch Tierarztl Wschr 2003;116(7-8): 328–32.

46. Nickel R, Schummer A, Seiferle E. In: Frewein J, Wille K-H, Wilkens H, editors. 7th edition, Lehrbuch der Anatomie der Haustiere. Bewegungsapparat, vol 1. Berlin: Parey; 2001. p. 15–27, 215–20, 230–82, 287–8, 407–554 [in German].

47. Sattler H, Harland U. In: Arthrosonographie. Berlin: Springer; 1988. p. 1–133.

48. Van Holsbeeck M, Introcaso JH. Musculoskeletal ultrasonography. Radiol Clin North Am 1992;30(5):907–25.

49. Chhem RK, Kaplan PA, Dussault RG. Ultrasonography of the musculoskeletal system. Radiol Clin North Am 1994;32(2):275–89.

50. Jurvelin JS, Räsänen T, Kolmonen P, et al. Comparison of optical, needle probe and ultrasonic technique for the measurement of articular cartilage thickness. J Biomech 1995;28(2):231–5.

51. Dik KJ. Ultrasonography of the equine stifle. Equine Vet Educ 1995;7(3):154–60.

52. Stanek C. Morphologische, funktionelle, chemische und klinische Untersuchungen zu den Erkrankungen der Fesselbeugesehnenscheide des Rindes. Wien Tierarztl Mschr 1987;74:397–412:1988;75:14–29, 46–58, 84–102, 127–38, 170–80 [in German].

53. Genovese RL, Rantanen NW, Hauser ML, et al. Diagnostic ultrasonography of equine limbs. Vet Clin North Am Equine Pract 1986;2(1):145–225.

54. Genovese RL, Rantanen NW. The superficial digital flexor tendon & the deep digital flexor tendon, carpal sheath, and accessory ligament of the deep digital flexor tendon (check ligament). In: Nyland TG, Mattoon JS, editors. Veterinary diagnostic ultrasound. Philadelphia: WB Saunders; 1998. p. 289–398 399–445.

55. Reef VB. Equine diagnostic ultrasound. Philadelphia: WB Saunders; 1998. pp. 39–186.

56. Dik KJ. Ultrasonography of the equine crus. Vet Radiol Ultrasound 1993;34(1): 28–34.

57. Reimers K, Reimers CD, Wagner S, et al. Skeletal muscle sonography: a correlative study of echogenicity and morphology. J Ultrasound Med 1993;12(2): 73–7.

58. Smith RKW, Dyson SJ, Head MJ, et al. Ultrasonography of the equine triceps muscle before and after general anaesthesia and in post anaesthetic myopathy. Equine Vet J 1996;28(4):311–9.

59. Léveillé R, Biller DS. Muscle evaluation, foreign bodies and miscellaneous swellings. In: Nyland TG, Mattoon JS, editors. Veterinary diagnostic ultrasound. Philadelphia: WB Saunders; 1998. p. 515–21.

60. Bonnaire F, Berwarth H, Paul C, et al. Einsatz der Sonographie zur Akut- und Verlaufsdiagnostik in der septischen Unfallchirurgie. Unfallchirurgie 1994;97(3): 164–70 [in German].

61. Walz M, Möllenhoff G, Josten C, et al. Die Bedeutung der Sonographie in der Erkennung von Wundheilungsstörungen nach chirurgischen Eingriffen. Orthopädische Praxis 1993;6(6):399–402 [in German].

62. Trent AM, Plumb D. Treatment of infectious arthritis and osteomyelitis. Vet Clin North Am Food Anim Pract 1991;7(3):747–78.

63. Dirksen G. Krankheiten der Bewegungsorgane. In: Dirksen G, Gründer H-D, Stöber M, editors. Innere Medizin und Chirurgie des Rindes. 4th edition. Berlin: Parey; 2002. p. 6–103, 187–9, 764, 773–9, 797–801, 816–8, 825, 834–5, 974–5 [in German].

64. Klee W, Hänichen T. Epidemiologische, klinische und pathologisch-anatomische Untersuchungen über die Entzündung der Karpalgelenkstrecker beim Rind. Schweiz Arch Tierheilkd 1989;131(3):151–7 [in German].

65. Anderson DE, St-Jean G, Morin DE, et al. Traumatic flexor tendon injuries in 27 cattle. Vet Surg 1996;25(4):320–6.
66. Sauer W, Grüner J, Jakober B, et al. Wertigkeit der Sonographie zur Erfassung eines Gelenk- und Weichteilempyems. Ultraschall Klin Prax 1987;2(2):175–7 [in German].
67. Nuss K, Ringer S, Meyer SW, et al. Lameness caused by infection of the subtendinous bursa of the infraspinatus muscle in three cows. Vet Rec 2007;160: 198–200 [in German].
68. Aufschnaiter M. Sonography of coagulated blood: experimental and clinical findings. Ultraschall 1993;4(2):110–3.
69. Bruns J, Lüssenhop S, Behrens P. Sonographische Darstellung von Weichteiltumoren der Extremitäten und gelenkassoziierten Weichteilveränderungen. Ultraschall in Med 1994;15(2):74–80 [in German].
70. Fornage BD, Touche DH, Segal P, et al. Ultrasonography in the evaluation of muscular trauma. J Ultrasound Med 1983;2(12):549–54.
71. Shepherd MC, Pilsworth RC. The use of ultrasound in the diagnosis of pelvic fractures. Equine Vet Educ 1994;6(4):223–7.
72. Reisinger R, Altenbrunner-Martinek B, Kofler J. Sternal recumbency after traumatic injury of the caudal thoracic spine with fracture of the dorsal spinous processes of the thoracic vertebrae 11 to 13 in a heifer. Wien Tierarztl Mschr 2008;95(3-4):72–9.
73. Howard CB, Einhorn M, Dagan R, et al. Ultrasound in diagnosis and management of acute haematogenous osteomyelitis in children. J Bone Joint Surg 1993;75-B: 79–82.
74. Braun U, Wild K, Merz M, et al. Percutaneous ultrasound-guided abdominocentesis in cows. Vet Rec 1997;140(23):599–602.
75. David F, Rougier M, Morisset S. Ultrasound-guided coxofemoral arthrocentesis in horses. Equine Vet J 2007;39(1):79–83.
76. Tucker R. Ultrasound-guided biopsy. In: Nyland TG, Mattoon JS, editors. Veterinary diagnostic ultrasound. Philadelphia: WB Saunders; 1998. p. 649–53.

Ultrasonography of the Bovine Female Genital Tract

Luc DesCôteaux, DMV, MSc[a,b,*], Giovanni Gnemmi, DVM, PhD[c],
Jill Colloton, DVM[d]

KEYWORDS

- Ultrasound • Bovine • Female • Reproduction
- Management • Diagnostic

Ultrasound examination of the bovine female reproductive tract opened the gateway for the use of ultrasound equipment on farms in the mid-1980s. Since that time, many research efforts have been devoted to developing practical applications in reproduction and diagnosis in bovine medicine. The literature on ultrasound use is in agreement that ultrasound examinations of the reproductive tract now offer practitioners one of the most rapid, precise, and cost-effective means of diagnosis in bovine reproductive medicine.[1–3]

Because this diagnostic tool has a wide variety of applications for herd and reproductive management, the objective of this article is to present the most common practical uses for bovine practitioners in the field. This article also considers other possible applications for more advanced practitioners and researchers using this technology to understand ovarian physiology better using color Doppler ultrasound, the specific applications of ultrasonography in embryo transfer programs, and the potential use of ultrasound examination in reproduction synchronization protocols for dairy cattle. Readers who would like more in-depth information and practical applications on these subjects are invited to consult the more detailed and interactive texts in the list of bibliographic references.[4]

This paper was translated and adapted with permission from Les Éditions du Point Vétérinaire (Wolters-Kluwer trademark).
[a] Department of Clinical Studies, Faculté de médecine vétérinaire, Université de Montréal, St-Hyacinthe, Québec J2S 7C6, Canada
[b] Food Animal Ambulatory Clinic, Faculté de Médecine Vétérinaire, Université de Montréal, St-Hyacinthe, Québec, Canada
[c] BovineVet Studio Veterinario Associato, Via Cadolini 9, Fr. Cuzzago, 28803 Premosello Chiovenda, Italy
[d] Bovine Services LLC, F4672 Highway 97, Edgar, WI 54426, USA
* Corresponding author. Department of Clinical Studies, Faculté de médecine vétérinaire, Université de Montréal, St-Hyacinthe, Québec, Canada.
E-mail address: luc.descoteaux@umontreal.ca (L. DesCôteaux).

PREPARING THE ANIMAL, RESTRAINT, REQUIRED MATERIALS

The cow must be adequately restrained to avoid injury and ensure that the user is in a comfortable position to carry out the examination. In a tie-stall operation in which cows have large stalls or in free-stall operations in which cows are examined in stalls, the assistant, usually the dairy producer or herd manager, should stand beside the cow to minimize its lateral movements and to hold the tail so that the practitioner can work unhindered (**Fig. 1**). In other situations in which cows are properly restrained and lateral movements are minimized (eg, palpation rail, headlocks), the herd manager is standing in front of the cows to identify cows for examination and completion of their reproduction records.

Manual emptying of the rectum is usually necessary to obtain the high-quality images needed for ovarian and uterine evaluations, early diagnosis of pregnancy, and fetal sexing.

On the farm, a 5-MHz linear rectal probe is the most versatile and commonly used probe for bovine reproductive examinations. Some practitioners prefer probes with a higher frequency (7.5–10 MHz), especially when examining the ovaries and for early diagnosis of pregnancy.[4] The more recent ultrasound units often include multifrequency probes that function between 5 and 10 MHz.

The image is viewed on a monitor or with binocular goggles. A monitor that needs to be set on a tabletop must be placed to the side where it can be easily viewed when the practitioner's arm is inside the cow; the angle and distance must also facilitate viewing and reading by the user. Portable ultrasound units that come with an over-the-arm strap, a harness, or a belt should be set on the side that is not used for palpation to visualize the monitor properly in an ergonomic and safe position (see **Fig. 1**).

A systematic and methodic examination of the reproductive tract should be performed in all cases. The authors recommend examining the ovaries first to help interpret the examination of the rest of the reproductive tract (eg, probability of pregnancy, diagnosis of twins, ovarian cyst) and to develop better diagnostic precision.

ULTRASOUND EXAMINATIONS OF THE OVARIES

Bovine ovaries are dynamic organs that produce anovulatory and ovulatory follicles and form corpora lutea (CLs) at regular intervals. The practitioner's challenge is to

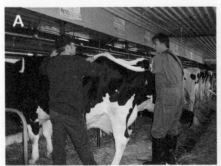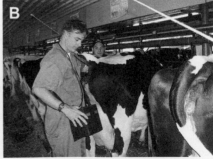

Fig. 1. (*A, B*) Ultrasound examination of the reproductive system. Photographs of a dairy producer assisting a bovine practitioner in performing an ultrasound examination using a portable unit that hangs by a strap over the user's arm. The assistant should stand beside the rear end of the animal to minimize lateral movements and hold the cow's tail so that the examiner is not hindered during the procedure.

interpret correctly the nature of the structures observed during the ultrasound examination at any given moment.

In dairy cows, the estrus cycle lasts between 18 and 24 days, and this allows two to three (and sometimes four) follicular waves to develop; at the end of these, a single dominant follicle 12 to 15 mm in diameter emerges.[4]

Follicles

Because of the several follicular waves and because follicles greater than 8 mm in size are nearly always present throughout the entire estrus cycle (except for the first few days), it is difficult, even in a research context with daily ultrasound examinations, to identify the dominant follicle, and thus predict when ovulation is going to occur.[4] This difficulty is even greater in the field, with a single ultrasound examination that could take place at any point during the cycle. In this situation, to identify cows that are edging toward heat (proestrus and estrus), the practitioner must rely on other signs, such as changes in the echotexture of the uterus, uterine tonus, and endometrial secretions (see section on ultrasound of the nongravid uterus), in addition to changes in behavior (**Fig. 2**).[4]

Corpus luteum

The presence of a CL on one of the ovaries provides evidence of sexual maturity in heifers and estrus cycling in cows.[4] In an inseminated cow, the position of the CL on one of the ovaries should alert the practitioner to the possibility of pregnancy in the ipsilateral uterine horn, which should be examined with special attention. The presence of a double ovulation (**Fig. 3**) in an inseminated cow should cause the practitioner to suspect a twin pregnancy, and this cow should be re-examined at a later date because of the increased risk for embryonic loss.[4]

It might be possible to estimate the age of CLs using ultrasound along with an examination of the uterus (see section on ultrasound of the nongravid uterus). Without a record of recent reproductive history, however, accurate diagnosis is a challenge because CLs can vary in morphology and ultrasonographic appearance.[4]

Transportable and portable ultrasound units used in bovine practice allow us to identify the contours of young CLs, starting from the third or fourth day of the estrus cycle.[4] As they age, the CLs become hypoechogenic (darker or blacker) compared

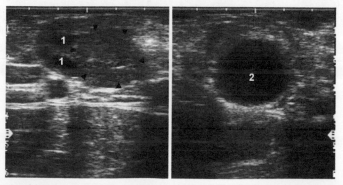

Fig. 2. Ultrasound image of a cow's ovaries in proestrus. This image shows two 0.5-cm follicles (1) on the left ovary and one 2.3-cm dominant follicle (2) on the right ovary. The CL is difficult to identify on the left ovary because it is isoechogenic with the surrounding ovarian stroma. ▶, edge of the corpus luteum.

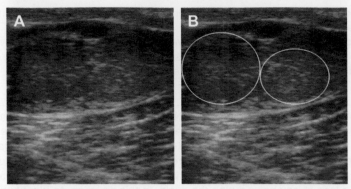

Fig. 3. (*A, B*) Ultrasound image of the left ovary in a twin pregnancy on day 28 (6-MHz linear probe, depth of 4 cm). Note the presence of 2 CLs (*double ovulation*) on this ovary.

with the surrounding ovarian stroma because of the greater concentration of blood vessels feeding this structure, which continues to develop until luteolysis occurs (**Fig. 4**).[5] The subtle signs of this on the ultrasound monitor are sometimes difficult to recognize in field conditions and in a well-lit environment.

For the first 10 days of the estrus cycle, between 30% and 50% of CLs are indented with a cavity that can easily be identified on the ultrasound image (**Fig. 5**).[6,7] A CL with a central cavity (CLc) is usually a young functional one, in spite of the fact that it can also be found, albeit rarely, after day 30 of gestation. CLcs are normal structures that produce a normal amount of progesterone. They do not change the length of the estrus cycle in cows, they do not reduce the probability of pregnancy, and they do not alter the risk for embryonic death in pregnant cows.[7,8]

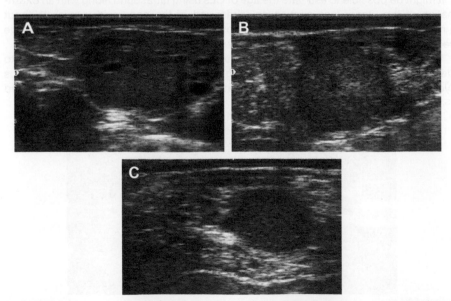

Fig. 4. Comparison of a CL on days 6, 9, and 11 of the estrus cycle in a cow (8-MHz linear probe, depth of 4 cm). Note that the CL from day 6 that was nearly isoechogenic with the adjacent ovarian stroma becomes hypoechogenic (darker) as it matures. CL on day 6 (*A*), CL on day 9 (*B*), and CL on day 11 (*C*).

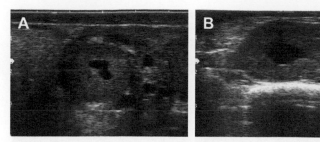

Fig. 5. Ultrasound images of a CLc between days 8 and 10 of the estrus cycle (10-MHz linear probe, depth of 4 cm).

Debates continue to persist as to how best to distinguish between a CL and a luteal cyst. The different types of CLcs and their progression are presented in another practical text that focuses on ultrasound examinations for ruminant reproduction.[4]

CLs that regress during proestrus are more difficult to identify in ultrasound examinations because they become isoechogenic with the surrounding ovarian stroma (see **Fig. 2; Fig. 6**).[4,5]

Ovarian Pathologic Conditions

Ovarian inactivity

Anovulatory anestrus occurs in between 10% and 64% of lactating dairy cows, with a mean of 20%.[9,10] The ovaries in these cows do not contain a CL or any large follicles; instead, small follicles less than 2 to 4 mm in diameter are present.[4] **Fig. 7** shows ultrasound images comparing an inactive ovary with an ovary from a cow in proestrus.

Ovarian cyst

Ovarian cysts are traditionally defined as follicular structures larger than 25 mm in diameter that persist for more than 10 days in the absence of a CL (**Fig. 8**). More recently, a diagnosis of ovarian follicular cyst was based on a diameter greater than 16 or 17 mm.[4,11,12]

The follicular cyst that undergoes partial luteinization becomes a luteal cyst that responds to prostaglandin F2α injection. Differentiation between a luteal cyst and a CLc is generally based on the thickness of the structure's luteal wall: it is generally, but not exclusively, greater than 3 mm in a CLc and less than 3 mm in a luteal cyst (**Fig. 9**).[4] This difference can be difficult to evaluate in the field with certain portable ultrasound units. This definition is mainly a theoretic one, however, because it is possible to encounter a CLc that is greater than 25 mm in diameter and does not persist longer than a normal CL. It should be noted that the ability to make a precise diagnosis of this type of ovarian structure does not involve any changes in the treatment plan for synchronizing ovulation in these cows.

ULTRASOUND EXAMINATION OF THE NONGRAVID UTERUS

Ultrasound examination of the uterus provides practitioners with one of the most rapid, most precise, and least invasive methods of evaluating uterine health.[4]

This section presents the principal ultrasound images of the uterus that can be obtained during the estrus cycle. The main disorders of the bovine uterus are also presented.

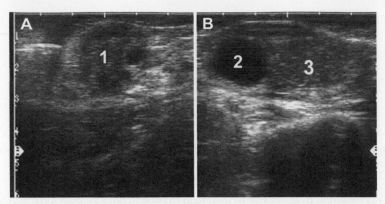

Fig. 6. The end-of-cycle CL (proestrus) is difficult to differentiate from the surrounding ovarian stroma because it is isoechogenic (8-MHz linear probe, depth of 6 cm). Left ovary with a small 0.3-cm follicle (*A*) and right ovary with a 1.5-cm follicle and a 2-cm CL that is isoechogenic with the ovarian stroma (*B*) are shown. 1, ovarian stroma; 2, 1.5-cm follicle; 3, CL.

Periestrus

This period extends from approximately 3 days before until 4 days after estrus and includes the phases of proestrus, estrus, and the beginning of metestrus. It is characterized by high estrogen levels in circulation and an increase in blood flow to the uterus.[4] On transrectal palpation, the uterus is turgid and the horns are less curved than during diestrus.[11] The cervix is partially opened, allowing the mucus produced by the endometrial glands to escape when estrus occurs.

These changes in the uterus are viewed by ultrasound as reduced uniformity in the gray tones and a swollen appearance of the uterine wall.[4,12] A more extensive surface of the uterus with dark anechoic zones corresponds to the edema and increased blood vessel activity under the endometrium that are also characteristic of this phase (**Fig. 10**). During estrus, the mucosa of the endometrium becomes more echogenic, and the interface between the endometrium and myometrium reveals a more extensive vascular bed lying between these two layers (**Fig. 11**).[4,12] Additionally, a greater accumulation of endometrial liquid can be seen in the uterine lumen during estrus (**Fig. 12**); this can be confused with early pregnancy examinations and lead to errors

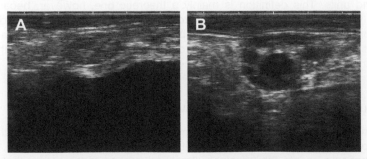

Fig. 7. Ultrasound images of an inactive ovary (*A*) and an ovary in proestrus (*B*). On the image to the right, note the presence of a 1-cm dominant follicle and some small follicles at the edges of the ovarian stroma (8-MHz linear probe, depth of 4 cm).

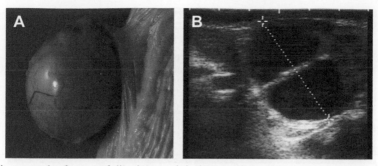

Fig. 8. Photograph of a 4-cm follicular cyst (*A*) along with its ultrasound image (*B*) obtained using an 8-MHz linear probe (depth of 5 cm). Note that the follicular cyst is divided into two cavities.

in diagnosis.[13] Ultrasound examination of the ovaries is used to ascertain the absence of a CL, which would confirm the absence of pregnancy.

Diestrus

During diestrus, high levels of circulating progesterone indicate the dominant hormonal state. The uterine wall is thinner than during the preceding period, and the uterus can be more difficult to view completely with sweeps of the ultrasound probe unless additional manipulations are performed using free fingers, because the horns are normally folded over ventrally during this phase.[13] The uterus is normally empty of endometrial liquid, and the ultrasound scan shows a more uniform appearance. The following images show the typical ultrasound appearance of a normal uterus during this phase of the estrus cycle (**Fig. 13**).

Uterine Pathologic Conditions

The main pathologic conditions of the uterus that can be viewed using ultrasound are infectious disorders.[4,13] These include puerperal metritis, clinical metritis, clinical and subclinical endometritis, and pyometra.[4] The definitions of these postpartum uterine infections have been addressed and proposed by Sheldon and colleagues[14] and are not by any means precise gold standards but rather suggestions to compare and improve studies in the future. Another noninfectious pathologic condition that can be diagnosed with ultrasonography is a mucometra.[4]

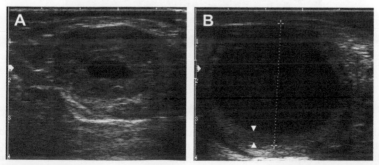

Fig. 9. Ultrasound differences between a CLc (*A*) and a luteal cyst (*B*) in a dairy cow (10-MHz linear probe, depth of 4 cm). A 2.8-cm CLc (*A*) and a 3.7-cm luteal cyst with a wall varying between 2 and 3 mm thick (*B*) are shown. ▶, luteinized wall of the cyst.

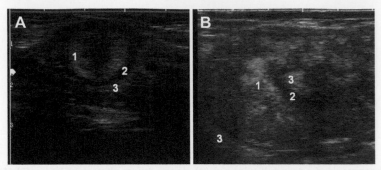

Fig. 10. Ultrasound images of transverse (*A*) and longitudinal (*B*) sections of the uterus during proestrus (8-MHz linear probe, depth of 4 cm). Note the significant nonuniform echogenicity and the swollen appearance of the uterine wall, particularly the endometrium. The anechoic vascular bed is easily identified under the endometrium of the transverse section of the uterus (black ring around the endometrium). 1, endometrium; 2, vascular zone; 3, myometrium.

Puerperal and clinical metritis (less than 21 days in milk)

A diagnosis of acute puerperal metritis (abnormally enlarged uterus and a fetid watery red-brown uterine discharge associated with signs of systemic illness [decreased milk yield, dullness, or other signs of toxemia] and fever >39.5 °C) is generally reserved for the first 10 to 15 days of lactation, although it is possible until 21 days in milk.[14] Ultrasound confirmation is not necessary for this acute infectious problem.

Ultrasound examination of clinical metritis (cow is not systemically ill but has an abnormally enlarged uterus and a purulent uterine discharge detectable in the vagina within 21 days post partum) usually shows a thick uterine wall with an extensive blood vessel network, without cotyledons; the liquid in the lumen has varying degrees of echogenicity (showing gray tones on the monitor) and contains many hyperechogenic particles (**Fig. 14**).[4]

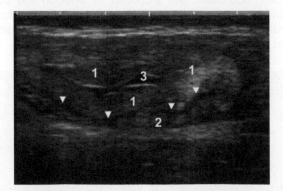

Fig. 11. Ultrasound image of an oblique longitudinal uterine section with a hyperechogenic endometrial mucosa and slight accumulation of mucus in the uterine lumen during estrus (8-MHz linear probe, depth of 4 cm). The prominent vascular zone under the endometrium and the swollen appearance of the uterine wall should also be noted. 1, endometrium; 2, myometrium; 3, accumulation of mucus in the uterus; ▶, vascular zone beneath the endometrium.

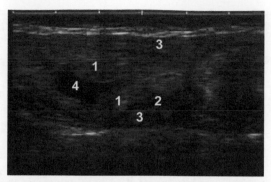

Fig. 12. Ultrasound image of a longitudinal section of the uterus with significant accumulation of endometrial liquid in the lumen during estrus (8-MHz linear probe, depth of 4 cm). 1, endometrium; 2, vascular zone; 3, myometrium; 4, uterine liquid.

Endometritis (clinical and subclinical) and pyometra

Clinical endometritis is characterized by the presence of purulent uterine discharge detectable in the vagina 21 days or more after parturition. In the absence of purulent discharge, an infectious uterus with accumulation of abnormal contents can be diagnosed as subclinical endometritis.

Pyometra is defined as the accumulation of purulent material within the uterine lumen in the presence of a persistent CL and a closed cervix.[14] This uterine infection is generally encountered beyond the voluntary waiting period (>50 days) in dairy cows. Ultrasound examination of this condition shows a variable accumulation of purulent liquid that is nonuniform in echogenicity, with hyperechogenic particles present (**Fig. 15**).[4] The diameter of the infected uterine horn generally varies between 5 and 20 cm.[4,15]

ULTRASOUND EXAMINATION OF THE GRAVID UTERUS

Early diagnosis of pregnancy in cows using ultrasound is a rapid, safe, and cost-effective procedure for dairy producers who would like to improve the reproductive performance of their herd. Ultrasound diagnosis of bovine pregnancy can be done with an excellent level of precision starting on day 27 after insemination.[2]

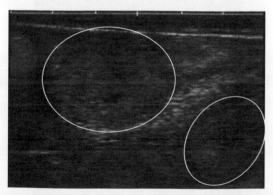

Fig. 13. Ultrasonogram of transverse sections of the uterus (*white circle*) during diestrus (8-MHz linear probe, depth of 4 cm). Note the highly uniform echogenicity of the uterus during this phase compared with the echogenic appearance of the uterus in periestrus in **Fig. 10A.**

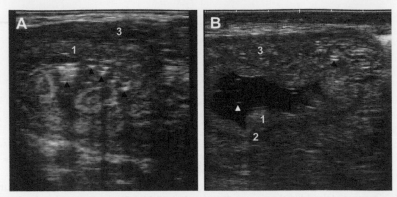

Fig. 14. Ultrasound images of clinical metritis in a cow between days 10 and 15 after calving (7.5–8-MHz linear probe, depth of 6 cm). Note the liquid with variable echogenicity on the image to the left, the presence of many hyperechogenic particles (▶), and a thick uterine wall. 1, endometrium; 2, vascular zone; 3, thickened myometrium (*B*) with an extensive vascular network (*A*).

In this section, the principal ultrasound indicators in making a diagnosis of normal pregnancy are presented, followed by some ultrasound images of twin pregnancies and embryonic death. Additionally, the most commonly reported fetal abnormalities during ultrasound checks of pregnancy in cows are presented.

Embryonic Period

The embryonic period is defined as the period between fertilization and the end of organogenesis on the 42nd day of gestation.[4]

Starting on the 26th day of gestation, ultrasound of early pregnancy shows a uterine lumen containing a variable quantity of anechoic liquid produced by the conceptus.

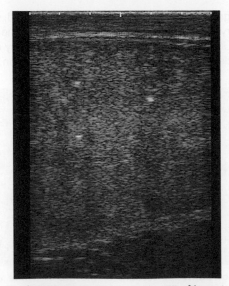

Fig. 15. Ultrasound image of pyometra in a cow on day 55 of lactation (8-MHz linear probe, depth of 9 cm). Note the nonuniform echogenic appearance of the uterine contents, which include several hyperechogenic particles.

The following ultrasound images show a few indicators of pregnancy that can be seen between days 28 and 42 (**Fig. 16**). Before day 27 or 28, there may not be enough liquid in the lumen of the uterus to confirm the diagnosis.[4,13] Visualization of the embryo in the amniotic liquid can be delayed until days 28 to 30 of gestation because it may be hidden behind endometrial folds. Starting on the 30th day, the amnion can be viewed as a highly echogenic envelope that produces specular reflections.[13,16]

Many ultrasound units come with a program that allows the practitioner to estimate the age of the bovine embryo or fetus using specific measurements. The distance between the crown of the head and the rump, the "crown-rump length" (CRL), is the easiest and most precise method of estimating gestational age up to day 55 (**Fig. 17, Table 1**).[4]

The reader is invited to consult the available figures and tables in the more specialized reference books that summarize the measurements of CRL and external skull, trunk, and eye diameters according to age; these references also present the main indicators in evaluating normal embryonic and fetal development up to day 140 of gestation.[4]

Fetal Period

Starting on day 45, fetal movement can be observed.[16] The fetus is active for approximately 60% of the time during an ultrasound examination.[17]

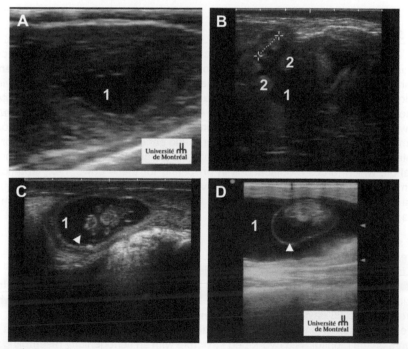

Fig. 16. Ultrasound images of a gravid uterus between days 28 and 42 (7.5–10-MHz linear probe). (*A*) Pregnancy on day 28 with accumulation of liquid only, because the embryo is not visible. (*B*) Embryo, aged 32 days (1.2 cm long), is well hidden behind the endometrial folds. (*C*) Embryo, aged 40 days (1.8 cm long), is surrounded by the amnion. The limbs and the head are visible. (*D*) Embryo, aged 42 days (2.4 cm in length) with an extremely echogenic amniotic membrane is shown. 1, allantoic liquid; 2, endometrial folds; ▶, amniotic membrane; X-X, the embryo lies between the two "X" marks. (*Courtesy of* the Université de Montréal; with permission.)

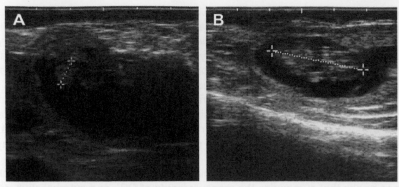

Fig. 17. Estimation of embryonic age by measuring the CRL. (A) CRL = 0.7 cm (estimated age: 30 days). (B) CRL = 2.7 cm (estimated age: 42 days).

The position of the fetus in the abdomen and the significant increase in its size begin to limit accessibility for transrectal ultrasound examination in the second half of gestation.[4] The following ultrasound images show a few of the indicators of pregnancy beyond day 42 in cows (**Fig. 18**). Other images are shown in the following section.

Fetal Sexing and Detection of Twins

Fetal sexing and detecting twin pregnancy are generally done during the second examination to confirm pregnancy after days 55 to 60.[4,13] This examination can be decisive for the future of the cow in the herd and for management before calving.[4] A dairy cow that is pregnant with a female fetus is more likely to retain her place in the herd than a cow carrying a male fetus in the event that a choice must be made. A cow that is pregnant with twins must undergo a careful ultrasound examination to determine fetal viability, normal development, and gender.[4] This last step is important in detecting potential freemartins. Cows that are pregnant with twins have a shorter gestation, which forces modifications in preparing for these cows' next lactation; it also means that the producer needs to be vigilant in monitoring problems associated with a twin pregnancy: dystocia, retained placenta, metritis, ketosis, and displacement of the abomasum.[18]

Fetal sexing

This examination can take place between days 56 and 100 of gestation, but the ideal time frame to facilitate ultrasound diagnosis is between days 60 and 70.[4,13,19,20] The genital tubercle, which is the fetal structure that develops into the penis or the clitoris, is visible starting on day 45 but does not reach its definitive location until somewhere between 55 and 58 days after insemination.[4,13,19,20]

The genital tubercle in the male and female cow is a highly echogenic structure that appears on the monitor as a two-lobed structure with an echogenicity resembling that of bone tissue.[4,13] The position of the tubercle relative to the fetal umbilicus and tail determines the diagnosis of fetal gender.[13,19,20]

The genital tubercle is located just caudal to the umbilicus in the male fetus, whereas in the female fetus, its final position is just under the tail (**Fig. 19**).[4,13,19,20]

After 70 days of gestation, the genital tubercle is covered by urogenital folds that eventually develop into the labia minora or the prepuce, which diminishes its echogenicity.[4,13] At this point, the ultrasound image reveals a four-lobed structure

Table 1
Principal physical and ultrasonographic characteristics of the bovine embryo and fetus during its development between 25 and 90 days of pregnancy

Stage of Pregnancy (Days)	Transverse Diameter of the Embryonic Vesicle (cm)	CRL (cm)	Some Observations
25	1.0	0.5–0.7	—
30	1.8–2.0	0.8–1.2	—
35	2.0–2.5	1.3–1.7	Digits recognizable on all four limbs
40	3.0–3.5	1.7–2.4	Embryonic movement begins
45	—	2.3–2.6	—
50	—	3.5–4.5	Migration of the genital tubercle in both genders
55	—	4.5–6.0	Fusion of the urogenital folds and the genital tubercle
60	—	6.0–7.0	External genital organs (clitoris, penis, scrotum) First centers of ossification in the skull and vertebrae
90	—	14–15	CRL measurement is beyond the length of most linear probes Other fetal measurements give better estimation of the fetal age Ossification of the limbs Differentiated stomach compartments

Data from DesCôteaux L, Colloton J, Gnemmi G. Practical atlas of ruminant and camelid reproductive ultrasonography. Ames (IA): Wiley-Blackwell; 2009.

(**Fig. 20**).[4,13] After day 70 of gestation, the term *genital tubercle* should therefore be replaced by *external genital organs*.[4]

Other indicators of fetal gender can also be identified. Among these are the teats that become visible on the female fetus beginning on days 75 to 80 of gestation. These structures remain rudimentary in the male fetus (**Fig. 21**).[4]

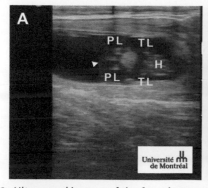
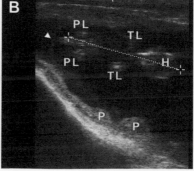

Fig.18. Ultrasound images of the fetus between days 45 and 53. (*A*) Fetus, aged 45 days, with all four limbs visible (thoracic limb [TL] and pelvis limb [PL]), the abdomen, and the head (H). (*Courtesy of* the Université de Montréal). (*B*) Fetus aged 53 days (CRL = 4.5 cm) with visible placentomes (P), the amnion (▶), the limbs (TL and PL), and the head (H) in a longitudinal section.

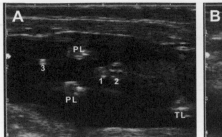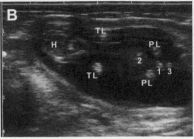

Fig. 19. Ultrasound images of a male fetus (A) and a female (B) fetus (10-MHz linear probe, depth of 4 cm). (A) Male 67-day-old fetus. Note the presence of the genital tubercle (1) caudal to the umbilicus (2). (B) Female 56-day-old fetus with genital tubercle (1) located under the tail (3). H, head; PL, pelvic limb; TL, thoracic limb.

Finally, it is interesting to note that the organs in the thoracic cavity (heart and lungs) and the abdomen (eg, liver, abomasum, rumen, kidneys, bladder) develop rapidly and are already easily visible after the second month of gestation.[4,17] A careful ultrasound examination of the fetus allows the practitioner to identify these developing organs and to diagnose certain fetal abnormalities. Information on the ultrasonographic appearance of the abdominal and thoracic fetal organs is available[4] but is beyond the scope of this review.

Twin pregnancy
The incidence of twin pregnancies in lactating dairy cows seems to be on the increase in the past few decades. One study shows that the rate increased from 4.54% in 1959 to 6.68% in 1997.[21] Today, many practitioners work with herds whose rate of twin pregnancies is greater than 8% to 10%. Dystocia and problems during the postpartum period are frequent consequences for cows that are pregnant with twins.[18] It is therefore important to identify these pregnancies so that follow-up and management of these cows can be improved before and after calving.

During the first ultrasound examination in early pregnancy, the uterus contains a greater quantity of liquid than is normal for that stage of gestation, in addition to

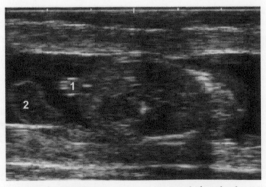

Fig. 20. Ultrasound image of a transverse section at penis level of a 73-day-old male fetus (8-MHz linear probe, depth of 4 cm). Note that an oblique longitudinal section of the umbilical cord can be seen (2) just to the left of the external male genital organs (1). This four-lobed hyperechogenic structure is composed of the penis in the center surrounded by the prepuce.

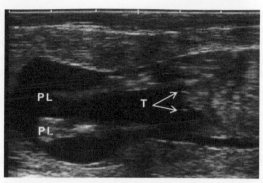

Fig. 21. Ultrasound image of a transverse section at the pelvic/pelvic limbs level of a 72-day-old female fetus (8-MHz linear probe, depth of 4 cm). The two pelvic limbs (PL) are easily visible, and two of the teats (T) can be detected between the limbs of the fetus.

more amniotic and allantoic membranes than can be anticipated for a single pregnancy (twin line) (**Fig. 22**).[4] The twin line is commonly encountered in twin pregnancies: it extends from one or both embryos or fetuses and corresponds to the chorioallantoic membrane shared by the twins.[4]

Embryonic and Fetal Death

The rate of embryonic death between days 28 and 42 of gestation is generally around 10% to 15%.[4,13,17] The fetal mortality rates are approximately 6% and 3%, respectively, for the periods between days 42 and 56 and days 56 and 98.[17] In ipsilateral twin pregnancies (in which both twins are in the same uterine horn), however, the mortality rate is 32%.[22] Therefore, it is important to do an ultrasound re-evaluation

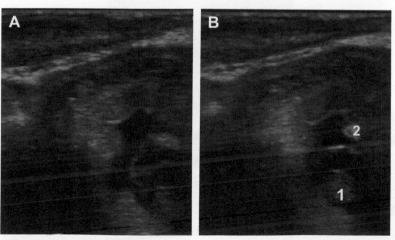

Fig. 22. Ultrasound images of a twin pregnancy in the left uterine horn on day 28 in a 3-year-old Holstein cow (6-MHz linear probe, depth of 4 cm). (*A*) Greater than normal quantity of liquid and allantoic membranes in a 28-day-old pregnancy are evident on this ultrasound image. (*B*) Two embryos are easily visible and separated by a chorioallantoic membrane commonly known as the "twin line."

of twin pregnancies to confirm the plan of action for the producer to use with these cows before the end of this more risky gestation (**Fig. 23**).[4]

The classic ultrasound images that allow the practitioner to diagnose embryonic or fetal death generally show at least one of the following signs: a significant quantity of extremely echogenic debris inside the amniotic or allantoic liquid, poor definition of the structures observed, and the absence of a fetal heartbeat.[4,13,17]

The following ultrasound images illustrate a few of the signs that are used to diagnose embryonic or fetal death (**Fig. 24**).

Fetal Abnormalities

The incidence of fetal abnormalities is low (0.07%), but most abnormal fetuses that make it to term cause dystocia.[17] It is therefore important to obtain as precise a diagnosis as possible of these abnormalities, with the objective of aborting abnormal fetuses.

The following fetal abnormalities are reported most often and can be easily identified with an attentive ultrasound examination: two-headed fetus (**Fig. 25**), hydrocephalus, hydropericardium, schistosomus reflexus, amorphus globosus (or fetal mole), and Siamese twins.[4,13,17]

OTHER APPLICATIONS

Ultrasound examination has become an essential tool in making important decisions relating to the specialized programs and techniques used in bovine reproduction. This section contains a brief presentation of the programs that benefit from judicious use of ultrasound examination to improve reproductive performances. The details and ultrasound images that illustrate the application of these techniques are beyond the scope of this review and can be consulted in the specialized references.[4,13,17]

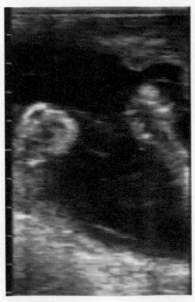

Fig. 23. Ultrasound image of twins in the same uterine horn on day 62 (5-MHz linear probe, depth of 10 cm). The twins' entire bodies are not visible in this image, but both heads can be identified.

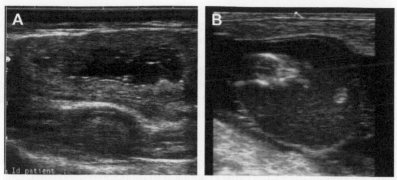

Fig. 24. Typical ultrasound images of embryonic and fetal death. (*A*) Embryonic death on day 45. Note the ill-defined contours and the irregular and highly echogenic allantoic membranes (10-MHz linear probe, depth of 5 cm). (*B*) Fetal death identified on day 68. Note the signs of fetal degeneration and a significant accumulation of hyperechogenic fetal debris in the amniotic liquid (7.5-MHz linear probe, depth of 5 cm).

Embryo Collection and Transfer Programs and In Vitro Fertilization

Bovine practitioners who collect and transfer embryos or perform specialized in vitro fertilization techniques need the information provided by ultrasound examinations of the genital tract to improve the reliability of their services.[4] Much practical research has been devoted to ultrasound evaluations in this context, and ultrasound is certainly justified when doing follow-up checks on superovulation protocols, on the day of

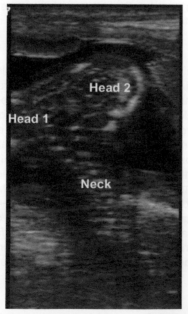

Fig. 25. Ultrasound image of a two-headed fetus on day 67 of pregnancy (6-MHz linear probe, depth of 7 cm). Note the presence of two cervical spines. (*Courtesy of* S. Buczinski, Dr. Vét, MSc, Quebec, Canada.)

insemination, and when the embryos are collected. Ultrasound examination of cows receiving the embryos leads to the selection of the most suitable cows and improved gestation rates for the transferred embryos.[4] Several ultrasonographic criteria have been tested (eg, follicle classifications, counting large ovulatory follicles before choosing expensive semen for donors, counting CLs before the collection or flush to justify repeated flushing until the CL and total ova count are close, evaluating the CLs in recipients) and proved over the past 2 decades, which now allows practitioners to offer innovative embryo transfer programs.[4]

Color Doppler Ultrasound

The color Doppler ultrasound technique shows hemodynamic changes in local ovarian circulation throughout the estrus cycle in addition to pathologic conditions. Examination of the uterus using this technique during the estrus cycle, during gestation, and in the postpartum period could possibly improve diagnostic precision and guide better treatment choices.[4] The added value of this supplemental ultrasound diagnostic method for the bovine uterus remains to be demonstrated. Only a few specialized references and research articles have presented its value in diagnosis; it should nevertheless become a valuable tool for avant-garde practitioners interested in developing the use of this type of ultrasound in the near future.[4,5,23,24]

Ultrasound use in Reproduction Synchronization Protocols for Dairy Cattle

The use of synchronization protocols has significantly changed breeding management for dairy cattle. The authors believe that ultrasound can be used to great advantage to improve results in synchronization programs by estimating the proportion of uterine problems and anovular cows before and at breeding time, thus indirectly assessing the early lactation nutritional balance at a herd level, by recommending rational synchronization protocols based on the presence or absence of CLs and by proposing early pregnancy examinations to resynchronize open cows efficiently.[4]

SUMMARY

Ultrasound is an economically valuable tool readily available to all veterinarians and producers. The ability of ultrasound to identify pregnant versus nonpregnant animals earlier allows nonpregnant animals to be returned to the breeding pool more quickly. More accurate identification of ovarian structures has become especially important with the advent of synchronization protocols. High rates of embryonic and fetal loss, particularly in dairy cattle, make the ability of ultrasound to evaluate fetal viability critical. Identification of twins helps producers to manage cows carrying them more effectively. Assessment of uterine pathologic conditions has always been difficult by rectal palpation, but ultrasound is a much more sensitive diagnostic tool. Even fetal gender determination, once considered useful only for those selling animals with high genetic value, has proved beneficial as a component of cull decisions for commercial herds. Ultrasound examination of the reproductive tract provides a "foot in the door" to help manage dairy herds (eg, nutrition, culling, business opportunity, reproduction) and to start offering other ultrasound medical services at the cow level.

REFERENCES

1. DesCôteaux L, Buczinski S. Examen échographique de l'appareil reproducteur et de la glande mammaire [Ultrasonographic examination of the reproductive tract and mammary gland]. In: Buczinski S, DesCôteaux L, editors. Échographie des

bovins [Bovine ultrasonography]. Paris: Les Éditions du Point Vétérinaire; 2009. p. 109–19 [in French].

2. DesCôteaux L, Fetrow J. Does it pay to use an ultrasound machine for early pregnancy diagnosis in dairy cows? In: Proceedings of the Annual Convention of the American Association of Bovine Practitioners. Spokane (WA); 1998. p. 172–4.

3. Oltenacu PA, Ferguson JD, Lednor AJ. Economic evaluation of pregnancy diagnosis in dairy cattle: a decision analysis approach. J Dairy Sci 1990;73: 2826–31.

4. DesCôteaux L, Gnemmi G, Colloton J. Practical atlas of ruminant and camelid reproduction ultrasonography. Ames (IA): Wiley-Blackwell; 2010.

5. Miyamoto A, Shirasuna K, Hayashi KG, et al. A potential use of color ultrasound as a tool for reproductive management: new observations using color ultrasound scanning that were not possible with imaging only in black and white. J Reprod Dev 2006;52:153–60.

6. Kito S, Okuda K, Miyazawa K, et al. Study on the appearance of the cavity in the corpus luteum of cows by using ultrasonic scanning. Theriogenology 1986;25: 325–33.

7. Pierson RA, Ginther OJ. Ultrasonic imaging of the ovaries and uterus in cattle. Theriogenology 1988;29:21–37.

8. Kastelic JP, Pierson RA, Ginther OJ. Ultrasonic morphology of corpora lutea and central luteal cavities during the estrous cycle and early pregnancy in heifers. Theriogenology 1990;34:487–98.

9. Opsomer G, Grohn YT, Hertl J, et al. Risk factors for post partum ovarian dysfunction in high producing dairy cows in Belgium: a field study. Theriogenology 2000; 53:841–57.

10. Walsh RB, LeBlanc SJ, Duffield TD, et al. Synchronization of estrus and pregnancy risk in anestrous dairy cows after treatment with a progesterone-releasing intravaginal device. J Dairy Sci 2007;90:1139–48.

11. Bonafos LD, Kot K, Ginther OJ. Physical characteristics of the uterus during the bovine estrous cycle and early pregnancy. Theriogenology 1995;43:713–21.

12. Pierson RA, Ginther OJ. Ultrasonographic appearance of the bovine uterus during the estrous cycle. J Am Vet Med Assoc 1987;190:995–1001.

13. Carrière PD, DesCôteaux L, Durocher J. Ultrasonography of the reproductive system of the cow. Faculté de médecine vétérinaire, Université de Montréal. St.-Hyacinthe, Québec, Canada: 2005. [CD-ROM audio-video-3D interactive learning environment and multilingual]. http://www.medvet.umontreal.ca/litiem/produits_fr.htm.

14. Sheldon M, Lewis GS, LeBlanc S, et al. Defining postpartum uterine disease in cattle. Theriogenology 2006;65(8):1516–30.

15. Barlund CS, Carruthers TD, Waldner CL, et al. A comparison of diagnostic techniques for postpartum endometritis in dairy cattle. Theriogenology 2008;69(6): 714–23.

16. Kastelic JP, Curran S, Pierson RA, et al. Ultrasonic evaluation of the bovine conceptus. Theriogenology 1998;29:39–54.

17. Ginther OJ. Ultrasonic imaging and animal reproduction: cattle. Wisconsin: Equiservices Publishing; 1998. p. 134–43.

18. Van Saun RJ. Comparison of pre-and postpartum performance of Holstein dairy cows having either a single or twin pregnancy. In: Proceedings of the Annual Convention of the American Association of Bovine Practitioners. British Columbia, Canada; 2001. p. 204.

19. Curran S. Fetal sex determination in cattle and horses by ultrasonography. Theriogenology 1992;37:17–21.
20. Stroud BK. Clinical applications of bovine reproductive ultrasonography. Compendium Continuing Education Practicing Veterinarian 1994;16:1085–97.
21. Day JD, Weaver LD, Franti CF. Association of twin pregnancy diagnosis and parturition with days open, days pregnant at diagnosis, parity, and milk production in dairy cattle. Bovine Practice 1997;31:25–8.
22. Lopez-Gatius H, Hunter. Spontaneous reduction of advanced twin embryos: its occurrence and clinical relevance in dairy cattle. Theriogenology 2005;63: 118–25.
23. Bollwein H, Meyer HH, Maierl J, et al. Transrectal Doppler sonography of uterine blood flow. Theriogenology 2000;53:1541–52.
24. Acosta TJ, Hayashi KG, Ohtani M, et al. Local changes in blood flow within the preovulatory follicle wall and early corpus luteum in cows. Reproduction 2003; 125:759–67.

Ultrasonographic Assessment of Late Term Pregnancy in Cattle

Sébastien Buczinski, DrVét, DÉS, MSc

KEYWORDS

• Fetal well-being • Ultrasonography • Late pregnancy
• High-risk pregnancy • Cloned pregnancy

After many years, the challenge of bovine production remains the ability to produce one healthy calf per cow per year. This statement is true for milk production and for replacement heifers in dairy industry.[1] The cow-calf productivity is also based on the maximum number of weaned calves produced per cow per year.[2] On the other side, assisted reproductive techniques such as embryo production or cloning have been developed as new technologies to improve genetic selection.[3] However, these techniques are expensive and accompanied with multiple complications and losses throughout the pregnancy especially for cloned fetuses.[4] In horses, the detection of any anomaly during the pregnancy can be a useful tool to anticipate pregnancy losses or to be prepared in dealing with high-risk pregnancies.[5] The terminology of high-risk pregnancies has been applied to the pregnancies in which a disease of the dam, the fetus, or adnexal anomalies can compromise the uterine and extra-uterine life.[4]

The transabdominal ultrasonography has become a widespread ancillary tool for assessing the fetus and its uterine adnexa in many veterinary species [5–8] and has been studied more extensively in human pregnancies.[9,10] Although the information available in the bovine pregnancy is not as developed as in human obstetric, interesting information can be obtained by the ultrasonographic assessment of the fetus and the uterine adnexa during the late pregnancy. This application of bovine ultrasound can be helpful in cases where the pregnancy may be compromised by a maternal disease or in cases of cloned pregnancies which are both high-risk pregnancies.[4] As in other species, the main objectives of the fetal ultrasonography are to

Clinique Ambulatoire Bovine/Bovine Ambulatory Clinic, Département des Sciences Cliniques, Faculté de Médecine Vétérinaire, Université de Montréal, CP 5000, Saint-Hyacinthe, QC, Canada J2S 7C6
E-mail address: s.buczinski@umontreal.ca

Vet Clin Food Anim 25 (2009) 753–765
doi:10.1016/j.cvfa.2009.07.005
0749-0720/09/$ – see front matter © 2009 Elsevier Inc. All rights reserved.

be able to detect any fetal growth restriction or abnormality,[9] any change in fetal biophysical profile,[10] and eventual congenital anomalies.[11]

THEORETICAL BASIS OF THE TRANSABDOMINAL ULTRASONOGRAPHY FOR ASSESSING THE FETUS AND UTERINE ADNEXA

Various maternal diseases or placental anomalies may adversely affect the fetus.[12] An extensive review of those interactions is out of the scope of this article but it is important to understand that the basis of the transabdominal ultrasound for assessing the pregnancies comes from the multiple interactions in the fetomaternal unit. The more common abnormalities include an abnormal uteroplacental perfusion, and decreased oxygen and nutrient delivery to the fetus.[13] Those processes have a detrimental impact on fetal health since they may affect fetal development and growth.[5,6,9,13] The placental insufficiency is responsible for intrauterine-growth restriction and has a detrimental impact on the cardiovascular and the central nervous system.[14] The consequences of fetal hypoxia are numerous. In cases of acute hypoxia (that can be found with maternal hemorrhage, respiratory distress, or shock) the fetal movements and the fetal heart rate (FHR) are decreased in ovine fetuses.[15] After 12 hours of maintained hypoxic conditions, ovine fetuses showed a back-to-normal FHR, then a higher FHR, than healthy fetuses because of increased catecholamine secretions.[15] However, the FHR variability is severely affected in these cases with absent or reduced FHR accelerations.[15] The fetal-movement patterns are also affected in cases of chronic hypoxic condition, since they return back to normal shortly after the hypoxic injury. They continue to decrease if hypoxic conditions are maintained and if they are concomitant with fetal acidemia.[16]

The ultrasonographic appearance of the placenta and the uterine fluids may also be affected by various conditions during the pregnancy.[17–19] Therefore, the assessment of the placentomes, and the uterine fluids and amniotic membrane may be informative when assessing the uteroplacental unit[4,19,20] especially in cloned pregnancies where abnormal number, shape, size, and appearance of the placentomes may be encountered.[20] Although much of the information coming from comparative medicine shows the usefulness of fetal well-being assessment, the practical applications for the bovine practitioner have been limited until now. However, information in studies performed in other species and studies in cattle have shown that information relevant for the clinician may be obtained when performing ultrasonography in late pregnancy.

TRANSABDOMINAL ULTRASOUND IN THE LAST TRIMESTER OF PREGNANCY IN THE COW

The ultrasonographic assessment of the conceptus on the last third of pregnancy is done with the cow standing and only attached by the head.[19] The examination (for a duration of about 30 minutes) begins by palpating the conceptus by ballottement of the abdomen to confirm the location of the fetus which is commonly located on the lower right flank. The ventral part of the right abdomen is then shaved caudally from the udder to the end of the milk vein cranially. The area is extended on the right to the horizontal lines 15 cm dorsally to the stifle and on the left to the linea alba (**Fig. 1**). The area can be extended if necessary to obtain a better view of the conceptus. The skin is then rinsed with water and ultrasonic gel is applied on the region of interest to improve the image quality. Owing to the size of the maternal abdomen and the fetus, a low-frequency probe (less than 5 MHz) is required to have a deep penetration.[6,18,19] A higher frequency probe (5 MHz) can be used for the assessment of the placentomes

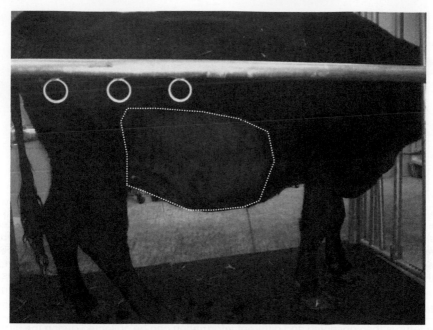

Fig. 1. The typical area (delimited by a dotted line) that is necessary to prepare to perform the ultrasonographic assessment of the fetomaternal unit in the last trimester of pregnancy. After locating the fetus by abdominal ballotment, the area from the udder to the xiphoid appendix cranially, up to the middle part of the flank can be shaved and extended during the examination if necessary.

and the uterine fluids.[20] However, it is difficult to observe the fetus consistently because of the low depth of penetration of these ultrasounds.

Placenta and Uterine Fluids Assessment

The procedure begins with the identification of fetal or placental structures. Most times, the placentomes are easily recognized by their specific aspect of an echogenic ovale to elliptic structure with a dimension of a chicken-egg (**Fig. 2**).[20] They are distributed on the uterine wall and are easily observed surrounded by anechoic-to-hypoechoic uterine fluids (see **Fig. 2**; **Fig. 3**). The amniotic fluid appeared as a hypoechoic fluid with various amounts of echoic particles (see **Fig. 3**).[19,21] The allantoic fluid is the most important uterine fluid in bovine pregnancy. It is easily recognized since its echogenicity is lower than the amniotic fluid and, therefore, it appears as an anechoic media. The echogenicity of the allantoic fluid slowly increases during the pregnancy.[20,21] Both uterine fluids are separated by a thin echoic membrane which is the amniotic membrane (see **Fig. 3**). The deepest pocket of fetal fluid has been mentioned as an interesting tool in the assessment of uterine fluid in other species.[4,22] A decreased amniotic fluid volume is diagnostic of oligohydramnios which is associated with adverse fetal outcomes in human.[22] The main indication for measuring the deepest pocket of uterine fluid in cattle is to detect hydrops of the uterine fluids.[5,19] In the last month of bovine pregnancy, the deepest pocket of uterine fluid is higher than 20 cm when using a 3.5 MHz probe and it is always possible to observe portions of the fetus when performing the transabdominal ultrasonography.[19]

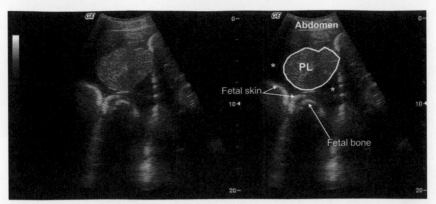

Fig. 2. Ultrasonographic appearance of a placentome (PL) in bovine late term pregnancy. The placentomes appear as echogenic ovoid structures surrounded by allantoic fluid (*asterisks*). The center area of the placentome is classically more echogenic than the peripheral area. The size of the placentomes is similar to a chicken egg. The fetal skin is also observed as an echogenic line. The fetal bones appear as a hyperechoic line stopping all ultrasounds with a shadow artifact.

Fetal Assessment

The fetus is then observed and different information can be collected during the ultrasonographic examination. Because of its large size, and despite low frequency probes, it is not possible to observe the whole fetus by contrast to the human[22] and ovine fetuses.[4] Therefore the assessment of specific fetal parts is limited. The fetal thorax is recognized by observing the heart beating (**Fig. 4**). The costal reverberations due to the bone or soft tissue interactions can also be seen when the thorax is observed in longitudinal plane (**Fig. 5**). The hypoechoic lung parenchyma is also observed. The fetal heart rate can therefore be calculated manually or being automatically obtained if an M-mode or a pulsed wave Doppler is available (**Fig. 6**). Previous studies have

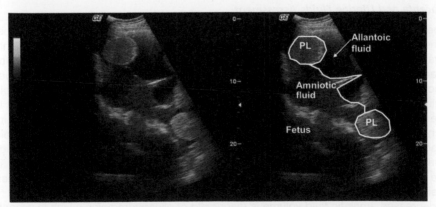

Fig. 3. Ultrasonographic appearance of the uterine fluids in a late-term pregnancy (8 months). Both allantoic and amniotic fluid are observed. The amniotic fluid is more echogenic than the allantoic fluid. It contains small, echoic particles to distinguish it from the allantoic fluid. The allantoic fluid is anechoic, similar to blood or urine. The amniotic and allantoic fluid are separated by a thin echogenic amniotic membrane (*yellow line*). Two placentomes (PL) are observed.

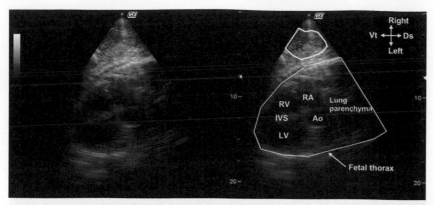

Fig. 4. The fetal heart can be imaged after the fetal thorax has been found. The calculation of the FHR can be done manually in counting the heartbeats during a 15 second period. The right (RV) and left ventricles (LV) are observed separated by the interventricular septum (IVS). The aortic root (Ao) and the right atrium (RA) are also observed. One placentome (PL) is squeezed between the fetus and the abdominal wall. Ds, dorsal; Vt, ventral.

shown that the FHR can be variable during the last days of pregnancy. The mean FHR varies from 114 beats per minute in bovine fetuses 3 weeks before birth, to 109 beats per minute during the last 2 weeks of pregnancy.[23] The variations of FHR during the last 2 weeks of pregnancy are from 90 to 125 beats per minute.[24] However, the fetus may infrequently experience episodes of severe tachycardia (more than 180 beats per minute) in the last 2 weeks of pregnancy without any problem.[25] Continuous monitoring of the FHR by Doppler and computer analysis of the FHR curves may be especially useful in determining FHR variability, which is an important indicator of fetal well-being.[9,15,16] However, continuous monitoring of FHR and computer analysis has only been done in healthy Holstein-Friesian cows, indicating that the mean number of FHR accelerations per hour was relatively constant during the last 3 weeks of

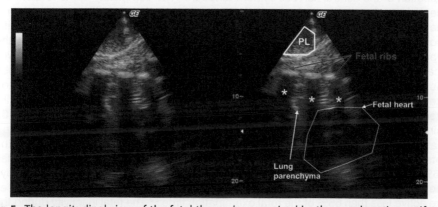

Fig. 5. The longitudinal view of the fetal thorax is recognized by the reverberation artifacts (*asterisks*) when the fetal ribs are imaged. The fetal ribs in transverse plane are characterized by hyperechoic surfaces displayed at a regular interval, since no ultrasounds can diffuse deeper than the osseous surface, shadows are observed after the echoic lines. The beating heart of the fetus can also be observed in this image, along with the hypoechoic lung parenchyma. PL, placentome.

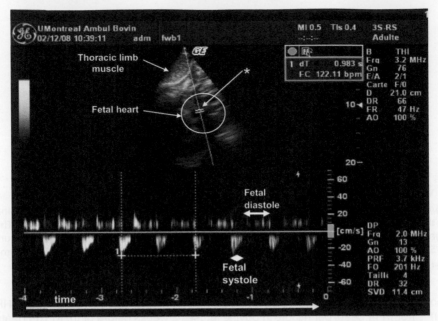

Fig. 6. Determination of the fetal heart rate by the pulsed-wave Doppler assessment. The fetal heart has been located and the volume sample (*) is observed on the beam path. The FHR is then determined in locating the distance between 3 heart beats (3 similar points on the sinusoidal curves). In this case the FHR (FC) has been calculated at 122 beats per minute.

pregnancy (4.4 to 5 h^{-1}).[23] Future work on FHR variability patterns in compromised pregnancies should therefore be obtained before being used in clinical settings.

The assessment of fetal movement or activity is also an important part of the biophysical profile in human[22] and equine fetuses.[6,18] The fetal activity is an interesting reflection of the central nervous system function.[5] The complexity of the fetal movements increase progressively during the pregnancy as the central nervous system is maturating.[26,27] The problem with large fetuses is that it is difficult to observe specific movements of the fetus. Therefore, most of time it is impossible to know exactly the type or the complexity of the fetal movement. For this reason, the fetal–global–activity scale introduced by Reef and colleagues[6] is a more practical technique to describe the fetal movements in cattle.[28] Briefly, the author used a scale of zero to four to grade the percentage of the examination time the fetus was moving. A score of zero is attributed to fetuses that did not move during the total examination time, which is about 30 minutes. A score of one is attributed to fetuses active less than 33% of the total examination time. A score of two is attributed to fetuses active during 33% to 66% of the total examination time. A score of three is attributed to fetuses active more than 66% of the total examination time. The last category concerns fetuses that are always moving during the examination period (score of four). The majority of healthy fetuses are active less than 66% of the total examination time.[29] The fetal inactivity during the examination period has never been observed in healthy bovine fetuses,[29] but has been reported in fetuses with a poor outcome.[28,29] However, although not described in healthy bovine fetuses, fetal inactivity or fetal sleeping periods are common findings in healthy human fetuses[3,10] and can be found less frequently in healthy equine fetuses.[30]

The fetal ultrasonography may be useful to anticipate an abnormal fetal growth.[5,9,13,14] Unfortunately the ultrasonographic tools that have been used in other species or in early pregnancy such as fetal head biparietal diameter, femoral length, or fetal abdominal circumference are not reliable in cattle because of the size of the fetus, the position of the fetus, and the size of the bones.[4] The fetal thoracic aortic diameter, which is used in the equine species to assess fetal growth,[5,6] has also been found to increase during the bovine pregnancy (**Fig. 7**).[31] This parameter is also correlated to the birth weight when measured in the last 10 days before calving with the relation $BW = 2.188Ao-0.667$ where BW is birth weight and Ao is thoracic aortic diameter (Correlation coefficient [R] = .062) (Buczinski and colleagues, unpublished data, 2008). Finally the metacarpal and metatarsal transversal thicknesses have been validated as interesting tools to anticipate large fetuses with a higher risk of dystocia.[32,33] The problem with this measurement is that it can be only obtained by transrectal ultrasonography when the fetus can be palpated and when the presentation of the fetus can be determined.[32,33] Therefore this technique may be only useful during the last weeks of pregnancy to anticipate calving problems.[32,33]

The fetal ultrasonography can also be informative concerning the assessment of the fetal organs. The abdominal organs can be easily recognized if the operator is used to bovine ultrasonography (**Fig. 8**). However, because of the position of the fetus, it can be difficult to systematically assess the fetal organs. The size of the equine fetal stomach increases as the gestation advances and is also correlated to fetal swallowing activity which is an indirect assessment of the fetal neurologic development.[5] To date, the ultrasonographic observation of the fetal organs may be of interest in the detection of congenital anomalies but has not been used for the assessment of fetal growth or well-being in bovine late pregnancy, despite its potential interest.

Vascular Assessment of the Uteroplacental Unit

Since the uteroplacental perfusion is a key factor of fetal development, the noninvasive assessment of the uterine perfusion has been described with Doppler ultrasonography in cows.[34] The Doppler ultrasonography of the uterine artery has been monitored during pregnancy in cows.[35,36] The uterine–blood-flow volume increased 17-fold when compared with day 30 of the pregnancy.[35] The uterine

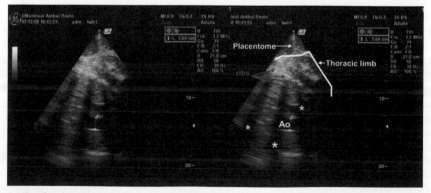

Fig. 7. The fetal aorta is recognized by its echoic wall and its size variation relative to the systolic and diastolic phase of the cardiac cycle. The thoracic aortic diameter (Ao here reported to be 1.64cm) can be an interesting tool to assess the fetal growth. The fetal ribs are also easily recognized because of the reverberation artifact (*asterisk*). The thoracic limb of the fetus is also observed in transverse section.

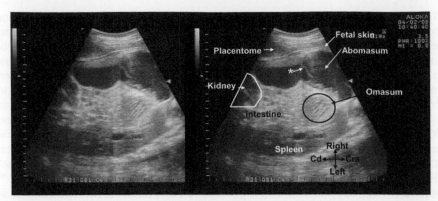

Fig. 8. The fetal ultrasonography can be useful to assess the fetal organs. In this picture, the major abdominal organs are represented. The fetal abomasum is filled by hypoechoic amniotic fluid and can be easily recognized by the presence of echoic abomasal folds (*asterisk*). The omasal lamellae are also observed as thin echoic lines. Cd, caudal; Cra, cranial.

arterial blood-flow ipsilateral to the pregnant horn was correlated with birth weight but the correlation was not strong (R = 0.34).[35] The resistance index decreased throughout the pregnancy until the eighth month of pregnancy and remained relatively constant until delivery.[36] This index was also negatively correlated with the birth weight (R = −0.45).[35] Unfortunately, there are no available reports concerning the usefulness of Doppler analysis of the uterine artery in high-risk or cloned pregnancies.

The Doppler analysis of fetal vessels may also be of interest in determining the patterns of the Doppler waves.[37] The Doppler signals of the human fetal vessels are affected by fetal anemia, intrauterine-growth restriction, and placental insufficiency.[37] However, the practical applications of these findings in cattle may be limited owing to the size and the position of the fetus by contrast to small ruminants.[38]

ABNORMAL FINDINGS IN THE ULTRASONOGRAPHIC ASSESSMENT OF THE LATE-TERM PREGNANCY

The main interest for assessing the bovine fetal well-being in late-term pregnancy is the management of high-risk pregnancies. Those pregnancies remain a clinical challenge in field or hospital settings because of the difficulty of knowing if maintaining the pregnancy is the better option than performing a caesarean section. There are two types of high-risk pregnancies that are observed in cattle. The first category consists of pregnancies that can be compromised because of a maternal or a fetal disease.[32,39,40] These types of pregnancy are the most frequently encountered in bovine practice. The second type of high-risk pregnancy is the cloned pregnancy. The cloning process is associated with losses throughout the pregnancy and in the neonatal period.[4,31,41]

Fetal Well-being Assessment in High-risk Pregnancy due to a Maternal or Fetal Disease

The maternal diseases that can affect the pregnancy are numerous.[42] However, the evidences of these relations have received less interest in cattle[4,29] than in horses.[5,6,43,44] The maternal diseases that include severe inflammatory process, maternal anemia, hypovolemic or septic shock or intoxications may all adversely affect the pregnancy.[4,29] A preliminary study in 10 high-risk pregnancies has shown that the transabdominal findings may be helpful in detecting a poor fetal outcome.[29] The absence of fetal heart beat is a specific sign of fetal death.[21,29] The fetuses that are always active during the examination period (30 minutes) and fetuses inactive throughout the examination period should be monitored, since their prognosis may be compromised.[28,29] Serial ultrasonographic examinations may be required to confirm those findings since hyperactivity or sleeping periods have been infrequently mentioned in healthy foals.[30] The punctual ultrasonographic assessment of the FHR did not appear to be an interesting tool for detecting fetal distress.[29] Unfortunately, no data are available concerning the FHR variability in those cases. The presence of large quantities of echoic particles in uterine fluids is also a sign of fetal distress or death.[21,29]

Multiple fetal anomalies can be encountered during bovine pregnancy.[45,46] However, the antenatal diagnosis of the fetal anomalies has been limited to an early ultrasonographic diagnosis.[47] The ultrasonographic assessment of the fetus may help in detecting congenital anomalies such as anasarca fetalis.[28] However, the position of the fetus may interfere with the diagnosis of existing fetal anomalies.[39]

Fetal Well-being Assessment in Cloned Pregnancies

Animal cloning is the latest assisted reproductive technology that has been developed in cattle.[4] Although the potential interest in cloning cattle is numerous,[48] the major problem with somatic cloning is accompanied with multiple losses throughout the pregnancy and in the early extrauterine life.[4,41,49,50] Although the majority of losses occur at the first trimester, losses can also occur later, which is uncommon in normal bovine pregnancies in the absence of an infectious agent.[31] The cloned pregnancies are therefore considered as high-risk pregnancy throughout the pregnancy period.[4,31,50] Moreover, the cloned calves may be affected by multiple congenital anomalies or adnexal anomalies such as hydrallantois.[41,51,52] For these reasons, the applications of the transabdominal ultrasonographic assessment may help in detecting the compromised pregnancies to manage the fetuses adequately.

As in other types of pregnancies, the absence of the fetal heart beat is a sign of fetal death.[28] The fetal inactivity or hyperactivity is also a clinical sign compatible with fetal demise.[28,29] However, the fetal activity has not been assessed in enough cases to be considered as a sensitive and specific sign of fetal distress.[40]

Abnormal growth patterns have also been recognized as a problematic issue in cloned pregnancy.[4,31] These problems are associated with various placental anomalies such as placentomegaly, a reduced number of placentomes, and fetal macrosomy.[52,53] These entities have been recently called large placenta, large offspring, or abnormal offspring syndrome.[4,52,53] The metacarpal or metatarsal thickness, and the thoracic aortic diameter should be useful for determining heavy calves with a higher risk of dystocia.[32,33]

The ultrasonographic findings may also be useful in cases of clinical suspicion of hydrallantois, which is frequently associated with fetal demise.[31] In those cases, the increased quantity of allantoic fluid lead to a permanent impossibility to image the fetal abdomen and fetal thorax.[31,40,52]

Other anomalies can also be observed in those cases such as abnormal placentomes (**Fig. 9**) or increased amniotic membrane thickness.[19,28,40,52] Other ultrasonographic abnormalities that have been mentioned in late-term cloned pregnancies are small placentomes (length <1 cm) which were not observed in control pregnancies.[20] A recent morphometric analysis of placentation in cloned and control pregnancies showed that large placentomes with a diameter of more than 11 cm are frequently

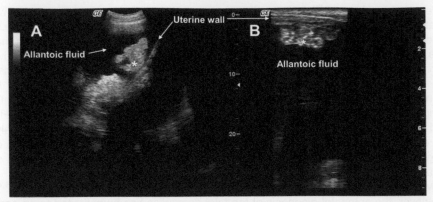

Fig. 9. Abnormal placentomes in a cloned pregnancy with hydrallantois in the seventh month of pregnancy. Some placentomes (*asterisks*) have an irregular shape and appear as lumpy structures (*A*). The echogenicity of other placentomes is different from normal. Hyperechoic and hypoechoic foci are observed (*B*), which contrasts with the normal echogenic aspect of normal placentomes. (*Modified from* Buczinski S. Echographie des Bovins, Les Éditions du Point Vétérinaire. France: Wolter-Kluwer; 2009. p. 161–8; with permission.)

found in cloned pregnancies in contrast to normal control pregnancies.[54] In the same study, the accessory placentomes (diameter less than 1 cm) were present in every cloned pregnancy and not in control pregnancies. However, there is no ultrasonographic study mentioning the placentomes size or number as a reliable indicator of suspicion of abnormal offspring syndrome or fetal demise. One should remember that grossly abnormal placental structures may not be systematically associated with a compromised fetus.[55] Therefore, the fetal assessment is also required for suspecting fetal demise.

SUMMARY

With a good knowledge of bovine anatomy and ultrasonography, the transabdominal ultrasonography of the fetomaternal unit can be performed and pertinent information can be obtained. Although the available data are limited concerning its use in the management of bovine high-risk pregnancy, hydrops or fetal death can be easily suspected. Measuring the thoracic aorta at the end of the pregnancy is an interesting tool for estimating birth weight. As in human obstetrics, care should be taken when interpreting the results of the ultrasonographic examination of the fetus and the uterine adnexa.[56] The repeatability of the ultrasonographic findings still needs to be achieved. Further studies are required to have a better comprehension of the ultrasonographic manifestations of the complex maternofetal interactions in cattle.

REFERENCES

1. Olynk NJ, Wolf CA. Economic analysis of reproductive management strategies on US commercial dairy farms. J Dairy Sci 2008;91(10):4082–91.
2. Dargatz DA, Dewell GA, Mortimer RG. Calving and calving management of beef cows and heifers in cow-calf operations in the United States. Theriogenology 2004;61(6):997–1007.
3. Vajta G, Gjerris M. Science and technology of farm animal cloning: state of the art. Anim Reprod Sci 2006;92(3–4):211–30.

4. Buczinski S, Fecteau G, Lefebvre RC, et al. Fetal well-being assessment in bovine near-term gestations: current knowledge and future perspectives arising from comparative medicine. Can Vet J 2007;48(2):178–83.

5. Bucca S. Diagnosis of the compromised equine pregnancy. Vet Clin North Am Equine Pract 2006;22(3):749–61.

6. Reef VB, Vaala WE, Worth LT, et al. Ultrasonographic assessment of fetal well-being during late gestation: development of an equine biophysical profile. Equine Vet J 1996;28:200–8.

7. England GC. Ultrasonographic assessment of the abnormal pregnancy. Vet Clin North Am Small Anim Pract 1998;28(4):849–68.

8. Ward VL, Estroff JA, Nguyen HT, et al. Fetal sheep development on ultrasound and magnetic resonance imaging: a standard for the in-utero assessment of models of congenital abnormalities. Fetal Diagn Ther 2006;21(5):444–57.

9. Lerner JP. Fetal growth and well-being. Obstet Gynecol Clin North Am 2004;31(1): 159–76.

10. Devoe LD. Antenatal fetal assessment: contraction stress test, nonstress test, vibroacoustic stimulation, amniotic fluid volume, biophysical profile, and modified biophysical profile-an overview. Semin Perinatol 2008;32(4):247–52.

11. Woodward PJ, Kennedy A, Sohaey R, et al. Diagnostic imaging: obstetrics. Salt-Lake City (UT): Amirsys; 2005.

12. Smith GC, Fretts RC. Stillbirth. Lancet 2007;370(9600):1715–25.

13. Cetin I, Boito S, Radelli T. Evaluation of fetal growth and fetal well-being. Semin Ultrasound CT MR 2008;29(2):136–46.

14. Barry JS, Rozance PJ, Anthony RV. An animal model of placental insufficiency-intrauterine growth restriction. Semin Perinatol 2008;32(3):225–30.

15. Bocking AD. Assessment of fetal heart rate and fetal movements in detecting oxygen deprivation in-utero. Eur J Obstet Gynecol Reprod Biol 2003;110(1): S108–12.

16. Richardson BS, Bocking AD. Metabolic and circulatory adaptations to chronic hypoxia in the fetus. Comp Biochem Physiol 1998;119(3):717–23.

17. Abramowicz JS, Sheiner E. Ultrasound of the placenta: a systematic approach. Part I: imaging. Placenta 2008;29(3):225–40.

18. Reef VB. Late term pregnancy monitoring. In: Samper JC, Pycock JF, McKinnon AO, editors. Current therapy in equine reproduction. St-Louis (MO): Saunders Elsevier; 2007. p. 410–6.

19. Buczinski S. Examen échographique du fœtus et de ses annexes dans le troisième tiers de gestation [Ultrasonography of the fetus and its adnexa in the last trimester of pregnancy]. In: Buczinski S, editor. Échographie des Bovins [Bovine ultrasonography]. Point Vétérinaire-Wolter-Kluwer; 2009. p. 161–8 [in French].

20. Kohan-Gadr HR, Lefebvre RC, Fecteau G, et al. Ultrasonographic and histological characterization of the placenta of somatic nuclear transfer-derived pregnancies in dairy cattle. Theriogenology 2008;69(2):218–30.

21. Jonker FH. Fetal death: comparative aspect in large domestic animals. Anim Reprod Sci 2004;82–3:415–30.

22. Manning FA. Fetal biophysical profile. Obstet Gynecol Clin North Am 1999;26(4): 557–77.

23. Breukelman S, Mulder EJH, Van Oord R, et al. Continuous fetal heart rate monitoring during late gestation in cattle by means of Doppler ultrasonography: reference values obtained by computer-assisted analysis. Theriogenology 2006; 65(3):486–98.

24. Jonker FH, Van Oord HA, Van Geijn HP, et al. Feasability of continuous recording of fetal heart rate in the near term bovine fetus by means of transabdominal Doppler. Vet Q 1994;16(3):165–8.
25. Jonker FH, Van Oord HA, Van der Weijden GC, et al. Fetal heart rate patterns and the influence of myometral activity during the last month of gestation in cows. Am J Vet Res 1993;54(1):158–63.
26. Romanini C, Rizzo G. Fetal behaviour in normal and compromised fetuses. An overview. Early Hum Dev 1995;43(2):117–31.
27. De Vries JI, Fong BF. Normal fetal motility: an overview. Ultrasound Obstet Gynecol 2006;27(6):701–11.
28. Buczinski S, Fecteau G, Comeau G, et al. Fetal well-being assessment, neonatal and postpartum findings of cloned pregnancies in cattle: a preliminary study on 10 fetuses and calves. Can Vet J 2009;50(3):261–9.
29. Buczinski S, Fecteau G, Lefebvre RC, et al. Ultrasonographic assessment of bovine fetal wellbeing during late pregnancy in normal, compromised and cloned pregnancies. In: 24th ACVIM forum, Louisville, J Vet Int Med 2006;20(3):722–23.
30. Reimer JM. Use of transcutaneous ultrasonography in complicated latter-middle to late gestation pregnancies in the mare: the 122 cases. In Proc Am Assoc Equine Pract 1997;43:159–61.
31. Heyman Y, Chavatte-Palmer P, LeBourhis D, et al. Frequency and occurrence of late-gestation losses from cattle cloned embryos. Biol Reprod 2002;66(1):6–13.
32. Takahashi M, Ueki A, Kawhata K, et al. Relationships between the width of the metacarpus or metatarsus and the birth weight in Holstein calves. J Reprod Dev 2001;47:105–8.
33. Takahashi M, Goto T, Tsuchiya H, et al. Ultrasonography monitoring of nuclear transferred fetal weight during the final stage of gestation in Holstein cows. J Vet Med Sci 2005;67(8):807–11.
34. Bollwein H, Meyer HHD, Maierl J, et al. Transrectal sonography of uterine blood flow in cows during the estrous phase. Theriogenology 2000;53(8):1541–52.
35. Panarace M, Garnil C, Marfil M, et al. Transrectal Doppler ultrasonography for evaluation of uterine blood flow throughout the pregnancy in 13 cows. Theriogenology 2006;66(9):2113–9.
36. Bollwein H, Baumgartner U, Stolla R. Transrectal Doppler sonography of uterine blood flow in cows during pregnancy. Theriogenology 2002;57(8):2053–61.
37. Mari G, Hanif F. Fetal Doppler: umbilical artery, middle cerebral artery and venous system. Semin Perinatol 2008;32(4):253–7.
38. Galan HL, Anthony RV, Rigano S, et al. Fetal hypertension and abnormal Doppler velocimetry in an ovine model of intrauterine growth restriction. Am J Obstet Gynecol 2005;192(1):272–9.
39. Buczinski S, Bélanger AM, Fecteau G, et al. Prolonged gestation in two Holstein cows: transabdominal ultrasonographic findings in late pregnancy and pathologic findings in the fetuses. J Vet Med A Physiol Pathol Clin Med 2007;54:624–6.
40. Buczinski S. Fetal well-being in late pregnancy (normal gestation, compromised and cloned pregnancies). In: DesCôteaux L, Gnemmi G, Colloton J. Editors. Practical atlas of ruminant and camelid reproduction ultrasonography. Ames, Iowa: Wiley-Blackwell; (in press).
41. Fecteau ME, Palmer JE, Wilkins PA. Neonatal care of high-risk cloned and transgenic calves. Vet Clin North Am Food Anim Pract 2005;21(3):637–53.
42. Creasy RK, Resnik R, Iams J, et al, editors. Creasy and Resnik's maternal-fetal medicine: principles and practice. 6th edition. Saunders Philadelphia: Elsevier; 2009. p. 1282.

43. LeBlanc MM. Identification and treatment of the compromised equine fetus: a clinical perspective. Equine Vet J Suppl 1997;24:100–3.
44. Vaala WE, Sertich PL. Management strategies for mares at risk of periparturient complications. Vet Clin North Am Equine Pract 1994;10(1):237–65.
45. Leipold HW, Huston K, Dennis SM. Bovine congenital defects. Adv Vet Sci Comp Med 1983;27:197–271.
46. Whitlock BK, Kaiser L, Maxwell HS. Heritable bovine fetal abnormalities. Theriogenology 2008;70(3):535–49.
47. Ginther OJ. Fetal anomalies. In: Ginther OJ, editor. Ultrasonic imaging and animal reproduction: cattle. Cross Plains (WI): Equiservices Publishing; 1998. p. 219–28.
48. Faber DC, Ferre LB, Metzger J, et al. Agro-economic impact of cloning. Cloning Stem Cells 2004;6(2):198–207.
49. Taverne MAM, Breukelman SP, Perenyi Z, et al. The monitoring of bovine pregnancies derived from transfer of in vitro produced embryos. Reprod Nutr Dev 2002;42(6):613–24.
50. Chavatte-Palmer P, Heyman Y, Renard JP. Clonage et physiopathologie de la gestation associée [Cloning and associated physiopathology of gestation]. Gynecol Obstet Fertil 2000;28(9):633–42 [in French].
51. Hill JR, Roussel AJ, Cibbelli JB, et al. Clinical and pathologic features of cloned transgenic calves and fetuses (13 cases studies). Theriogenology 1999;51(8): 1451–65.
52. Constant F, Guillomot M, Heyman Y, et al. Large offspring or large placenta syndrome? Morphometric analysis of late gestation bovine placentomes from somatic nuclear transfer pregnancies complocated by hydrallantois. Biol Reprod 2006;75(1):122–30.
53. Farin PW, Piedrahita JA, Farin CE. Errors in development of fetuses and placentas from in-vitro-produced bovine embryos. Theriogenology 2006;65(1):178–91.
54. Miglino MA, Pereira FTV, Visintin JA, et al. Placentation in cloned cattle: structure and microvascular architecture. Theriogenology 2007;68(4):604–17.
55. Hill JR, Edwards JF, Sawyer N, et al. Placental anomalies in a viable cloned calf. Cloning 2001;3(2):83–8.
56. Lalor JG, Fawole B, Alfirevic Z, et al. Biophysical profile for fetal assessment in high-risk pregnancies. Cochrane Database Syst Rev 2008;(1):CD000038.

Ultrasound Imaging of the Bull Reproductive Tract: An Important Field of Expertise for Veterinarians

Giovanni Gnemmi, DVM, PhD[a],*, Réjean C. Lefebvre, DMV, PhD[b]

KEYWORDS

- Bull genital tract examination • Ultrasound evaluation
- Testicle • Vesiculitis

Reproductive management in bovine intensive and extensive farming of both dairy and beef industries represents one of the most critical points in animal production. Over the past 40 years, the reproductive performance of dairy cows has progressively deteriorated because of poor heat detection. In the United States alone, reproductive inefficiency costs between $1 and $2 billion per year.[1] Faced by this tendency, farmers, veterinarians, and scientists have tried to promote a series of strategies (eg, synchronization protocol) aimed at reducing losses in terms of days open and improving pregnancy rates. However, these strategies focus on the reproductive management of females only. Considering the male aspect in future strategies would be helpful for the cattle industry.

Taking into account the enormous value of bulls for the artificial insemination industry in terms of money and genetic improvement, the male/female ratio in beef production, and the worrisome reintroduction of bulls on dairy farms, it is imperative to consider maintaining optimal bull fertility as a key factor in the success of the entire cattle industry. Surprisingly, bull fertility is normally the last factor to be considered when a decrease in reproductive performance is measured in a herd. Despite the incontestable importance of bull fertility, a complete clinical evaluation of their reproductive system, also known as a breeding soundness evaluation (BSE), is rarely performed. This is routinely observed on farms, where no BSEs are performed before and following a breeding period. Artificial insemination centers also rarely examine bulls by ultrasonography before and after puberty.

[a] Bovinevet Studio Veterinario Associato, Via Cadolini 9, Fr. Cuzzago 28803, Premosello Chiovenda (VB), Italy
[b] Département des Sciences Cliniques, Faculté de Médecine Vétérinaire, Université de Montréal, 3200 Rue Sicotte, Saint-Hyacinthe, Québec J2S 2M2, Canada
* Corresponding author.
E-mail address: giovanni.gnemmi@bovinevet.com (G. Gnemmi).

Vet Clin Food Anim 25 (2009) 767–779
doi:10.1016/j.cvfa.2009.07.006
0749-0720/09/$ – see front matter © 2009 Elsevier Inc. All rights reserved.

vetfood.theclinics.com

A breeding soundness evaluation is a reliable and effective clinical method of differentiating bulls with a high fertility potential from those that are clearly unsatisfactory. This allows the culling of poor potential breeders before they are sent to pasture with cows, or before the commercial exploitation of their semen. The BSE is not a fertility test, but rather a systematic clinical approach for recognizing bulls with poor fertility potential. The routine BSE is mainly based on seminal characteristics (semen quality), scrotal circumference, and manual testicular palpation; however, other techniques are often needed to pursue a specific diagnosis. One such complementary technique is ultrasonography. Compared with other specialized examination techniques, such as the biopsy, ultrasonography is a noninvasive[2–5] technique that does not involve risks to the reproductive potential of the bull. This technique helps to further characterize pathologies of the male reproductive tract by specifying the localization and nature of tissue changes associated with anomalies, which help in the determination of the prognosis. Whether in the context of a BSE or for the investigation of a case of bull infertility, real-time ultrasonography presents significant advantages for the diagnosis of male reproductive tract anomalies affecting external and internal reproductive organs.

Ultrasonography, whether used on a routine basis or as a complementary technique, should always be preceded by a partial BSE, at the least. A meticulous evaluation of the semen should be performed should alterations in the quantity and/or quality of the semen be observed (azoospermia, oligospermia, pyospermia, morphologic alteration, low concentration, low survival rate after freezing).[4–6] The morphologic alteration of a reproductive organ (testis, epididymis, pampiniform plexus, seminal vesicles, prostate, deferent ducts, or the bulbourethral glands) and the presence of unexplained pain also call for further investigation. The early and precise diagnosis of an anomaly decreases its negative consequences on the future fertility of the bull and the economic losses[6] incurred.

The objective of this article is to provide an overview of the use of ultrasound imaging for evaluating the bull's reproductive tract, and to discuss its trends and future applications.

EQUIPMENT

Today, about 15% to 20% of buiatricians use ultrasonography[7] on a routine basis in their practice. A portable, sturdy, and battery-operated unit (powered by long-life lithium batteries) weighing between 850 and 2000 g and possessing a "5–7" LCD screen is advantageous for use on the farm, and most can withstand field conditions. For bovine practice, a B-mode (brightness modality) real-time scanner is used with a 5.0- to 7.5-MHz linear-array transducer designed for intrarectal use. A sectorial transducer is not the best choice for studying testes because of their round shape.[4–6] As for the ultrasonographic unit, choosing the most appropriate transducer is important because it determines the tissue penetration of the sound waves as well as the image resolution. For most uses, the 5.0- to 7.5-MHz linear transducer is recommended.[4–6]

TECHNIQUES

The bull has to be suitably restrained to ensure a safe examination. Light sedation (xylazine 0.01–0.02 mg/kg intravenously) may be necessary for aggressive and/or anxious bulls. In some cases, semen collection can be performed before the physical and genital examinations, allowing the bull to relax.[4–6]

External Examination

A visual evaluation of the bull and its scrotum is performed while the animal is relaxed by approaching it from behind using the same precaution as for transrectal examinations. From the posterior approach, the transducer is applied directly to the surface of the testis in a delicate, slow, and continuous movement. A sufficient amount of high-quality ultrasonographic gel is necessary to generate good images.[4–6] Contact between the probe and the skin can be improved by moistening the skin with warm (35–40°C) water.

While one thumb pushes a testis upwards, out of the transducer's ultrasound wave, the other hand pushes the testis to be examined toward the bottom of the scrotum. This stretches the scrotal wall and allows for better contact between the transducer and the scrotum.[4–6] The transducer is applied longitudinally on the external face of the testis halfway between the head and tail of the epididymis. Once both testes have been individually assessed, the spermatic cords of both testicles are seized at its dorsal pole and pushed down toward the bottom of the scrotum (**Fig. 1**). The transducer is then moved transversally on both testes simultaneously. This allows the echotexture of both testicles to be compared rapidly (**Figs. 2** and **3**).

Evaluation of the testicles always includes two projections[4]:

1. Sagittal: parallel to the principal axis of the testis (**Fig. 4**)
2. Transversal: perpendicular to the principal axis of the testis (**Figs. 5** and **6**)

These projections reveal the following:

- Length and thickness of the testis
- Quality of parenchyma (echogenicity and structure of the tissue, identification of blood vessels)
- Characteristics of the testicular tunics (thickness and presence of edema)
- Epididymis (echogenicity and structure of the tissue) (**Figs. 7** and **8**)

Ultrasonographic examination of the spermatic cords, particularly the pampiniform plexus, completes the assessment of the external genital tract.

The free end of the penis can be visualized while erect and is readily palpated through the skin of the prepuce. Caudally, the sigmoid flexure can also be palpated.

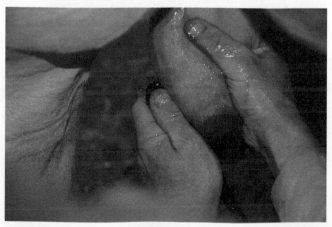

Fig.1. Ultrasound testicle examination: sagittal view. The probe is parallel to the long axis of the testicle.

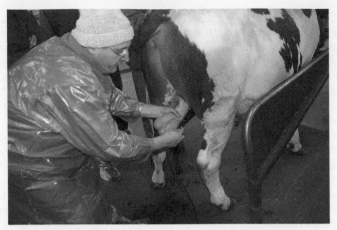

Fig. 2. Ultrasound testicle examination: sagittal view of both testicles. The probe is parallel to the long axis of the testicles. This view allows comparison of the parenchyma of both testicles.

Contrarily to the testicles, the long hair found in this area must be shaved before ultrasound gel is applied to the skin.

Transversally, a hyperechoic urethra appears surrounded by an echoic corpus spongiosum and corpus cavernosum. The corpus cavernosum is surrounded by the tunica albuginea, a dense hyperechoic membrane.

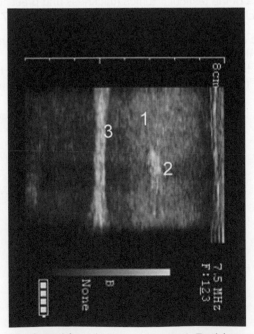

Fig. 3. Sagittal view of both testicles: ultrasound image. 1. Testicle parenchyma, 2. mediastinum testis, 3. scrotal septum.

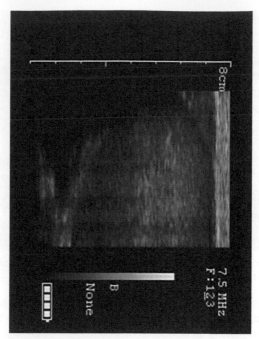

Fig. 4. Sagittal view of the testicle: ultrasound evaluation. The normal testicle parenchyma appears hypoechoic, but homogeneous. In the center of the parenchyma, the rete testis is observed as an echoic and bright structure.

Internal Examination

Before transrectal palpation, feces must be removed from the rectum to facilitate the introduction of the transducer and ensure the proper visualization of the internal reproductive organs. A preliminary examination of the topography, the size, and the consistency of the internal reproductive organs needs to be performed before proceeding to ultrasonographic examination. For biosecurity reasons (Johne's, bovine leukosis virus

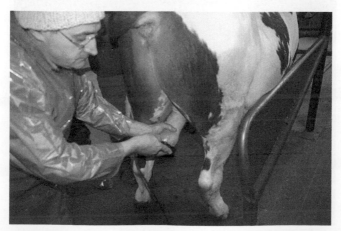

Fig. 5. Ultrasound testicle examination: transversal view. The probe is perpendicular to the long axis of the testicle.

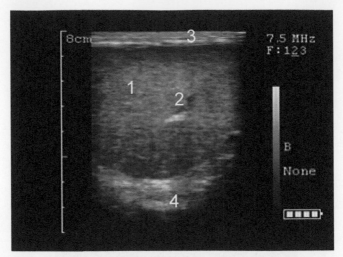

Fig. 6. Transversal view of the testicle: ultrasound image. 1. Testicle parenchyma, 2. rete testis, 3. scrotum septum, 4. skin of the scrotum.

[BLV], bovine viral diarrhea [BVD]), the transducer should be placed in a plastic sleeve (such as a rectal palpation sleeve) containing gel. Alternatively, the transducer should be cleaned thoroughly using an adequate disinfectant solution (eg, VirkonS) between animals. The seminal vesicles (**Fig. 9**), the ampullae (**Fig. 10**), the prostate gland (**Fig. 11**), the bulbourethral glands (**Fig. 12**), and the urethral pelvis are identified and evaluated.

PATHOLOGIES OF THE EXTERNAL REPRODUCTIVE SYSTEM
Anomalies of the Testis

Ultrasonography is the mainstay of diagnostic modality for identification and localization of intrascrotal lesions like cysts[8] and for differentiating testicular from

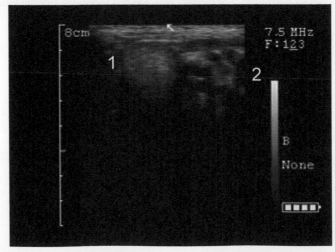

Fig. 7. Ultrasonographic view of the head of the epididymis. 1. Head of epididymis, 2. pampiniformis plessus.

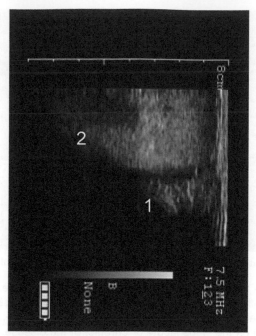

Fig. 8. Ultrasonographic view of the tail of the epididymis. 1. Tail of epididymis, 2. testicle parenchyma.

paratesticular lesions. It is performed with minimum restraint and discomfort for the animal and provides highly sensitive information with a low occurrence of false positives (<5%, Kaiper 1989).[9] It is used primarily for determining the location and nature of palpable lesions and to demonstrate non palpable lesions. The more common reported anomalies are orchitis, testicular cyst, testicular degeneration, hematoma, testicular abscess, hydrocele, hematocele, testicular hypoplasia, and neoplasia.

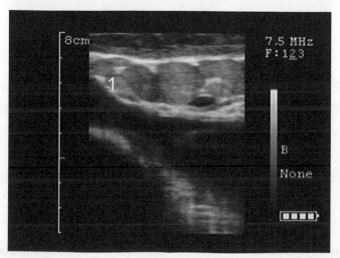

Fig. 9. Ultrasonographic evaluation of the vesicular gland. 1. Vesicular gland.

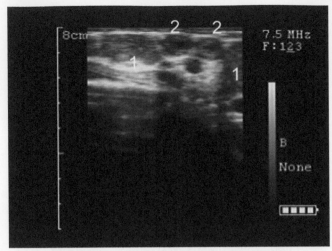

Fig. 10. Anatomy of internal reproduction apparatus: the ampulla. 1. Vesicular gland, 2. ampulla.

1. Orchitis is a rare and unilateral pathology of the testicular tissue. Although a single testicle is normally affected early on in the disease, the resulting local and systemic hyperthermia can cause the second testicle to degenerate. Ultrasonographic findings depend on the stage (acute or chronic) of the disease. The acute form is characterized by a painful, hot, edematous, and swollen scrotum on physical examination. Ultrasonography reveals testicular tissue that has lost its homogeneous appearance. In the chronic form of the disease, testicular echotexture increases with echogenic (fibrosis) or hyperechoic (mineralization) zones scattered throughout the testis and displaying acoustic shadowing.

2. Testicular cyst: ultrasonography is the diagnostic modality of choice for identification and localization of intrascrotal (intratesticular or extratesticular) cystic lesions. Cystic lesions in testes and epididymis have been reported in numerous species including bovine (Matuszewska and Sysa[10]). They appear as a well-defined

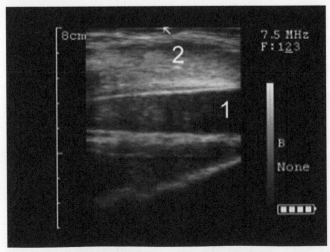

Fig. 11. Anatomy of internal reproduction apparatus: prostata and urethralis muscle. 1. Disseminate prostata, 2. urethralis muscle.

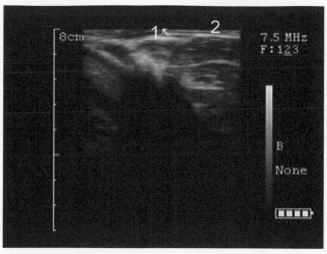

Fig.12. Anatomy of internal reproduction apparatus: bulbo urethralis gland and Bulbo spongiosus muscle. 1. Bulbo urethralis gland, 2. bulbo spongiosus muscle.

hypoechogenic or anechoic area a few millimeters to a few centimeters (1–2 cm) in diameter. In many cases, these cystic structures do not alter testicular function and/or semen quality.

3. Testicular degeneration is an acquired condition characterized by the loss of testicular parenchyma integrity, eventually leading to a decrease in size. It is an important cause of infertility in bulls and increases progressively with age. Diagnosis is based on history, scrotal examination, semen analysis, and ultrasonography. Ultrasonographically, the testicular tissue loses its architecture and become hyperechoic (fibrosis) with time and characterized by shadow artifacts (**Fig. 13**).

4. Hematoma is a rare condition that is always related to a traumatic event. Ultrasonographically, a hematoma appears as a round anechoic or hypoechoic structure depending on its stage of organization. Over time, ultrasonographic examination reveals a multilobed mass of mixed echogenicity with a defined echoic capsule.

5. Testicular abscesses have a very heterogeneous appearance on ultrasonography, related to stage of organization. Testicular abscesses often may have a metastatic origin.

6. Hydrocele: an accumulation of fluid within the tunica vaginalis that surrounds the testis, causing painless swelling of the scrotum. It occurs secondary to a spermatic cord torsion or compression of the pampiniform plexus (lymphatic tissue hyperplasia, granulomatous epididymitis). Normally, the cavum vaginalis (space between the *tunica vaginalis lamina visceralis* and *tunica vaginalis lamina parietalis*) is a virtual space (<2 mm).[4] In the case of a hydrocele, the space between the tunica layers increases in volume and can reach a few centimeters (**Fig. 14**). The fluid within a hydrocele may be simple (serous) or complex (hematocele or pyocele). A hydrocele may be idiopathic, the result of a persistent communication between the scrotum and the peritoneal cavity. Ultrasonographically, the space appears anechoic with echogenic points.

7. Hematocele is defined by the presence of blood within the *cavum* vaginalis The space appears anechoic and becomes hyperechoic over time.

8. Hypoplasia is defined as smaller testis (one or two testes) than normal for age and it is presumed congenital associated with abnormalities of germinal cells. Testicular

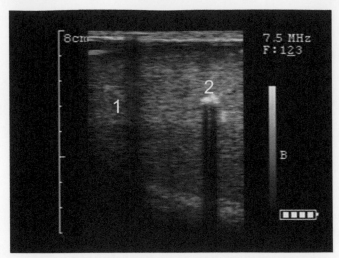

Fig. 13. Ultrasonographic aspect of testicle pathologies: testicular degeneration. 1. Testicle parenchyma, 2. shadow.

hypoplasia is probably the most common reproductive abnormality in young bulls and is generally considered to have a large heritable component. Ultrasonographically, the testicular parenchyma appears hypoechoic when compared with its normal echogenicity.

9. Neoplasia: despite being reported in bulls, it is often overlooked during a rapid evaluation. The animal is normally presented with a unilateral enlargement of the scrotum. Tumors may be hyperechoic (calcification or fibrosis), anechoic, or composed of a mixture of echogenicities, and are usually easy to distinguish from the normal testicular parenchyma.

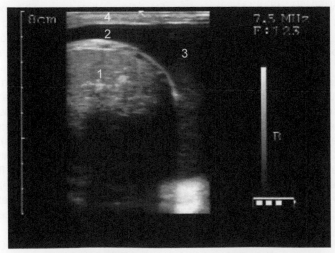

Fig. 14. Ultrasonographic aspect of testicle pathologies: hydrocele. 1. Testicle parenchyma, 2. internal vaginal tunica, 3. vaginal cavity increased in size for the presence of liquid, 4. external vaginal tunica.

Anomalies of the Epididymis

1. Epididymitis: Acute epididymitis is characterized by hypoechogenicity caused by the presence of exudates. In chronic form, the testicular parenchyma becomes more heterogeneous and echoic.

Anomalies of the Spermatic Cord

1. Varicocele is a dilation of the pampiniform plexus caused by the dysfunction of the valves located in the tortuous veins of the testicular vascular cone. Small varicocele are asymptomatic and associated with decreased fertility and poor semen quality in old bulls. Pathologic varicocele is characterized by the presence of edema inside the pampiniformis plexus. Ultrasonographically, varicocele appears as irregular hypoechoic or anechoic areas.
2. Lymphatic tissue hyperplasia can be present in cases of infectious viral diseases (BLV), and can cause the compression of the pampiniform plexus (leading to a hydrocele). Ultrasonographically, the lymphatic tissue will appear hypoechoic.
3. Inguinal hernia: an enlarged scrotal neck is very indicative of an inguinal hernia. The ultrasonographer can distinguish intestinal loops with a mobile content within the tunica vaginalis. On rare occasions, intraluminal gas is also observed[4] and the omentum appears as a more hyperechoic area.
4. Torsion of the spermatic cord (>180°) occurs when a portion of the spermatic cord rotates around its vertical axis. Ultrasonographically, ipsilateral hypoechoic dilation of the spermatic cord is observed ventral to the torsion. There is an increase or decrease in testicle echogenicity, which becomes similar to that of a corpus luteum. Scrotal edema and hydrocele are present.

Anomalies of the Penis

1. Hematoma: traumatic rupture of the dorsal surface of the tunica albuginea allows blood to exit the corpus cavernosum.[4] This pathology often causes a prepucial prolapse, swelling anterior to the scrotum, and the bull become reluctant to mate. Secondary abscess is common following the injury. It is characterized ultrasonographically by a heterogeneous mass of variable size with a thin hyperechoic wall.[4]

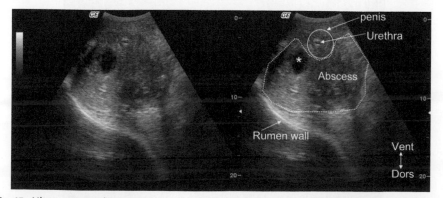

Fig. 15. Ultrasonographic aspect of the penial pathologies: abscess. Transverse ultrasonogram of the penis in a bull with a swollen ventral area. An heterogenic mass surrounding the penis is seen with anechoic (*) to echoic content. This findings were compatible with an abscess near the penis that were confirmed by puncture of the abscess. Vent, ventral; Dors, dorsal. (*Courtesy of* S. Buczinski, Dr. Vét, MSc, Université de Montréal, QC.)

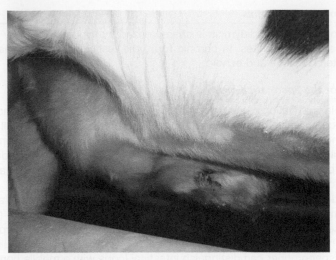

Fig. 16. Penis pathologies: abscess.

2. Abscess often occurs secondary to a hematoma. Its ultrasonographical structure varies with time. Young abscesses have a thin hyperechoic wall with a typical heterogeneous snowstorm appearance on the monitor. Older abscesses have a much thicker hyperechoic wall and an echoic (fibrosis) to hyperechoic (calcification) content (**Figs. 15** and **16**).

PATHOLOGIES OF THE INTERNAL REPRODUCTIVE SYSTEM
Anomalies of the Seminal Vesicles

1. Vesiculitis: the seminal vesicles are the most frequently affected accessory glands of the male reproductive tract.[11] Their infection is always accompanied by an increase in leucocytes, and often by pyospermia. The infection can be unilateral or bilateral. It is most frequent in young bulls having recently reached puberty.[2]

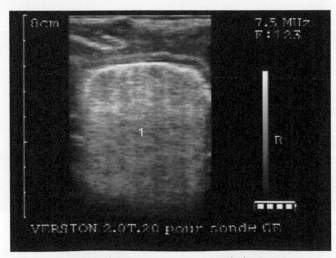

Fig. 17. Ultrasonographic aspect of the vesicular glands pathologies: abscess.1. Abscess of the vesicular gland.

In the acute form, the gland is hypertrophic and pus can be observed within the gland. The gland is also hypertrophic in chronic form, but fibrosis makes it appear echoic or hyperechoic when compared with the contralateral gland (**Fig. 17**).
2. Hypertrophy: paraphysiological in older bulls, it is not associated with alterations in semen quality. Conversely, hypertrophy in young bulls is pathologic and associated with semen leukocytosis. The gland appears enlarged and increased in echogenicity, resembling luteinic tissue.

SUMMARY

Diagnosing male reproductive system pathologies can often be frustrating because of the challenge involved in precisely determining their site, severity, and prognosis. The introduction of complementary ultrasonographic examination enables clinicians to address these important questions. This procedure should be performed not only on bulls destined to artificial insemination, but on all farm bulls. The examination is easy to perform with a versatile ultrasonographic unit designed for bovine theriogenology. To recognize abnormal tissues, however, the operator must have an excellent knowledge of the ultrasonographic anatomy of the reproductive system.

REFERENCES

1. Pursley JR. Practical ovsynch programs. Presented at the 40th Annual Convention of the American Association of Bovine Practitioners. Vancouver, British Columbia, Canada, September 20–22, 2007.
2. Gilbert R, Fubini S. Surgery of the male reproductive tract. In: Fubini SL, Ducharme NG, editors. Farm animal surgery. Philadelphia: WB Saunders; 2004. p. 352.
3. Larson LL. Examination of the reproductive system of the bull. In: Morrow DA, editor. Current therapy in theriogenology. 2nd edition. Philadelphia: WB: Saunders; 1986. p. 101–16.
4. Gnemmi G, Lefebvre R. Bull anatomy and ultrasonography of the reproductive tract. In: Luc DesCôteaux, Gnemmi G, Colloton J. practical atlas of ultrasonography for ruminant reproduction. Black Well; in press.
5. Gnemmi G. Place de l'échographie du taureau en pratique. Point Vét 2007;275: 51–4 [in French].
6. Gnemmi G. Ultrasonografia dell'apparato riproduttore maschile: applicazioni in campo. Summa 2006;9:43–9 [in Italian].
7. Gnemmi G, Maraboli C, Colloton J. Ultrasonografia in ginecologia buiatrica. Summa 2006;9:11–16 [in Italian]
8. Brunereau L, Fauchier F, Fernandez P, et al. Sonographic evaluation of human male infertility. J Radiol 2000;81:1693–701.
9. Kaiper G. The clinical value of scrotal sonography. Z Urol Nephrol 1989;82: 419–24.
10. Matuszewska M, Sysa PS. Epididymal cysts in European bison. J Wildl Dis 2002; 38:637–40.
11. Bagshaw PA, Ladds PW. A study of the accessory sex glands of the bulls in abattoirs in northern Australia. Aust Vet J 1974;50:489–95.

Ultrasonographic Assessment of Umbilical Disorders

Adrian Steiner, Dr med vet, MS, Dr Habil*, Beatrice Lejeune, Dr med vet

KEYWORDS

• Umbilical • Sonography • Urachus • Calf • Bovine

Umbilical disorders are of great clinical relevance in calves during the early postnatal period. Umbilical disorders may be classified as (1) noninfectious disorders such as hernias and urachal cysts, (2) infectious disorders involving extra- and intra-abdominal umbilical structures, or (3) combinations thereof. Infections are mainly caused by *Arcanobacterium pyogenes*, Streptococci, and Staphylococci, but also by *Pasteurella* spp, *Proteus* spp, *Bacteroides* spp. and *E coli*. The latter is most likely to cause systemic infection and septic polyarthritis.[1] The risk of systemic infection is negatively correlated with the amount and quality of colostrum ingested during the first 12 hours of life. Clinical symptoms of umbilical infections may include reduced appetite, weakened general condition, hyperthermia, and swelling of the umbilicus with fistula formation and purulent discharge. Disorders of the urachus or the umbilical arteries are characterized by pollakiuria.[2] Diagnostic procedures for differentiation of the various umbilical pathologies include general clinical examination focusing on urination, the respiratory tract, and the joints, followed by clinical examination of the extra-abdominal umbilical structures (ie, umbilicus) and deep bimanual palpation of the intra-abdominal remnants.[1] During the past decade, ultrasonographic examination of umbilical structures has markedly gained importance as a diagnostic and prognostic aid when assessing calves suffering from umbilical disorders. Ultrasonography is valuable mainly for visualization of (1) intra-abdominal remnants not accessible to deep external manual palpation and (2) non- or partially reducible umbilical hernias. Intra-abdominal infections of umbilical structures may occur without any external signs of inflammation.[3,4] After retrospective analysis of 32 cattle with umbilical abnormalities, it was shown that concordance between ultrasonographic and physical (surgical or postmortem) findings was good-to-excellent for all umbilical structures. Intra-abdominal adhesions were found intraoperatively in 47% of animals with umbilical abnormalities; adhesions, however, were not detected ultrasonographically in any of the cases.[4] Many umbilical pathologies require surgical intervention.

Clinic for Ruminants, Vetsuisse-Faculty of Bern, 3012 Bern, Switzerland
* Corresponding author.
E-mail address: adrian.steiner@knp.unibe.ch (A. Steiner).

Vet Clin Food Anim 25 (2009) 781–794
doi:10.1016/j.cvfa.2009.07.012
0749-0720/09/$ – see front matter © 2009 Elsevier Inc. All rights reserved.

vetfood.theclinics.com

Sonography of the ventral abdomen makes the surgeon aware of the dimensions of internalized abscesses and the potential involvement of organs such as urinary bladder or liver before surgery. This is particularly true for adolescent or even adult animals in which the limitations of physical examination are even more evident.[2,4,5] Meticulous preoperative planning is essential, because some conditions may require marsupialization instead of the routine surgical resection of the abscess.[6-8] Ultrasonography brought about a reduction of complications that occurred during the subsequent surgical resection. Additionally, in particular cases with poor prognosis, attempts at surgical repair were abandoned beforehand for economic reasons, based on sonographic findings.[9]

PREPARATION OF THE CALF

The umbilicus and abdomen must be clipped from the pubis laterally to the inguinal region and cranially to the sternum and to the costal arch on the right abdominal wall. The right flank over the liver field is also clipped if involvement of the umbilical vein and the liver is suspected. An adequate amount of coupling gel is administered to the clipped skin to allow for sufficient contact to accurately image the structures. Proper restraint of the calf will result in a stress-free, thorough examination of the intra-abdominal umbilical remnants.[4,10-12]

TECHNIQUE OF SONOGRAPHIC EXAMINATION

The ultrasonographic examination is best performed from the right side with the animal in standing position.[4,10-12] This allows the abdominal viscera to push potentially involved umbilical cord remnants close to the ventral abdominal wall. The standard examination procedure consists of two or three steps, depending on the involvement of the umbilical vein.[13] Imaging starts at the umbilicus and includes visualization of the umbilical structures caudal to the umbilicus (step 1); it is followed by the structures cranial to the umbilicus (step 2), and completed by the standard sonographic examination of the liver from the right flank (step 3), if involvement of the liver is suspected.[14-16] Step 1: The extra-abdominal umbilical structures are assessed caudally with the probe positioned transversely to the long axis of the umbilicus. The probe is slowly moved from the apex of the umbilicus to the base; there it is tilted to a vertical position and then moved in the midline toward the prepubic area. Thereby, a transverse view is presented with the probe centered over potential intra-abdominal umbilical remnants (urachus or umbilical arteries), which are tracked to their very end. Sections parallel to the longitudinal axis of pathologic structures are then presented at the discretion of the examiner to better identify the area of potential involvement of the urinary bladder and/or intra-abdominal structures such as intestinal organs. Step 2 is similar to step 1, but assesses the cranial aspects of the umbilicus in a transverse plane to its long axis. It further involves the intra-abdominal aspects of umbilical vein remnants. The probe is slowly moved cranially and to the right of the midline with the transducer oriented perpendicularly to the long axis of the umbilical vein, until the hilus of the liver can be visualized, where the scanner is oriented transversely to the body wall. Sections parallel to the longitudinal axis of pathologic structures are then presented at the discretion of the examiner to better identify the area of potential involvement of the liver and/or other intra-abdominal structures. Step 3 consists of a standard ultrasonographic assessment of the liver and is added to better define the extent of the potential involvement of liver tissue into the infectious process (see the article by Braun elsewhere in this issue).

The types of probes being used depend on the age of the animal and the dimension of intra-abdominal masses involved. They may range from 13 mHz for superficial structures of small diameter in young calves to 3.5 mHz for structures with a large dimension that extend into the depth of the abdomen.[9] Either a sector scan or a linear array probe may be used.

PHYSIOLOGIC INVOLUTION OF THE UMBILICAL STRUCTURES

After rupture of the umbilical cord, the two umbilical arteries retract actively, and the urachus is pulled back passively by these vessels into the abdomen. Smooth-muscle contraction brings about luminal closure. The umbilical arteries ultimately become the lateral ligaments of the urinary bladder. Ultrasonographically, urachal remnants may not be identified in healthy calves at any time. At 1 week after birth, the umbilical arteries abruptly terminate at the apex of the bladder. They may be identified laterally to the urinary bladder for more than 3 weeks as circular structures with wall and center. Echogenicity of the lumen varies from anechoic to hypoechogenic compared with surrounding tissues. Some arteries may exhibit a central hyperechogenic focus.[10,11] The umbilical vein, which is paired externally and covered by the amnionic membrane, does not retract, but collapses in association with some minor smooth-muscle contraction. Intraluminal coagulated blood is resorbed within a few weeks. Intra-abdominally, the umbilical vein finally becomes the round ligament of the liver, suspended in the falciform ligament. Ultrasonographically, in the postpartum period, the umbilical vein can be traced from the body wall to the liver. The lumen is generally larger near the body wall with a diameter ranging from 10 mm to 25 mm. It appears as a round-to-oval anechoic to hypoechogenic structure (**Fig. 1**). Within 3 weeks after birth, ultrasonographic identification of the intra-abdominal umbilical vein becomes impossible in up to 50% of the healthy calves. If still visible, the vein appears hypoechogenic to the surrounding tissue and indistinctly marginated.[10,11] The umbilical sheath shrinks and dries within 3 days postpartum. It is normally fully eliminated at 2 to 3 weeks of age and the skin scar has healed by 4 weeks of age. The body wall closes completely around the umbilical structures within days to a few weeks.

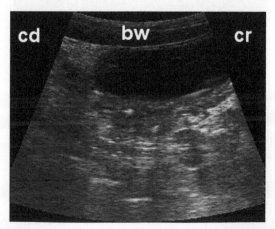

Fig. 1. Physiologic appearance of the umbilical vein of a 2-day-old Holstein-Friesian calf. The vein appears as an anechoic structure. The sonogram is taken cranial to the umbilicus, with the probe held perpendicular and in a section parallel to the long axis of the vein. bw, body wall; cd, caudal; cr, cranial.

Ultrasonographically, the umbilicus is mostly hypoechogenic, and at that time, the paired umbilical veins may no longer be definitively identified.[10]

ULTRASONOGRAPHIC APPEARANCE OF UMBILICAL PATHOLOGIES

The following ultrasonographic appearances of umbilical structures should be considered abnormal: (1) presence of hyperechogenic structures in the umbilicus (**Fig. 2**); (2) identification of urachal remnants in calves of any age; (3) presence of umbilical arteries increasing in diameter over time or extending cranially over the tip of the urinary bladder after the age of 1 week (see **Fig. 2**); (4) identification of the umbilical vein in its complete length after the age of 3 weeks, or (5) presence of hyperechogenic focuses within the intra-abdominal parts of the umbilical vein at any age.[11]

Umbilical Hernia

Defects of the abdominal wall in the area of the umbilicus may occur either as simple hernias or hernias with concomitant umbilical cord remnant infections or subcutaneous abscessation. Abdominal structures protruding through the defect of the body wall into the hernial sac are manually reducible and the circumferential hernial ring can be palpated. This manipulation is characterized by an extremely high diagnostic sensitivity for this pathology, which represents a congenital defect.[17] Ultrasonographic examination allows for the visualization of the hernial ring as an abrupt discontinuity of the abdominal wall (**Fig. 3**). Furthermore, the hernial contents such as abdominal fluid, parts of the omentum maius (epiplocele), parts of the abomasum (abomasocele), small intestinal loops (enterocele), or combinations thereof may be identified.[18] Peritoneal fluid presents as completely anechoic and is accumulated in the ventral aspects of the hernial sac (**Fig. 4**). The abomasum is characterized by floating hyperechogenic folds that protrude into the lumen of this hollow organ, while

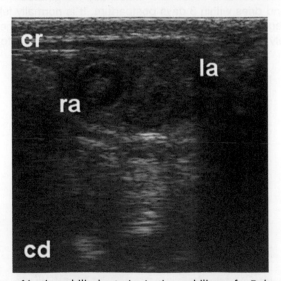

Fig. 2. Cross-section of both umbilical arteries in the umbilicus of a 5-day-old Holstein-Friesian calf with omphaloarteritis. The right artery depicts a hyperechogenic center and the left artery a hypoechogenic center. The sonogram is taken at the base of the umbilicus, with the probe positioned cranially to the umbilicus and in a transverse plane to the long axis of the umbilicus. cd, caudal; cr, cranial; la, left artery; ra, right artery.

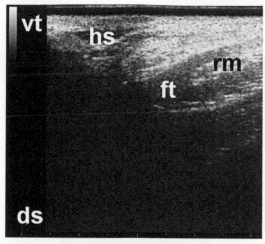

Fig. 3. Sagittal section of the defect in the body wall of a 13-month-old Red Holstein heifer. The body wall ends abruptly and is characterized by the hypoechogenic fibrous tissue covering the hyperechogenic rectus muscle. The probe is situated at the caudal border of the hernial ring and held perpendicular to the body wall. ds, dorsal; ft, fibrous tissue; hs, hernial sac; rm, rectus muscle; vt, ventral.

the contents appear mostly anechoic with interspersed mobile, hyperechogenic clumps (curdled milk) in milk-fed calves. The small intestinal loops, imaged in longitudinal- and cross-sections exhibit the characteristic contractions, liquid contents, and double layer appearance of the wall (**Fig. 5**). The omentum maius presents as noncontractile structure of disordered, hyperechogenic, interconnected areas. If concurrent

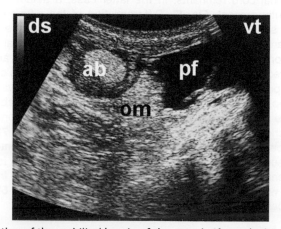

Fig. 4. Sagittal section of the umbilical hernia of the same heifer as depicted in **Fig. 3**. A well-demarcated abscess is present at the cranial base of the hernia. Omentum maius protrudes into the caudal aspects of the hernial sac. Anechoic peritoneal fluid is accumulated in the ventral aspects of the hernial sac. The probe is situated at the cranial wall of the umbilicus and held in a vertical position. ab, abscess; ds, dorsal; om, omentum maius; pf, peritoneal fluid; vt, ventral.

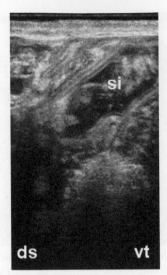

Fig. 5. Sagittal section of the umbilical hernia of a 6-week-old Holstein-Friesian calf. Several empty and fluid-filled small intestinal loops are visualized within the umbilicus. The probe is situated at the cranial wall of the umbilicus and held in a vertical position. ds, dorsal; si, small intestinal loops; vt, ventral.

infection of the umbilical stalk is present, this is characterized by one or more hyperechogenic centers each surrounded by a hypoechogenic wall (see **Fig. 4**).

Abscessation of the Umbilicus

Simple umbilical abscesses are restricted to the subcutaneous tissue in the area of the umbilicus and are nonreducible. Otherwise, umbilical abscesses may involve intra-abdominal umbilical cord remnants. In the latter case, a defect in the abdominal wall is concurrently present (**Fig. 6**). Differentiation of the different pathologies is crucial, because surgical measures may vary from simple drainage of the accumu-lated pus to laparotomy with resection of intra-abdominal umbilical cord remnants. Therefore, ultrasonographic examination of the body wall and the abdominal cavity must be performed with great care. Subcutaneous abscessation is characterized by the presence of pus, surrounded by a hypoechogenic capsule of varying thickness. The ultrasonographic appearance of the contents of the umbilical abscess may vary depending on the cellularity and consistency of the pus. Watery contents appear as multiple, hyperechogenic particles on an anechoic background (**Fig. 7**). Pus of creamy consistency appears as multifocal, hyperechogenic particles interspersed with extremely hyperechogenic areas (**Fig. 8**). Pus of cheesy consistency is often of homo-geneous echodensity. If the abscess contains gas, the fluid–gas interface can be visualized nicely with the probe held in a vertical position (see **Fig. 8**). Combinations of umbilical abscesses and umbilical hernias do exist (see **Fig. 4**).

Disorders of the Urachus

Diseases of the urachus may be classified as infectious, such as urachal abscess formation with or without involvement of the urinary bladder; or noninfectious, which includes persistent urachus and urachal cyst.[12,19,20] The extent of the urachal abscess is of clinical importance, because surgical excision of abscesses exceeding 10 cm in

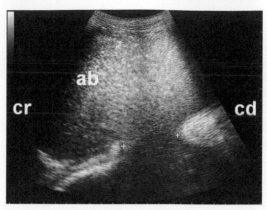

Fig. 6. Sagittal section of the umbilical abscess of a 12-month-old Holstein-Friesian heifer, involving intra-abdominal umbilical cord remnants. A defect in the abdominal wall is concurrently present. The probe is positioned at the tip of the umbilicus and directed toward the abdominal wall. ab, abscess; cd, caudal; cr, cranial; +, caudal delineation of the defect in the body wall; +1, cranial delineation of the defect in the body wall.

diameter prove difficult and may require preoperative percutaneous lancing and draining.[12,20] Urachal abscess formation is characterized by a cord containing one or more abscesses and running from the tip of the urinary bladder to the umbilicus. Abscesses appear as granular, hyperechogenic material within a defined cavity. The appearance of the material may vary depending on the cellularity and consistency of the pus (see "Abscessation of the umbilicus," above). In the view parallel to the longitudinal axis,

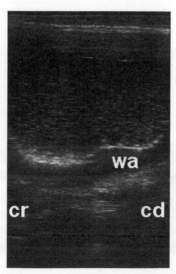

Fig. 7. Cross-section of the subcutaneous umbilical abscess of a 10-week-old Red Holstein calf. The abscess contents are of watery consistency and appear as hyperechogenic particles on an anechoic-to-hypoechogenic background. The sonogram is taken from the right side, halfway between the base and the tip of the umbilicus, with the probe positioned transversely to the long axis of the umbilicus. cd, caudal; cr, cranial; wa, wall of abscess.

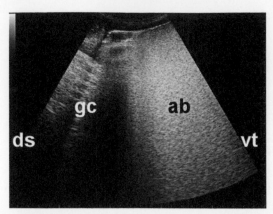

Fig. 8. Sagittal section of the extra-abdominal umbilical abscess of a 3-month-old Holstein-Friesian calf. Creamy pus is depicted in the ventral aspect of the abscess, while the dorsal gas cupule is characterized by reverberation artifacts. The probe is positioned at the cranial wall of the abscess and held in vertical position. ab, abscess of creamy contents; ds, dorsal; gc, gas cupule; vt, ventral.

the urinary bladder appears as a tubular or conical structure with anechoic contents (**Fig. 9**). The wall at the tip of the urinary bladder may appear remarkably thickened, indicating persistent inflammation in this area (**Fig. 10**). This contrasts to the normal situation, in which the blind end of the bladder appears roundish.[21] In cases with persistent communication between the abscess and the tip of the bladder, the appearance of the contents of the bladder is similar to that of the attached abscess. The site of communication may be visualized in the view parallel to the longitudinal axis (**Fig. 11**).

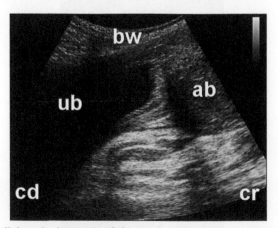

Fig. 9. Section parallel to the long axis of the urachus abscess in the area of the attachment to the tip of the urinary bladder of a 5-week-old Red-Holstein calf. The anechoic urine is separated from the abscess by the hyperechogenic wall of the urinary bladder. Signs of fistula formation from the abscess to the urinary bladder are not present. The probe is positioned in the midline and held perpendicular to the body wall. ab, abscess of the urachus; bw, body wall; cd, caudal; cr, cranial; ub, urinary bladder.

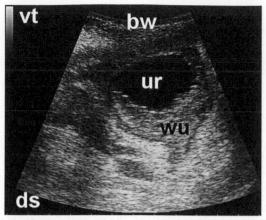

Fig.10. Section transverse to the long axis of the urachus at the tip of the urinary bladder of the same calf as **Fig. 9**. The wall of the urinary bladder, which has an increased thickness at the dorsal aspect, surrounds the anechoic urine. The probe is positioned in the midline and held perpendicular to the body wall. bw, body wall; ds, dorsal; ur, urine within urinary bladder; vt, ventral; wu, wall of urinary bladder.

Persistent urachus rarely occurs in calves and is clinically characterized by the presence of a fistula at the tip of the umbilicus with dripping of urine. Ultrasonographically, in cross-section, it appears as a round structure with a hypoechogenic wall and an anechoic center. It is continuous from the urinary bladder to the umbilicus (**Fig. 12**).[12,20] Urachal cyst is defined as a persistent urachus, the distal end of which

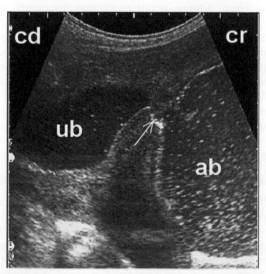

Fig.11. Section parallel to the long axis of the urachus at the tip of the urinary bladder of a 3-month-old Brown Swiss calf. Fistula formation (*arrow*) is visible between the abscess and the urinary bladder. The urine is mixed with pus evidenced by hyperechogenic particles on a hypoechogenic background. The probe is positioned in the midline and held perpendicular to the body wall. ab, abscess; cr, cranial; cd, caudal; ub, urinary bladder.

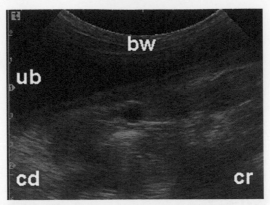

Fig. 12. Section parallel to the long axis of the persistent urachus at the tip of the urinary bladder of a 4-week-old Holstein-Friesian calf. The tip of the urinary bladder is continuous with the persistent urachus, running as a thin anechoic structure toward the umbilicus. The probe is positioned in the midline and held perpendicular to the body wall. bw, body wall; cr, cranial; cd, caudal; ub, urinary bladder.

is sealed in the area of the umbilicus.[19] Ultrasonographically, the appearance of the cyst is similar to the persistent urachus. In the area of the umbilicus, however, the diameter of the anechoic lumen increases, reaching several centimeters, and it ends blind at the tip of the umbilicus; toward the abdominal wall, the diameter of the lumen decreases to a few millimeters. From there, the cyst can be traced along its course back to the tip of the urinary bladder.[19]

Disorders of the Umbilical Arteries

Disorders of the umbilical arteries occur much less frequently as compared with disorders of the urachus. They include periarterial hematoma formation and infection/abscessation.[22] Clinical differentiation of abscessation between artery and urachus may prove difficult, because clinical signs of disorders such as pollakiuria are similar. Differentiation, however, is important, because abscesses of the umbilical arteries may extend far toward the internal iliac artery, making complete surgical excision extremely difficult. Marsupialization may be the surgical intervention of choice in such cases.[7] Disorders of the urachus and of one or both umbilical arteries often occur simultaneously. Purulent umbilical artery is diagnosed if the center of this structure depicts as hyperechogenic, the diameter exceeds 15 mm, and/or this vessel is visible cranial to the tip of the urinary bladder (**Fig. 13**). Definitive diagnosis is only possible if the affected artery is observed lateral to the urinary bladder.[12]

Disorders of the Umbilical Vein

Infections of the umbilical vein may be classified as such with or without involvement of the liver. If the liver is involved, it is important to differentiate between a single abscess continuous with the umbilical vein abscess or multiple solitary abscesses. If the liver is not involved, the affected vein may be resected in toto with protection of the liver tissue. Marsupialization is performed in cases of a single abscess continuous with the umbilical vein,[6,8] while the prognosis is poor and no treatment advised in cases of formation of multiple abscesses dispersed within the liver tissue. The latter also holds true for a single abscess involving the portal vein. Involvement of the liver is determined by imaging the area of entrance of the umbilical vein into the sulcus

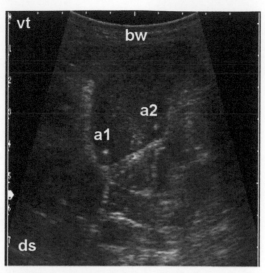

Fig. 13. Section transverse to the long axis of the umbilical arteries cranial to the tip of the urinary bladder of a 3-week-old Holstein-Friesian calf. The umbilical arteries are characterized by their hyperechogenic center, embedded in a hypoechogenic structure representing fibrous tissue. The probe is positioned in the midline and held perpendicular to the body wall. a1, a2, umbilical arteries; bw, body wall; ds, dorsal; vt, ventral.

venae umbilicalis at the caudoventral margin of the liver with the probe positioned at the costal arch on the right abdominal wall. Standard examination of the liver from the right flank completes the procedure.[14–16]

Abscesses appear as granular, hyperechogenic material within a defined cavity, the wall of which depicts as hypoechogenic and varies in thickness. The appearance of the material may vary depending on the cellularity and consistency of the pus.

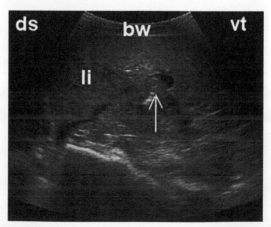

Fig. 14. Visualization of the liver from the tenth intercostal space of an 8-week-old Red Holstein calf. The lumen of the portal vein is severely reduced by an infectous thrombus (*arrow*) protruding into this vessel. The probe is held in vertical position and perpendicular to the body wall. bw, body wall; ds, dorsal; li, liver tissue; vt, ventral.

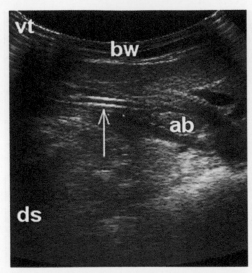

Fig. 15. Section longitudinal to the long axis of the umbilical vein of the same calf as **Fig. 14**. A silicone catheter (*arrow*) is introduced into the umbilical vein and the tip advanced to the proximal end of the isthmus, where the liver abscess is clearly visible. The probe is positioned cranial to the umbilicus to the right of the midline and held perpendicular to the umbilical vein. ab, abscess; bw, body wall; ds, dorsal; vt, ventral.

Involvement of the liver is evident if, in the transverse view to the longitudinal axis, the purulent vein is completely surrounded by hepatic tissue.[12] Rotating the probe to visualize the umbilical vein parallel to its longitudinal axis will then allow one to determine the proximal delineation of the purulent process and the potential involvement of the portal vein. Involvement of the portal vein may also be visualized by standard examination of the liver from the right flank (**Fig. 14**). If a draining tract is present at the

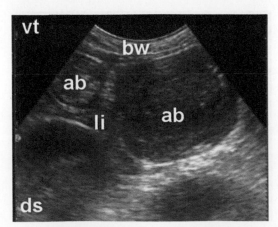

Fig. 16. Section transverse to the long axis of the umbilical vein of a 7-week-old Red Holstein calf. Two abscesses are visible within the liver tissue. The probe is positioned cranial to the umbilicus and to the right of the midline close to the costal arch and held perpendicular to the body wall. ab, abscess; bw, body wall; ds, dorsal; li, liver tissue; vt, ventral.

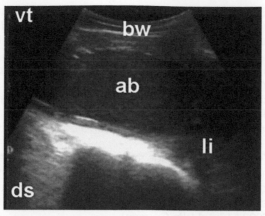

Fig.17. Section at 45° to the long axis of the umbilical vein of a 4-month-old Holstein-Friesian calf. One abscess is visible, involving the main part of the depicted liver tissue. The probe is positioned cranial to the umbilicus and to the right of the midline close to the costal arch. ab, abscess; bw, body wall; ds, dorsal; li, liver; vt, ventral.

tip of the umbilicus, the pus-filled lumen of the umbilical vein may be very small, making identification of the exact extent of the purulent process difficult. For this purpose, physiologic saline solution may be carefully instilled through the fistula to clearly visualize the expansion of the lumen. The same procedure may be performed during postoperative care after marsupialization of the umbilical vein abscess to monitor the progress of healing and determine the correct starting time for the second surgical intervention (**Fig. 15**).[6] Multiple solitary abscesses of the liver are characterized by multifocal hyperechogenic spots dispersed in the liver parenchyma, exhibiting only minimal wall formation or by several hyperechogenic areas well delineated by a thin hypoechogenic wall (**Fig. 16**).[12] Some abscesses may be huge and involve major parts of the liver (**Fig. 17**).

SUMMARY

Umbilical ultrasonography should be performed according to a given protocol with the calf in standing position from the right side. It is readily performed under conditions in a rural practice. Umbilical ultrasonography allows one to identify the structures involved and differentiate between various disorders with a high diagnostic sensitivity. It does not replace the clinical examination but supplements it. A specific diagnosis of the umbilical disorder is very important, because the treatment regimen, the prognosis, and the treatment costs completely depend upon the extent of the disease process and the structures involved.

REFERENCES

1. Nuss K. Erkrankungen der inneren Nabelstrukturen beim Rind. Tierarztl Prax 2007;35(G):149–56 [in German].
2. Trent AM, Smith DF. Pollakiuria due to urachal abscesses in two heifers. J Am Vet Med Assoc 1984;184:984–6.
3. Steiner A, Baumann D, Fluckiger M. [Urachal abscess without pathologic changes in the extra-abdominal navel in a cow. Case report]. Tierarztl Prax 1988;16:33–6 [in German].

4. Staller GS, Tulleners EP, Reef VB, et al. Concordance of ultrasonographic and physical findings in cattle with an umbilical mass or suspected to have infection of the umbilical cord remnants: 32 cases (1987–1989). J Am Vet Med Assoc 1995; 206:77–82.

5. Braun U, Nuss K, Wapf P, et al. Clinical and ultrasonographic findings in five cows with a ruptured urachal remnant. Vet Rec 2006;159:780–2.

6. Steiner A, Lischer CJ, Oertle C. Marsupialization of umbilical vein abscesses with involvement of the liver in 13 calves. Vet Surg 1993;22:184–9.

7. Lopez MJ, Markel MD. Umbilical artery marsupialization in a calf. Can Vet J 1996; 37:170–1.

8. Edwards RB, Fubini SL. A one-stage marsupialization procedure for management of infected umbilical vein remnants in calves and foals. Vet Surg 1995;24:32–5.

9. Flock M. [Ultrasonic diagnosis of inflammation of the umbilical cord structures, persistent urachus and umbilical hernia in calves]. Berl Munch Tierarztl Wochenschr 2003;116:2–11 [in German].

10. Watson E, Mahaffey MB, Crowell W, et al. Ultrasonography of the umbilical structures in clinically normal calves. Am J Vet Res 1994;55:773–80.

11. Lischer CJ, Steiner A. Ultrasonography of umbilical structures in calves. Part I: ultrasonographic description of umbilical involution in clinically healthy calves. Schweiz Arch Tierheilkd 1993;135:221–30.

12. Lischer CJ, Steiner A. Ultrasonography of the umbilicus in calves. Part 2: ultrasonography, diagnosis and treatment of umbilical diseases. Schweiz Arch Tierheilkd 1994;136:227–41.

13. Lischer CJ, Steiner A. Nabel. In: Braun U, editor. Atlas und Lehrbuch der Ultraschalldiagnostik beim Rind. 1st edition. Berlin: Parey Buchverlag; 1997. p. 227–52 [in German].

14. Braun U. Ultrasonographic examination of the liver in cows. Am J Vet Res 1990; 51:1522–6.

15. Braun U, Pusterla N, Wild K. Ultrasonographic findings in 11 cows with a hepatic abscess. Vet Rec 1995;137:284–90.

16. Braun U. Leber. In: Braun U, editor. Atlas und Lehrbuch der Ultraschalldiagnostik beim Rind. 1st edition. Berlin: Parey Buchverlag; 1997. p. 35–68 [in German].

17. Priester WA, Glass AG, Waggoner NS. Congenital defects in domesticated animals: general considerations. Am J Vet Res 1970;31:1871–9.

18. Baxter GM. Umbilical masses in calves: diagnosis, treatment, and complications. Compend Contin Educ Pract Vet 1989;11:505–13.

19. Lischer CJ, Iselin U, Steiner A. Ultrasonographic diagnosis of urachal cyst in three calves. J Am Vet Med Assoc 1994;204:1801–4.

20. Steiner A, Fluckiger M, Oertle C, et al. [Urachal disorders in calves: clinical and sonographic findings, therapy and prognosis]. Schweiz Arch Tierheilkd 1990; 132:187–95 [in German].

21. Braun U. Harnblase. In: Braun U, editor. Atlas und Lehrbuch der Ultraschalldiagnostik beim Rind. 1st edition. Berlin: Parey Buchverlag; 1997. p. 147–8 [in German].

22. Rademacher G. Von den Nabelarterien ausgehende periarterielle Hämatome beim Kalb—Diagnose, Prognose, Therapie [Perivascular hematomas of the navel arteries in calves. Diagnosis, prognosis and treatment]. Tierarztl Umsch 2006;61: 3–15 [in German].

Postscript

The following article is an addition to Alpaca and Llama Health Management, the July 2009 issue of Veterinary Clinics of North America: Food Animal Practice (Volume 25, Issue 2).

Nutritional Diseases of Llamas and Alpacas

Robert J. Van Saun, DVM, PhD

KEYWORDS

- Llamas • Alpacas • Nutritional disease • Vitamin D
- Rickets • Cu toxicity

Literature citations of specific nutrient deficiency or toxicity diseases of camelids are limited, but they suggest similar pathologic mechanisms and presentation compared with other species.[1–3] A lack of published reports does not suggest llamas and alpacas are less susceptible to nutritional disease, but rather reflect a situation of underreporting. Case reports of hepatic lipidosis, Cu toxicity, polioencephalomalacia, plant poisonings, and urolithiasis account for the greatest number of disease-related citations.[4] This article will review commonly encountered nutritional diseases, based on literature reports and clinical experience, in llamas and alpacas as well as basic nutritional diagnostics for the veterinary practitioner.

ENERGY BALANCE–ASSOCIATED DISEASES

Camelids, like all other animals and humans, are susceptible to either a deficient or excessive intake of energy relative to requirements, resulting in variable stages of malnutrition or obesity, respectively. Unique to camelids, however, is their greater susceptibility to hepatic lipidosis, a disease often, but not necessarily, associated with negative energy balance (refer to the article concerning metabolic diseases elsewhere in this issue for a complete discussion).

Protein-Energy Malnutrition

Starvation is defined as a prolonged and complete deprivation of feed intake. True starvation cases are the exception rather than the rule, but are most likely underreported. More typically encountered is a situation of protein-energy malnutrition (PEM) where energy, protein, or both are deficient in the diet over a period of time. Body weight loss and a decline in body condition score are the most common clinical signs.[5] Growing animals will also show a slowing or near complete cessation in gain. Pregnant and lactating females experiencing PEM may be prone to hepatic lipidosis.[6]

This article was originally planned to appear in the July 2009 issue of *Veterinary Clinics of North America: Food Animal Practice*.

Department of Veterinary and Biomedical Sciences, 115 W.L. Henning Building, Pennsylvania State University, University Park, PA 16802-3500, USA

E-mail address: rjv10@psu.edu

Because of greater requirements, young growing animals, late pregnant females, and lactating females are the first to show clinical signs. Time frame and severity of body weight and condition loss will be dependent upon the degree of dietary energy and protein deficiency.

Beyond physiologic state and its impact on increasing requirements, environmental conditions, especially extreme cold, will increase energy needs. Camelids raised in northern regions of North America are exposed to environmental temperatures much lower than their native habitat. In these cold conditions, camelids will expend additional energy to maintain body temperature. Data for other species suggest maintenance energy is increased 1% for every 1°C below an animal's lower critical temperature.[7] Based on data from sheep and assuming a full fleece, lower critical temperature for llamas and alpacas would be approximately 0 to 10°C.[7] If animals are wet, mud covered, or exposed to wind chill, then maintenance energy may be increased as much as 75%. Clearly, PEM is a potential risk for llamas and alpacas raised in extreme northern climates.[5]

Routine body condition scoring or body weight estimates can be used to diagnose potential problems. A thick fleece can readily hide body weight and condition changes from view, thus requiring a hands-on condition score or body weight measure. Serum nonesterified fatty acids (NEFA; >0.6 mEq/L) and β-hydroxybutyrate (BHB; >5 mg/dL) concentrations may or may not be elevated depending on severity and duration of the dietary deficiency and presence of secondary hepatic lipidosis. Hypoalbuminemia and hypoproteinemia are often observed, but total protein concentration as well as other serum chemistry parameters can be variable depending on underlying or secondary conditions. Anemia, neutropenia, and lymphopenia often are associated with PEM, although altered white blood cell number and differential count may reflect underlying chronic infectious or parasitic disease.

Once unexplained body weight or condition score loss has been identified, one needs to determine a cause. Chronic infectious, parasitic, and dental diseases can induce body weight and condition losses similar to PEM.[5] However, most animals afflicted with an infectious or parasitic disease have reduced appetites despite their energy deficit. In contrast, PEM animals maintain a healthy appetite until near terminal stages. Protein-energy malnutrition is often a secondary process to chronic disease conditions. Animals identified early in the disease process can be recovered with appropriate feeding therapy and supportive care, although those becoming weak and recumbent have a very poor prognosis even with aggressive therapy.

The most common reason for PEM is poor-quality forages coupled with the animal's inability to consume sufficient amounts of the forage or an increased requirement.[5] Under South American conditions, animal body weight and condition score changes will mimic seasonal forage growth patterns. Camelids will gain significant body weight and condition and will give birth during the rainy season in concert with high-quality forage availability. During the dry season, animals will lose considerable weight and condition and be in various stages of malnutrition.[8] Animals giving birth during the dry season are much more prone to PEM and secondary infectious and parasitic disease problems, often leading to their demise.

Llamas and alpacas raised in North America are exposed to a greater diversity of environmental conditions ranging from extreme hot and humid environments (Southern United States) to extremely cold winter conditions (Northern United States, Canada, and Alaska). Average winter daily temperature in northern North America may fall below −15°C and may decline to −35°C.[5] These are environmental extremes llamas and alpacas never experience in their native environment. Cold, wet conditions have the challenges associated with providing effective protective shelter and increased energy intake to compensate for additional maintenance requirements. Alternatively, hot and humid environments bring challenges of preventing heat stress, a significant health risk for llamas and alpacas. Either environmental extreme can result in a situation of potential PEM with poor quality forage.

Prevention of PEM is based on appropriate feeding regimes where forage quality is matched to nutrient needs of the animal. Where forage quality is insufficient, feeding of supplemental feeds is necessary. To achieve such feeding programs, forage quality will need to be evaluated by chemical analysis. Routine assessment of an animal's energy status by body weight or condition scoring is a recommended practice, especially for those individuals with higher energy requirements and before and during the cold weather season. Important times to assess body condition score would be during early to mid pregnancy, early to mid lactation, and periodically (4–6 times per year) to other animals of the herd to assess energy status.[9]

Obesity

Obesity is considered one of the more prevalent nutritional problems in North American llamas and, less commonly, alpacas.[10,11] Feeding too high quality of forage relative to requirements as well as overfeeding of additional supplements are the primary contributors to obesity. Many commercial supplements available in North America are touted as low-energy feeds, but contain substantial amounts of cereal grains or readily fermentable fiber as energy sources. The noted discrepancy in feed intake expectations between North and South American data might also be a contributor to the greater obesity issues for camelids in North America. Deleterious effects of obesity include greater susceptibility to heat stress, metabolic derangements, infertility, and associated locomotive problems.

To prevent obesity one has two options, either increase energy expenditure or reduce energy intake. An animal's energy requirement is primarily a function of lean body weight (3.0 out of 5.0 condition score weight) and physiologic state (maintenance, growth, pregnancy, lactation). Packing or hiking and other activities will increase energy expenditure, but this is not always a viable option. Reducing energy intake is the most readily adapted and obvious approach. Energy-dense supplements should be limited. Forage intake, quality, or both need to be reduced for obese animals. Feed lower-quality forages exclusively or before grazing to minimize pasture intake. Segregate obese animals so they cannot "steal" food from others. Increase stocking density or grazing intensity to reduce intake. Graze obese animals only on mature pastures. There is much individual animal variation in the propensity for obesity. Body weight or condition score must be routinely assessed to achieve the appropriate nutritional balance to maintain optimum condition for a given animal.

MINERAL-ASSOCIATED DISEASES

Although there are limited published studies documenting classic mineral deficiency diseases in camelids, circumstantial evidence based on veterinary teaching hospital cases in the United States would suggest camelids are susceptible to all potential mineral deficiency diseases. Based on clinician experiences, hypocalcemia and hypomagnesemia in camelids present with similar clinical signs, diagnostic criteria, and therapeutic response to that of other ruminants.[1,2] Most published reports have characterized trace mineral deficiency or toxicity diseases of llamas and alpacas.

Copper Deficiency and Toxicity

Copper (Cu) deficiency is a concern with ruminant animals because of the unique interaction between molybdenum (Mo), sulfur, and dietary Cu that results in reduced availability. Often Cu deficiency is associated with anemia, altered hair coloration, impaired immune response, and poor growth.[12] Two llamas (10 and 23 months of age) with low serum Cu concentrations (<0.14 µg/mL; deficiency < 0.29 µg/mL [Llama and alpaca reference values, Clinical Nutrition Laboratory, Animal and Population Diagnostic Center, Michigan State University, E. Lansing, MI]) and responding to Cu supplementation had presented with anemia and poor condition.[13] Other reports had linked Cu deficiency to neurologic deficits (hind limb ataxia, posterior paresis) similar to the disease "swayback" observed in neonatal sheep.[1,14,15] Reported serum Cu concentrations were not considered deficient and the affected animals did not respond to Cu therapy, thus questioning the role of Cu in the observed disease process. In only one case, a 6-month-old llama with ascending paralysis was found to have 5 and 0 µg/g Cu in liver and kidney, respectively; consistent with a deficient (<16 µg/g dry weight [Llama and alpaca reference values, Clinical Nutrition Laboratory, Animal and Population Diagnostic Center, Michigan State University, East Lansing, Michigan]) status.[1] More evidence is required to determine if there is a role for Cu deficiency in neurologic disease of camelids, similar to that described for sheep.

Published studies[16–19] as well as anecdotal field cases suggest llamas and alpacas to be sensitive to Cu toxicity, although not as keenly sensitive as sheep. In contrast to the hemoglobinuria and hemoglobinemia observed in sheep Cu toxicity cases,[12] hepatic necrosis without hemolysis typifies Cu toxicity lesions in llamas[16] and alpacas.[19] Elevated hepatic enzymes may be associated with toxicity cases, but not consistently. As with sheep, excessive Cu intake results in chronic hepatic accumulation until a saturation point is reached and Cu ions are released, thus inducing the hepatocellular damage. Across studies, affected llamas and alpacas had serum Cu concentrations ranging between 2.2 and 5.7 µg/mL (reference range: 0.4 to 0.5 µg/mL [Llama and alpaca reference values, Clinical Nutrition Laboratory, Animal and Population Diagnostic Center, Michigan State University]), indicating excessive Cu concentration. Hepatic Cu content ranged from 640 to 1700 µg/g dry weight. Reported dietary Cu content ranged from 33 to 36.6 mg/kg.[16,19] In all cases of perceived Cu toxicity, dietary ratio of Cu-to-Mo was greater than 16:1. Based on these reports, llamas and alpacas are prone to Cu toxicity on diets with greater than 20 mg/kg Cu and 16:1 Cu-to-Mo ratio. A dietary Cu-to-Mo ratio between 6- and 10-to-1 is recommended.[20]

Iron Deficiency

Three llamas (14–29 months of age) presenting with characteristic microcytic, hypochromic anemia and poor growth were considered to have iron deficiency.[21] Serum iron concentrations in these cases were between 20.1 and 59.7 µg/dL, below established reference range (61.4 to 162 µg/dL) for adult llamas[22] and the animals responded to parenteral Fe (iron dextran) supplementation. Although not determined in these cases, iron deficiency potentially results from either inadequate intake, typical of growing animals on milk-based diets, or chronic blood loss.[23] Anemia is a commonly reported disease in llamas and alpacas and these reports suggest the pathogenesis associated with iron deficiency is similar across species.

Selenium Deficiency and Toxicity

Nutritional myodegeneration (ie, white muscle disease) resulting from clinical selenium (Se) deficiency has been reported in dromedary camels.[24] Although there are no published reports of Se deficiency disease in llamas and alpacas, it has been empirically diagnosed and is a disease of concern in many regions of North America.[1,2,11,25] Any age animal can be affected, although younger animals most commonly experience clinical disease. Severe Se deficiency results in pathologic degeneration of skeletal muscle fibers with secondary fibrosis.[12] Affected clinical animals will show signs reflective of specific muscles affected and severity of degenerative changes to muscle fibers. Typically both hind legs are symmetrically affected; however, tongue and heart muscles are commonly involved in newborn or young growing animals. With skeletal muscle damage, affected young or older animals will show various degrees of lameness, weakness, or difficulty moving. Acute death can occur in those younger animals where the heart muscle is damaged. Newborn animals with tongue lesions will have difficulty nursing and may be diagnosed as a "dummy" animal. Severe Se deficiency has been associated with abortion and stillbirth. All of these clinical presentations have been documented in most domesticated species and believed to occur in llamas and alpacas.

Diagnosis of Se deficiency can be achieved through assessment of Se status using serum, whole blood, or liver Se concentrations, or whole blood glutathione peroxidase activity. Llamas and alpacas are different compared with cattle, sheep, and goats with respect to blood Se distribution having a lesser difference between serum and whole blood concentrations. Llamas and alpacas have a greater amount of Se-dependent glutathione peroxidase activity in serum rather than being concentrated primarily in red blood cells. Deficient whole blood Se concentrations are defined as less than 120 ng/mL with adequate between 150 and 220 ng/mL for either llamas or alpacas (Llama and alpaca reference values, Clinical Nutrition Laboratory, Animal and Population Diagnostic Center, Michigan State University). Serum Se concentrations less than 80 or less than 110 ng/mL are considered deficient for adult alpacas and llamas, respectively. Criteria defining adequacy and deficiency are variable with age.

Selenium toxicity is of concern in llamas and alpacas, although not typically an issue with most ruminant animals because of the low dietary availability observed with inorganic Se sources. Injectable Se has high biologic availability, is readily absorbed, and is most often the cause of Se toxicosis. There is no antidote for acute Se toxicity. In such cases the animal will show signs of distressed breathing, salivation, and cardiovascular collapse. This all may occur within minutes to an hour following an injection of an excessive amount of Se. Toxic dosages have not been well defined for all species, but more than 0.5 mg/kg body weight is considered toxic for sodium selenite injections, which is about 20 times the suggested label dose.

A number of veterinary diagnostic laboratories are finding very high concentrations of Se (>12 μg/g dry weight) in llama and alpaca liver samples, suggesting an excessive level of supplementation. Some laboratories have identified Se toxicosis as a potential contributor to the death of the animal in a number of these cases, based solely on liver mineral content and no definable pathologic lesions. Whether the high liver Se concentration is a result of injection or oral Se supplementation has not been clearly defined. In some of these "toxicity" cases, no injectable Se supplementation was documented, suggesting excessive oral supplementation. Use of the newer organic selenomethionine supplements may result in higher liver and tissue Se concentrations. Further investigation is required to better define camelid Se requirements and assessment of Se status.

Zinc Deficiency

Zinc deficiency and its relationship to skin lesions is another disease process of great concern with camelids. A group of llamas and alpacas fed grass hay and commercial supplement feed containing 15.8 and 51.3 mg/kg zinc, respectively, had a reported 25% incidence of skin lesions.[26] Mean serum zinc concentrations were 0.22 and 0.17 μg/mL for llamas and alpacas, respectively, and affected animals responded to zinc supplementation.[26]

This report is consistent with a described nonpruritic, idiopathic hyperkeratosis syndrome recognized in 1- to 2-year-old male and female llamas and alpacas.[27] Colored fleeced animals are seemingly more susceptible.[11,27] Lesions are mostly noted on hairless areas of the body (ventral abdomen, axilla, medial thighs, and inguinal region) and are characterized by a thickening of the skin with tightly adhering crusts. Histologic changes of epithelial and follicular orthokeratotic hyperkeratosis are characterized in the lesions.[27] Although parakeratotic hyperkeratosis is typically associated with zinc deficiency, zinc-responsive orthokeratotic hyperkeratosis has been recognized in other ruminants.[12,27] Affected animals seem to respond to supplemental zinc gradually over a 2- to 3-month period. Zinc supplementation can be achieved with daily supplementation with either 1 g zinc sulfate (36.3% zinc) or 2 to 4 g zinc methionine (10% zinc). Zinc methionine is often recommended for supplementation, as it is believed to be more available in the face of interfering dietary agents such as high calcium intake. These zinc supplements are not very palatable and would need to be incorporated into a supplement or masking vehicle rather than top-dressed. A maintenance intake of 1 g zinc methionine is suggested for preventive measures in susceptible populations.[27] Whether or not this condition is truly a zinc deficiency is debated, but these data support the hypothesis that zinc is a primary factor in the disease.

VITAMIN-ASSOCIATED DISEASES

One published report has documented a vitamin E–related muscular disease in a llama, with musculoskeletal lesions similar to what is seen in other species.[28] No reports of vitamin A deficiency or toxicity have been published.

Vitamin D Deficiency

Llamas and alpacas are seemingly different compared with other ruminants relative to vitamin D physiology. Growing llamas and alpacas between 3 and 6 months of age are susceptible to a seasonal vitamin D deficiency resulting in a hypophosphatemic rickets syndrome.[29–32] Greatest prevalence in northern latitudes of North America occurs between December and March and crias born between September and February are at greatest risk.[33] Crias born between March and August had significantly greater serum vitamin D concentrations through the first 7 months of life compared with crias born between September and March.[33] Fall-born crias may never obtain vitamin D reserves from summer sunshine, compared with spring-born crias. Fall-born crias will have lowest concentrations of vitamin D and phosphorus during the period of rapid growth compared with spring-born crias.

Affected crias show a slower rate of growth, reluctance to move, humped-back stance, and shifting leg lameness. On physical examination, joints were enlarged, most obviously the carpus. Hypophosphatemia (<3.0 mg/dL) is the most consistent diagnostic finding in addition to radiographic bone changes consistent with widened and irregular growth plates typical of rachitic changes.[29,30,32] Seasonal variation in blood vitamin D concentrations has also been implicated with susceptibility of long bone fractures.[34] Vitamin D is required not only to support bone mineralization, but to facilitate intestinal absorption of phosphorus.

Serum vitamin D and phosphorus concentrations show a seasonal pattern where lowest values occur during December to March and highest values during June to

September.[33] Intensity and angle of the sun at the most distant latitudes within Northern or Southern hemispheres may be insufficient during winter (Northern hemisphere) or summer (Southern hemisphere) months to maintain adequate vitamin D status without dietary supplementation. Vitamin D is naturally synthesized in nonpigmented areas of the skin upon exposure to sunlight. More darkly colored and heavily fleeced camelids have lower vitamin D concentrations, but shearing increases skin exposure and subsequently, vitamin D concentration.[33]

Treatment and prevention of this syndrome can be accomplished with therapeutic or preventive vitamin D supplementation.[32,35,36] Vitamin D can be effectively supplemented by injection, oral dosing, or increasing dietary levels. Injections of vitamin D_3 between 1000 and 1500 IU/kg body weight have been shown to maintain adequate serum vitamin D concentrations for up to 3 months.[35,36] Oral gels delivering vitamin D_3 at 33,000 IU every 2 weeks or 100,000 IU once monthly have also been used successfully.[32] Both of these methods can be used to effectively treat an affected cria or used as a preventive measure. Recommendations for daily vitamin D intake (30 IU/kg body weight) are higher than other species as a result of lower oral vitamin D bioavailability in llamas and alpacas.[3,37] One must also recognize that vitamin D is one of the more potentially toxic nutrients and therefore, care must be taken in not exceeding recommendations with indiscriminate supplementation.

Polioencephalomalacia

Polioencephalomalacia is a metabolic disorder of all ruminant animals resulting from inadequate thiamin availability induced by elevated thiaminase activity, insufficient bacterial thiamin synthesis, production of antithiamin metabolites, or some combination.[38] The disease condition can also be induced by excessive dietary sulfur or overdose of amprolium,[38,39] although excess sulfur has not been implicated in camelid cases as reported in cattle and sheep. A rapid change from high forage to high-concentrate, low-fiber diet leading to reduced ruminal pH and altered microbial flora is often associated with polioencephalomalacia conditions.[38] Clinical signs include depression, seizures, opisthotonos, blindness, hyperesthesia, and sudden death. Observed neurologic signs are attributed to induced cerebrocortical necrosis resulting from reduced transketolase activity impairing glucose use by neural tissues.

Polioencephalomalacia has been reported in young and adult llamas and alpacas.[1,40–42] In all reported cases, affected animals presented with classical neurologic clinical signs associated with polioencephalomalacia. Diagnosis was presumptively made by presenting signs and rapid response to thiamin therapy (10 to 20 mg/kg body weight) or definitively by presence of microscopic lesions consistent with polioencephalomalacia on necropsy. Inciting dietary causes in these reported cases were all associated with either increased access to grain or abrupt dietary changes where fiber intake was reduced. Specifically, clinical cases were associated with excessive oat grain consumption,[1] free access to a hay and grain diet with additional concentrates being available approximately 3 days before onset,[42] or an abrupt change from a hay-based to pelleted diet.[40] Prevention is based on proper feeding management practices in minimizing abrupt dietary changes and reducing access to readily fermented grain ingredients.

OTHER NUTRITION-ASSOCIATED DISEASES
Lactic Acidosis (Grain Overload)

Ruminal acidosis is a well-defined disease process in ruminant animals resulting from excessive accumulation of volatile fatty acids and lactic acid within the rumen as a result of large amounts of rapidly fermentable carbohydrates being ingested. This process has been recognized in llamas and alpacas[1,2,11] and pathophysiology in camelids is similar to that of ruminants.[43] Affected animals will present as dehydrated, lethargic, and depressed. Forestomach motility is reduced and diarrhea may be present. Compartment 1 (C-1) pH will be 5.0 or less with accompanying metabolic acidosis and electrolyte disturbances. Affected animals responded favorably to fluids and alkalizing agent therapy with no observed long-term problems.

Amount of grain required to induce acidosis in camelids may be less than for ruminants, possibly because of the greater fermentation capacity and longer retention time of C-1. In reported cases,[43] documented grain intake in an affected individual was 500 g. Amount of offered grain to animal groups having clinical presentation ranged from 150 g/d to 1 kg/d, suggesting social hierarchy and feeding management are important factors in disease risk. Mixtures of cracked corn, oats, and barley were most often associated with clinical cases of acidosis. This cereal grain mixture would contain more than 60% fermentable starch. Prevention mainly revolves around maintaining animal-safe storage facilities to minimize accidental exposure and good feeding management practices. Grain products should be evaluated relative to their starch content, preferably via chemical analysis at a commercial feed analysis laboratory. Feed tag information provided on commercial grain products can be used to screen products. Products having cereal grains, namely corn, oats, barley, or wheat, as the first three ingredients and low crude fiber content (<12%) have the highest potential risk of inducing acidosis in an inappropriate feeding situation.

Urolithiasis

Similar to other male ruminants, male llamas and alpacas are at risk for blockage of the urethra as a result of its smaller diameter and presence of a sigmoid flexure compared with females.[1,44] In male cattle, sheep, and goats, struvite (magnesium-ammonia-phosphate) crystal secondary to high grain feeding and low dietary calcium-to-phosphorus ratio is the most common cause of urolithiasis. Various calcium salts, phosphatic complexes, silica, and oxalates are all potential mineral sources causing uroliths.[44] Although not a common disorder in llamas and alpacas, silicate and struvite crystals have been reported.[45,46]

Clinical signs associated with urolithiasis will depend on the degree of blockage and severity of surrounding tissue reactions. If blockage is complete, retrograde pressure will build in the bladder to the point of rupture and subsequent death of the animal. Bladder rupture secondary to urethral blockage has been reported in camelids,[47,48] although mineralized stones were not specifically identified. Incomplete blockage results in variable stages of stranguria, exaggerated and prolonged urination posture, urine dribbling, and blood-tinged urine.[44] Affected animals may be depressed and lethargic, grind their teeth, and show signs of abdominal distention and pain. Therapeutic approach will depend on severity of blockage, duration, and secondary complications.

Little is known about how urolithiasis occurs in llamas and alpacas and it is assumed that the disease process is similar to other ruminants.[44] Problems associated with struvite crystals have been diagnosed in several male camelids grazing in lush grass pastures (Van Saun, personal observations, 2004–2006). These pastures were heavily fertilized and nutrient content analysis showed excessive potassium (>3% dry matter), high phosphorus (>0.5% dry matter), and low calcium (<0.6% dry matter). Removal from the pasture with supplementation of calcium to the diet prevented further obstructive problems. Certain plants and mature grasses may contain large amounts of oxalates and silicates, respectively, which can potentially contribute to urolith formation.

Nutritional alterations are the primary concern and focus of prevention. Goals of a dietary prevention program are to increase water consumption with addition of salt to the diet and maintain appropriate amounts of calcium and phosphorus in the diet with a calcium-to-phosphorus ratio between 2.0-to-4:1.[44] Struvite crystals can be prevented by dietary modification to induce urine acidification. Traditionally, dietary supplementation (5–10 g/kg of dry matter) of ammonium chloride has been used. More palatable commercial products capable of acidification are available as they are commonly used in dairy cattle rations before calving to prevent milk fever. However, little data are available to validate the efficacy and safety of prolonged feeding of such products to llamas and alpacas.

FEED TOXICITIES
Poisonous Plants

Camelids are potentially susceptible to the wide variety of poisonous plants identified for other animals; however, few reports are found in the literature.[1,11,49] Ornamental rhododendrons and azaleas (Ericaceae family) are most often associated with camelid intoxications.[1,50,51] Sierra laurel (Leucothoe davisiae) was implicated in the intoxication of two llamas.[52] The identified toxic principle in these plants is a diterpenoid compound called grayanotoxin, formally termed andromedotoxin.[53] Typical clinical signs include vomiting, anorexia, abdominal pain, salivation, weakness to paresis, muscle fasciculations, cardiac arrhythmia, and bradycardia. Signs occur within 6 hours of ingestion and recovery may occur within 2 to 3 days. Toxic dose for ruminants is considered between 0.15% and 0.6% of body weight. There is no known antidote and symptomatic therapy is recommended.

Other observed plant intoxications in llamas and alpacas have been associated with death camas (Zigadenus sp),[49] oleander (Nerium oleander),[49] and dumb cane (Dieffenbachia seguine).[1] Death camas contain steroid alkaloids, including zygacine, in all parts of the plant.[53] Lethal dose varies between 0.6% and 6.0% of body weight. Intoxicated llamas showed rapid breathing, weakness, salivation, and vomiting. Acute death in five alpacas was attributed oleander consumption.[49] Oleander contains a number of toxins, most importantly compounds with cardiac glycoside activity.[53] This is an extremely lethal toxin, requiring only 0.005% of body weight for cattle or horses. Llamas consuming dumb cane showed immediate signs of intense oral cavity irritation with salivation, spitting, coughing, and shaking of the head.[1] Dumb cane contains calcium oxalate crystals that cause severe irritation.[53] Irritation of the mouth resulted in swelling of the tongue and pharynx and subsequent problems with swallowing and breathing.

Camelids seemingly are sensitive to a range of potential poisonous plants similar to other ruminants and horses. Although only previously reported in horses, hemolytic anemia with Heinz body and methemoglobin formation was reported in alpacas consuming red maple leaves (Acer rubrum).[54] Secondary hepatogenous photosensitization was diagnosed in a llama grazing a tropical grass, Brachiaria decumbens, pasture in Brazil.[55] Intoxication of alpacas from endophyte (Neotyphodium lolii)-infected perennial ryegrass (Lolium perenne L) has been reported.[56,57] The primary toxic agent is lolitrem-B, a neurogenic alkaloid that induces tremors, incoordination, head shaking, and staggers in afflicted animals.[53] Removal of the offending forage will result in a gradual recovery. In contrast, there are no published reports of camelid intoxication from endophyte-infected tall fescue, although there are many reports involving cattle and horses. There are differences of opinion among clinicians and producers as to the prevalence of ryegrass or fescue toxicosis in llamas and alpacas with some suggesting the problem to be prevalent in their geographic region, whereas others have observed a sporadic problem.

Feed Supplements

Ionophore agents are commonly used as a feed additive in ruminant diets. Derived from fungi, they have selective antimicrobial activity through altered ion exchange in the bacterial cell membrane. Ionophores are approved for use in coccidiosis control or to improve feed efficiency. There are a number of ionophore compounds, but only monensin sodium and lasalocid are approved for use in goats and sheep, respectively.[37] Horses are well documented to be sensitive to toxicity of ionophore compounds, although toxicity disease can result from feeding ionophores to nontarget species or at an excessive dosage owing to mixing errors.[58,59]

In spring of 2003, more than 1000 alpacas were exposed to salinomycin at the approved poultry (66 ppm) incorporation rate through a feed mill mixing error.[60] Estimated intake of salinomycin in affected animals was between 0.5 and 1.5 mg/kg of body weight. Within 3 days of consuming the contaminated feed, affected animals showed clinical signs of diarrhea, muscle tremors, weakness, and acute death as a result of severe acute rhabdomyolysis from salinomycin intoxication. Myocardial failure and pulmonary edema accounted for continued death loss over a period of 2 weeks following exposure to the contaminated feed. Death loss in alpacas occurred up to 3 months following exposure. Because llamas and alpacas are not approved target species for any of the available ionophore agents, sensitivity to toxicosis is unknown.

Nonprotein Nitrogen, Nitrate, and Nitrite Toxicity

Nonprotein nitrogen (NPN) toxicosis is primarily a disease of ruminant animals as a direct result of rumen microbial production of toxic compounds from excessive amounts of NPN consumption. Compounds of concern to ruminants are urea, nitrates, and nitrites and a risk to camelids is presumed. Urea is a common lawn fertilizer and ruminant feed supplement. Nitrates and nitrites are NPN compounds found in plants and water. Certain forage plants (ie, corn, oats, barley, sorghum, Sudan grass) and weeds (ie, pigweed, nightshade, Johnson grass), under extreme environmental conditions such as drought, can accumulate nitrates or nitrites and potentially pose a serious problem.[53] Potential accumulating plants should be evaluated for nitrate or nitrite concentrations.

Dietary NPN sources are eventually reduced to ammonia, which can be used by rumen microbes for protein synthesis. This is a unique feature of the ruminant animal and is a primary reason for their ability to use poor-quality feeds. Urea is rapidly cleaved into CO_2 and two ammonia molecules. To assimilate ammonia into microbial protein, energy derived from microbial fermentation of dietary carbohydrate is required. Poor-quality forages do not provide sufficient amounts of energy in synch to support NPN use by rumen microbes. If ammonia is not used by the rumen microbes, it will diffuse across the rumen wall into portal blood circulation. Ammonia is a potent cellular toxin disrupting energy metabolism and potassium homeostasis. The liver normally converts excess ammonia back into urea for recycling or excretion. In NPN toxicosis the liver is overwhelmed with excess ammonia, blood ammonia concentrations will increase dramatically, resulting in subsequent clinical signs. Urea toxicosis occurs rapidly within 30 to 60 minutes of excess consumption. Clinical signs include frothy salivation, bruxism, colic, muscle tremors, incoordination, and recumbency, followed by death. Treatment is unrewarding for the most part unless identified very early in toxicity. Diagnosis is based on history, smell of ammonia to the animal, and quantification of ammonia in either blood or rumen contents.

Nitrates and nitrites induce their toxic effects through a different mechanism. Nitrate is reduced to nitrite, which is a very rapid reaction in the rumen. Nitrite is reduced to ammonia for microbial use, although presence of ammonia can inhibit this reaction. Nitrite accumulation, as a result of either excess ammonia or nitrate presence, is absorbed across the rumen wall into portal circulation. In the blood, nitrite reacts with hemoglobin to produce methemoglobin, which reduces oxygen carrying capacity. Clinical signs of nitrate or nitrite intoxication are similar to those seen with urea poisoning and include dyspnea, cyanosis, and death depending on the amount of methemoglobin formation. Abortions may also occur following exposure to nitrate intoxication. Diagnosis is based primarily on history of exposure and quantification of nitrate in aqueous humor. Classically, nitrate intoxication cases are associated with "chocolate-colored" blood (>30% methemoglobin). Methylene blue is a specific antidote that can be used for treating early cases.

Prevention of inappropriate exposure to NPN sources is the best method of control. Rumen microbes can be adapted to NPN sources by slowly increasing their incorporation rate in the diet and ensuring adequate fermentable carbohydrate sources, although use of NPN in camelid diets is not common. Forages that contain high concentrations of NPN sources should be diluted out with other feeds not containing NPN sources. When environmental or plant-growing conditions are conducive to nitrate accumulation, feeds should be analyzed for nitrate content.

SUMMARY

Published reports and empiric clinical evidence would suggest llamas and alpacas share similar risks to other ruminant animals relative to most nutrient deficiency or toxicity disease problems. Camelids have unique metabolic differences compared with other ruminants resulting in greater susceptibility to hepatic lipidosis and diseases related to vitamin D and zinc deficiency. Relative to Cu toxicity, camelids seem intermediate between sheep and other ruminants. Because of their greater fermentation efficiency, camelids seemingly are more sensitive to inappropriate dietary changes resulting in polioencephalomalacia or acidosis. A better understanding of camelid nutrient requirements and metabolism are needed to prevent continued problems with nutritional diseases.

REFERENCES

1. Smith JA. Noninfectious diseases, metabolic diseases, toxicities, and neoplastic diseases of South American camelids. Vet Clin North Am Food Anim Pract 1989; 5(1):101–43.
2. Belknap EB. Medical problems of llamas. Vet Clin North Am Food Anim Pract 1994;10(2):291–307.
3. Van Saun RJ. Nutritional diseases of South American camelids. Small Rumin Res 2006;61:153–64.
4. Anonymous. Information resources on the South American camelids: llamas, alpacas, guanacos, and vicunas 1943–2006. Bibliographic index, USDA National Agricultural Library, 2001 (Updated February 2006). Available at: http://www.nal.usda.gov/awic/pubs/llama.htm. Accessed October 17, 2008.
5. Carmalt JL. Protein-energy malnutrition in alpacas. Comp for Cont Ed for Pract Vet 2000;22(12):1118–24.

6. Tornquist SJ, Van Saun RJ, Smith BB, et al. Histologically-confirmed hepatic lipidosis in llamas and alpacas: 31 cases (1991–1997). J Am Vet Med Assoc 1999;214(9):1368–72.
7. National Research Council. Effect of environment on nutrient requirements of domestic animals. Washington, DC: National Academy Press; 1981. p. 152.
8. Lopez A, Maiztegui J, Cabrera R. Voluntary intake and digestibility of forages with different nutritional quality in alpacas. Small Rumin Res 1998;29:295–301.
9. Hilton CD, Pugh DG, Wright JC, et al. How to determine and when to use body weight estimates and condition scores in llamas. Vet Med 1998;93(11): 1015–8.
10. Johnson LW. Llama nutrition. Vet Clin North Am Food Anim Pract 1994;10(2): 187–201.
11. Fowler ME. Feeding and nutrition. Medicine and surgery of South American camelids: llama, alpaca, vicuna, guanaco. 2nd edition. Ames (IA): Iowa State University Press; 1998. p. 12–48.
12. Underwood EJ, Suttle NF. The mineral nutrition of livestock. 3rd edition. New York: CABI Publishing; 1999. p. 614.
13. Andrews AH, Cox A. Suspected nutritional deficiency causing anemia in llamas (Lama glama). Vet Rec 1997;140:153–4.
14. Palmer AC, Blakemore WF, O'Sullivan B, et al. Ataxia and spinal cord degeneration in llama, wildebeeste and camel. Vet Rec 1980;107:10–1.
15. Morgan KL. Ataxia and head tremor in an alpaca (Lama pacos). Vet Rec 1992; 131:216–7.
16. Junge RE, Thornburg L. Copper poisoning in four llamas. J Am Vet Med Assoc 1989;195(7):987–9.
17. Mullaney TP, Slanker MR, Fitzgerald SD, et al. Copper toxicosis in llamas. Proc Am Assoc Vet Lab Diag 1996. p. 36 (Abstract).
18. Weaver DM, Tyler JW, Marion RS, et al. Subclinical copper accumulation in llamas. Can Vet J 1999;40:422–4.
19. Carmalt JL, Baptiste KE, Blakley B. Suspect copper toxicity in an alpaca. Can Vet J 2001;42:554–6.
20. Pugh DG. Copper nutrition in llamas. Llamas 1993;7(2):77–9.
21. Morin DE, Garry FB, Weiser MG, et al. Hematologic features of iron deficiency anemia in llamas. Vet Pathol 1992;29:400–4.
22. Smith BB, Van Saun RJ, Reed PJ, et al. Blood mineral and vitamin E concentrations in llamas. Am J Vet Res 1998;59(8):1063–70.
23. Morin DE, Garry FB, Weiser MG. Hematologic responses in llamas with experimentally-induced iron deficiency anemia. Vet Clin Pathol 1993;22(3):81–6.
24. Hamliri A, Khallaayoune K, Johnson DW, et al. The relationship between the concentration of selenium in the blood and the activity of glutathione peroxidase in the erythrocytes of the dromedary camel (Camelus dromedarius). Vet Res Commun 1990;14:27–30.
25. Pugh DG. Selenium nutrition for llamas: an overview. Llamas 1993;7(3):43–5.
26. Clauss M, Lendl C, Schramel P, et al. Skin lesions in alpacas and llamas with low zinc and copper status—a preliminary report. Vet J 2004;167(3):302–5.
27. Rosychuk RAW. Llama dermatology. Vet Clin North Am Food Anim Pract 1994; 10(2):228–39.
28. Chauvet AE, Shelton GD, Darien BJ. Vitamin E deficiency associated with myopathy in a llama. Prog Vet Neurol 1996;7(4):149–52.
29. Fowler ME. Rickets in llamas and alpacas. Llamas 1990;4(2):92–5.
30. Fowler ME. Rickets in alpacas. Alpacas Fall 1992;10–3.

31. Hill FI, Thompson KG, Grace ND. Rickets in alpacas (*Lama pacos*) in New Zealand. N Z Vet J 1994;42:75 [Abstract].
32. Van Saun RJ, Smith BB, Watrous BJ. Evaluation of vitamin D status of llamas and alpacas with hypophosphatemic rickets. J Am Vet Med Assoc 1996;209(6):1128–33.
33. Smith BB, Van Saun RJ. Seasonal changes in serum calcium, phosphorus and vitamin D concentrations in llamas and alpacas. Am J Vet Res 2001;62(8): 1187–93.
34. Parker JE, Timm KI, Smith BB, et al. Seasonal interaction of vitamin D and bone density in the llama. Am J Vet Res 2002;63:948–53.
35. Smith BB, Van Saun RJ. Hypophosphatemic rickets in South American camelids: interaction of calcium, phosphorus, and vitamin D. In: Gerken M, Renieri C, editors. Proceedings of the second European symposium on South American camelids. Italy: Universita Degli Studi Di Camerino; 1996. p. 79–94.
36. Judson GJ, Feakes A. Vitamin D doses for alpacas (*Lama pacos*). Aust Vet J 1999;77(5):310–5.
37. National Research Council. Nutrient requirements of small ruminants (sheep, goats, cervids and New World camelids). Washington, DC: National Academy Press; 2007. p. 324.
38. Cebra C, Loneragan G, Gould D. Polioencephalomalacia (cerebrocoritcal necrosis). In: Smith B, editor. Large animal internal medicine. 4th edition. St. Louis (MO): Mosby Elsevier; 2009. p. 1021–6.
39. Gould D. Update on sulfur-related polioencephalomalacia. Vet Clin North Am Food Anim Pract 2000;16(3):481–96.
40. Pugh DG. Polioencephalomalacia in a llama herd. Equine Pract 1993;15(2):24–6.
41. Beck C, Dart AJ, Collins MB, et al. Polioencephalomalacia in two alpacas. Aust Vet J 1996;74:350–2.
42. Kiupel M, Van Alstine W, Chilcoat C. Gross and microscopic lesions of polioence-phalomalacia in a llama (*Lama glama*). J Zoo Wildl Med 2003;34:309–13.
43. Cebra CK, Cebra ML, Garry FB, et al. Forestomach acidosis in six New World camelids. J Am Vet Med Assoc 1996;208(6):901–4.
44. Gerros TC. Recognizing and treating urolithiasis in llamas. Vet Med 1998;93(6): 583–90.
45. Kock MD, Fowler ME. Urolithiasis in a three-month-old llama. J Am Vet Med Assoc 1982;181:1411.
46. Kingston JK, Stäempfli HR. Silica urolithiasis in a male llama. Can Vet J 1995;36: 767–8.
47. McLaughlin BG, Evans NC. Urethral obstruction in a male llama. J Am Vet Med Assoc 1989;195(11):1601–2.
48. Dart AJ, Dart CM, Hodgson DR. Surgical management of a ruptured bladder secondary to a urethral obstruction in an alpaca. Aust Vet J 1997;75(11):793–5.
49. Hoffman E. Poisons. In: Hoffman E, editor. The complete alpaca book. 2nd edition. Santa Cruz (CA): Bonny Doon Press; 2003. p. 485–502.
50. Crawford JE. Rhododendron poisoning in alpacas. Vet Rec 1999;144:680.
51. Miller RM. Azalea poisoning in a llama: a case report. Vet Med Small Anim Clin 1981;76:104.
52. Fowler ME. Plant poisoning in two pack llamas. Calif Vet 1985;39(3):17–20.
53. Cheeke PR. Natural toxicants in feeds, forages, and poisonous plants. 2nd edition. Danville (IL): Interstate Publishers; 1998. p. 479.
54. DeWitt SF, Bedenice D, Mazan MR. Hemolysis and Heinz body formation associated with ingestion of red maple leaves in two alpacas. J Am Vet Med Assoc 2004;225(4):578–83.

55. Birgel Junior EH, dos Santos MC, de Ramos JA, et al. Secondary hepatogenous photosensitization in a llama (*Lama glama*) bred in the state of Sáo Paulo, Brazil. Can Vet J 2007;48(3):323–4.

56. Holmes LA, Frame NW, Frame RK, et al. Suspected tremorgenic mycotoxicosis (ryegrass staggers) in alpacas (*Llama pacos*) in the UK. Vet Rec 1999;145(16): 462–3.

57. Mackintosh C, Orr M. Ryegrass staggers in alpacas? Vet Rec 1993;132(5):120.

58. Roder JD, McCoy CP. Ionophore toxicoses. In: Howard JL, editor. Current veterinary therapy (food animal practice). 4th edition. Philadelphia: WB Saunders; 1999. p. 244–5.

59. Hall JO. Ionophore use and toxicosis in cattle. Vet Clin North Am Food Anim Pract. 2000;16:497–505.

60. Kosal ME, Anderson DE. An unaddressed issue of agricultural terrorism: a case study on feed security. J Anim Sci 2004;82:3394–400.

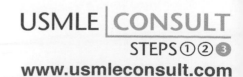

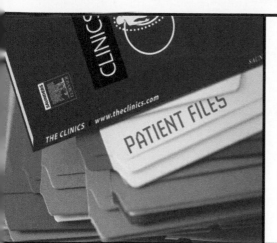
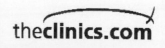

Moving?

Make sure your subscription moves with you!

To notify us of your new address, find your **Clinics Account Number** (located on your mailing label above your name), and contact customer service at:

Email: journalscustomerservice-usa@elsevier.com

800-654-2452 (subscribers in the U.S. & Canada)
314-447-8871 (subscribers outside of the U.S. & Canada)

Fax number: 314-447-8029

**Elsevier Health Sciences Division
Subscription Customer Service
3251 Riverport Lane
Maryland Heights, MO 63043**

*To ensure uninterrupted delivery of your subscription, please notify us at least 4 weeks in advance of move.

Printed and bound by CPI Group (UK) Ltd, Croydon, CR0 4YY

03/10/2024

01040463-0006